# EAI/Springer Innovations in Communication and Computing

**Series Editor**

Imrich Chlamtac, European Alliance for Innovation, Ghent, Belgium

**Editor's Note**

The impact of information technologies is creating a new world yet not fully understood. The extent and speed of economic, life style and social changes already perceived in everyday life is hard to estimate without understanding the technological driving forces behind it. This series presents contributed volumes featuring the latest research and development in the various information engineering technologies that play a key role in this process.

The range of topics, focusing primarily on communications and computing engineering include, but are not limited to, wireless networks; mobile communication; design and learning; gaming; interaction; e-health and pervasive healthcare; energy management; smart grids; internet of things; cognitive radio networks; computation; cloud computing; ubiquitous connectivity, and in mode general smart living, smart cities, Internet of Things and more. The series publishes a combination of expanded papers selected from hosted and sponsored European Alliance for Innovation (EAI) conferences that present cutting edge, global research as well as provide new perspectives on traditional related engineering fields. This content, complemented with open calls for contribution of book titles and individual chapters, together maintain Springer's and EAI's high standards of academic excellence. The audience for the books consists of researchers, industry professionals, advanced level students as well as practitioners in related fields of activity include information and communication specialists, security experts, economists, urban planners, doctors, and in general representatives in all those walks of life affected ad contributing to the information revolution.

Indexing: This series is indexed in Scopus, Ei Compendex, and zbMATH.

**About EAI**

EAI is a grassroots member organization initiated through cooperation between businesses, public, private and government organizations to address the global challenges of Europe's future competitiveness and link the European Research community with its counterparts around the globe. EAI reaches out to hundreds of thousands of individual subscribers on all continents and collaborates with an institutional member base including Fortune 500 companies, government organizations, and educational institutions, provide a free research and innovation platform.

Through its open free membership model EAI promotes a new research and innovation culture based on collaboration, connectivity and recognition of excellence by community.

More information about this series at http://www.springer.com/series/15427

Sandeep Kautish • Sheng-Lung Peng
Ahmed J. Obaid
Editors

# Computational Intelligence Techniques for Combating COVID-19

Springer

EAI
RESEARCH MEETS INNOVATION

*Editors*
Sandeep Kautish
LBEF Campus
Kathmandu Nepal; (In Academic Collaboration with Asia Pacific University of Technology & Innovation)
Kuala Lumpur, Malaysia

Sheng-Lung Peng
Taoyuan Campus
National Taipei University of Business
Taoyuan, Taiwan

Ahmed J. Obaid
Faculty of Computer Science and Mathematics
Department of Computer Science
University of Kufa
Najaf, Iraq

ISSN 2522-8595 ISSN 2522-8609 (electronic)
EAI/Springer Innovations in Communication and Computing
ISBN 978-3-030-68935-3 ISBN 978-3-030-68936-0 (eBook)
https://doi.org/10.1007/978-3-030-68936-0



This Springer imprint is published by the registered company Springer Nature Switzerland AG
The registered company address is: Gewerbestrasse 11, 6330 Cham, Switzerland

# Preface

Since the beginning of year 2020, human society has been going through a very tough phase globally, that is, an unexpected medical emergency where more than 200 countries of the world have been affected by the coronavirus (COVID-19). As of November 25, 2020, 1.4 million people have lost their lives across the world due to the COVID-19 outbreak. The death toll is still climbing. The USA, despite being the most developed country in the world, has already recorded the deaths of more than 260,000 people, which clearly shows that the most developed countries are also unable to control the COVID-19 pandemic. The coronavirus, which is a highly infectious and pathogenic virus, originated from Wuhan in December 2019, travelled the whole of China and spread around the world within 3 months of its origination. Genome analysis of the virus revealed that bats could be the possible reservoirs, which caused the spread of COVID-19.

Artificial intelligence (AI) and machine learning (ML) techniques have a great potential to serve as prevailing tools for combating COVID-19. AI, along with machine learning, computer vision applications, augmented reality and virtual reality (AR and VR) techniques, deep learning, and natural language processing, is capable of creating data science models and algorithms for pattern recognition, clarification, and accurate predictions in genome patterns of COVID-19. These functions can guide accurate recognitions, diagnosis patterns, predictions, and treatment of COVID-19 infections.

The primary aim of this book is to foster the need for extensive computational researches for combating COVID-19 in terms of adaptive computational modeling, synthesis, and analysis of biological systems using evolutionary methods and algorithms of computational intelligence. The book covers all computational approaches, that is, in silico methods ranging from all allied fields of data sciences and computational intelligence–oriented techniques. This book attempts to assert all relevant research, that is, key themes, complex adaptive systems, metrics, and paradigms, dedicated towards COVID-19, enabled with evolutionary methods of computational sciences. Also, this book lays emphasis on a digitally enabled fight back against the pandemic. In short, this book is a state-of-the-art document on the latest research in the field of computational intelligence and computational biological approaches related to combating COVID-19.

This book comprises well-structured chapters written by academic and industry researchers from across the world, and all of them are experts in their respective field of research. All the chapters have a common focus, that is, how computational intelligence techniques can help human society in combating COVID-19. The chapters cover a variety of topics such as the Internet of Things (IoT), machine learning, deep learning, big data analytics for modeling COVID-19, AI-enabled social distancing, bioinformatics approaches for vaccine development, AR-/VR-aided techniques, Chatbots for virtual assessments and diagnosis, and many more.

Kuala Lumpur, Malaysia Sandeep Kautish
Taoyuan, Taiwan Sheng-Lung Peng
Najaf, Iraq Ahmed J. Obaid

# Acknowledgment

We, the editors of *Computational Intelligence Techniques for Combating COVID-19*, wish to acknowledge the efforts of the authors who have submitted their wonderful chapters to our edited textbook in the stipulated time.

Further, we would like to convey our special thanks to Eliska Vlckova, Managing Editor at the European Alliance for Innovation (EAI), for her consistent support and guidance at each stage of the book's development.

We wish to bestow our best regards to all reviewers for providing constructive comments to the authors to improve their chapters with respect to quality, coherence, and content presentation. Without the support from reviewers, this book would not have become a reality. Also, we wish to convey our gratitude to our co-editors, Dr. Sheng Lung Peng and Dr. Ahmed J. Obaid, for their consistent support and faith.

At personal a side, I (Sandeep Kautish) wish to say thanks to my wife Yogita and son Devansh, who motivated me to initiate this book project in April 2020 during the very early days of the never-seen-before COVID-19 pandemic.

We believe that "cooperation, coordination, and commitment can make any project a success." For the successful completion of this edited book, we, the editors, acknowledge everyone who helped us directly and indirectly.

Sandeep Kautish

# Contents


**1 South Asian Countries Are Less Fatal Concerning COVID-19: A Hybrid Approach Using Machine Learning and M-AHP** . . . . . . . . . . 1
Soham Guhathakurata, Sayak Saha, Souvik Kundu, Arpita Chakraborty, and Jyoti Sekhar Banerjee

**2 Application of Deep Learning Strategies to Assess COVID-19 Patients** . . . . . . . . . . 27
V. Ramasamy, Chhabi Rani Panigrahi, Joy Lal Sarkar, Bibudhendu Pati, Abhishek Majumder, Mamata Rath, and Sheng-Lung Peng

**3 Applications of Artificial Intelligence (AI) Protecting from COVID-19 Pandemic: A Clinical and Socioeconomic Perspective** . . . . . . . . . . 45
Ritwik Patra, Nabarun Chandra Das, Manojit Bhattacharya, Pravat Kumar Shit, Bidhan Chandra Patra, and Suprabhat Mukherjee

**4 COVID-19 Risk Assessment Using the C4.5 Algorithm** . . . . . . . . . . 61
Sarmistha Nanda, Chhabi Rani Panigrahi, Bibudhendu Pati, Mamata Rath, and Tien-Hsiung Weng

**5 Recent Diagnostic Techniques for COVID-19** . . . . . . . . . . 75
Rajeshwar Kamal Kant Arya, Meena Kausar, Dheeraj Bisht, Deepak Kumar, Deepak Sati, and Govind Rajpal

**6 COVID-19: AI-Enabled Social Distancing Detector Using CNN** . . . . . . . . . . 95
K. Anitha Kumari, P. Purusothaman, D. Dharani, and R. Padmashani

7 **IoT-Enabled Applications and Other Techniques to Combat COVID-19** ... 117
N. Renugadevi, S. Saravanan, C. M. Naga Sudha, and Parul Tripathi

8 **Optimum Distribution of Protective Materials for COVID−19 with a Discrete Binary Gaining-Sharing Knowledge-Based Optimization Algorithm** ... 135
Said Ali Hassan, Prachi Agrawal, Talari Ganesh, and Ali Wagdy Mohamed

9 **Developing COVID-19 Vaccines by Innovative Bioinformatics Approaches** ... 159
Renu Jakhar, Neelam Sehrawat, and S. K. Gakhar

10 **Big Data Analytics for Modeling COVID-19 and Comorbidities: An Unmet Need** ... 185
Sushil K. Shakyawar, Sahil Sethi, Siddesh Southekal, Nitish K. Mishra, and Chittibabu Guda

11 **AR and VR and AI Allied Technologies and Depression Detection and Control Mechanism** ... 203
S. B. Goyal, Pradeep Bedi, and Navin Garg

12 **Machine Learning Techniques for the Identification and Diagnosis of COVID-19** ... 231
A. Gasmi

13 **Factors Associated with COVID-19 and Predictive Modelling of Spread Across Five Urban Metropolises in the World** ... 257
Arvind Chandra Pandey, Bikash Ranjan Parida, Shubham Bhattacharjee, Tannu Priya Wasim, Munizzah Salim, and Rahul Kashyap

14 **Chatbots for Coronavirus: Detecting COVID-19 Symptoms with Virtual Assessment Tool** ... 275
Aasma Chouhan, Supriya Pathak, and Reshma Tendulkar

15 **Enabled IoT Applications for Covid-19** ... 305
A. Gasmi

16 **Impact of Covid-19 Infodemic on the Global Picture** ... 333
Tapash Rudra and Sandeep Kautish

17 **COVIDz: Deep Learning for Coronavirus Disease Detection** ... 355
Mohammed Anis Oukebdane, Samir Ghouali, Emad Kamil Hussein, Mohammed Seghir Guellil, Amina Elbatoul Dinar, Walid Cherifi, Abd Ellah Youcef Taib, and Boualem Merabet

**Index** ... 379

# Chapter 1
# South Asian Countries Are Less Fatal Concerning COVID-19: A Hybrid Approach Using Machine Learning and M-AHP

**Soham Guhathakurata, Sayak Saha, Souvik Kundu, Arpita Chakraborty, and Jyoti Sekhar Banerjee**

## 1.1 Introduction

On 30 January 2020, the outbreak of COVID-19 [1] was declared a Public Health Emergency of International Concern by the World Health Organization, i.e., WHO, which later went on to declare COVID-19 as pandemic in 11 March. On 9 January 2020, the first confirmed death was in Wuhan. The first death outside of China occurred on 1 February 2020 in the Philippines, and the first death outside Asia was in France in 14 February [2]. So far, more than 188 countries and territories have recorded a minimum of one case of COVID-19. Many countries have imposed many containment measures like quarantines and curfews to restrict the spread of the virus. Many European countries had around 300 million people under lockdown by late April, while the United States had around 200 million people under some form of lockdown. However, there has been a constant rise in the death toll in the United States, with over 89,000 deaths as of 17 May 2020. Similarly, the First World nations in Europe and Asia have recorded a high ratio of confirmed cases to deaths compared to the SAARC countries. Approximately 1.5% of the total coronavirus cases worldwide have been accounted in South Asia and even a lower percentage of deaths among all the nations.

The South Asian Association for Regional Cooperation (SAARC) includes India, Afghanistan, Bangladesh, Maldives, Nepal, Pakistan, Bhutan, and Sri Lanka. These nations account for one-fifth of the world's population. In spite of the high population

S. Guhathakurata · S. Saha
Department of CSE, Bengal Institute of Technology, Kolkata, India

S. Kundu
Department of Electrical and Computer Engineering, Iowa State University, Ames, IA, USA

A. Chakraborty · J. S. Banerjee (✉)
Department of ECE, Bengal Institute of Technology, Kolkata, India



S. Kautish et al. (eds.), *Computational Intelligence Techniques for Combating COVID-19*, EAI/Springer Innovations in Communication and Computing,
https://doi.org/10.1007/978-3-030-68936-0_1

and average health facilities, the death rate has been significantly low in these parts of the world. India has 90,927 confirmed cases and 2872 deaths, which has accounted to be the highest among the SAARC nations as of 31 April 2020. In contrast, the death tolls for France, Italy, Spain, the United Kingdom, and Russia are all above 25,000.

Table 1.1 portrays the vast difference in the transformation of confirmed cases to death when it comes to comparing between the SAARC nations and the other developed countries. Taking into consideration that India's population is equivalent to 17.7% of the total world population and Dhaka, the capital of Bangladesh, accounts for the sixth most populated city in the world, the number of deaths has been low.

The paper highlights the factors which are the prime cause for such a low death toll in SAARC nations. It is a fact that SAARC countries account for one-fifth of the world population, and the transmission rate of such a high transmissible virus-like COVID-19 is relatively low in these nations. The factors [3] include:

(I) The average temperature, high humidity, and warmer weather in the South Asian region can reduce the transmission of the disease.
(II) The *Bacillus* Calmette-Guerin (BCG) vaccine, which is offered in these countries primarily for the protection against tuberculosis, creates a strong immune response against the virus.
(III) Critical days, which implies the least number of days taken by the government authority to impart action after the first report or confirmation of COVID-19 case in that country.
(IV) Average age of the country – the youth of any country responds significantly better compared to the aged population which has a crucial part to play for the death count of the countries.
(V) The herd immunity, which provides a resistance against deadly diseases that occur when a significantly large amount of population has become affected by the virus leading to the development of resistance against that infection.

Observations and reports have conveyed the idea that these factors have been the prime reasons for the low death rate of the SAARC nations. Using the analytical

**Table 1.1** Statistical data of COVID-19 for (a) countries with the highest deaths and (b) SAARC countries as of 15 May 2020 [25]

| (a) | | | (b) | | |
|---|---|---|---|---|---|
| Countries | Confirmed | Deaths | Countries | Confirmed | Deaths |
| USA | 14,97,244 | 89,420 | India | 90,927 | 2,872 |
| Russia | 2,81,752 | 2,631 | Pakistan | 40,151 | 873 |
| Spain | 2,77,719 | 27,650 | Bangladesh | 22,268 | 328 |
| UK | 2,40,161 | 34,466 | Afghanistan | 6,664 | 169 |
| Brazil | 2,33,511 | 15,662 | Sri Lanka | 960 | 9 |
| Germany | 2,24,760 | 31,763 | Maldives | 1,078 | 4 |
| Turkey | 1,48,067 | 4,096 | Nepal | 292 | 2 |
| France | 1,42,291 | 27,625 | Bhutan | 21 | 0 |

hierarchy process, logical weights have been assigned to these factors in order to calculate the susceptibility risk index for each and every country taken into consideration for this study. Finally, we have applied hierarchical clustering in order to have a proper visualization of the distribution of death rate of the respective countries corresponding to their risk index.

This paper is constructed as follows. In Sect. 1.2, the paper deals with related studies. Section 1.3 presents the causes of less disastrous effect of COVID-19 in South Asian countries. The experimental results and discussion are displayed in Sect. 1.4 followed by the conclusion in Sect. 1.5.

## 1.2 Related Studies

In the recent past, a lot of work in the field of data processing, market research, image processing, bioinformatics, etc. has been performed with the help of hierarchical clustering algorithm. A brief review is presented here.

Ying Zhao, George Karypis, and Usama Fayyad in [4] clustered documents by using hierarchical clustering [5]. The authors combined the features from both partitional and agglomerative approaches to remove the early-stage error and also improve the quality of clustering solutions. The result of this paper stated that for significantly high cases, constrained agglomerative methods result in better solutions than agglomerative methods alone.

Feng Luo, Kun Tang, and L Khan in [6] proposed to obtain gene expression pattern and find the number of clusters dynamically by using a new hierarchical clustering which constructs a hierarchy from top to bottom. This algorithm works efficiently in extracting patterns with different abstraction levels, thus recognizing features in complex gene expression.

Deng Cai et al. [7] proposed a hierarchical clustering method that uses textual, visual, and link analysis to cluster the web image search results into different semantic clusters. The representations comprise of textual feature-based representation, graph-based representation, and visual feature-based representation.

Seema Bandyopadhyay and E.J. Coyle in [8] proposed a randomized clustering and distributed algorithm. The algorithm can organize the sensors in a wireless sensor network (WSN) into the cluster. The authors observed that when the number of levels in the hierarchy increases, the energy savings also increase, so the authors applied the algorithm to produce a hierarchy of clusterheads.

Richard Cheng and Glenn W. Milligan in [9] mapped influence regions with the help of hierarchical clustering. They simulated core group data structures and went on to present three-dimensional response surface plots for several hierarchical clustering methods. They represented the relative influence of the corresponding coordinate location by the response surface in the bivariate data space on the clustering of the core groups. The study revealed by the substantial plot marked the differences between clustering methods.

Twinkle Tiwari and Nihar Ranjan Roy in [10] sensed the physical parameters like pressure, humidity, temperature, motion, etc. in heterogeneous wireless sensor networks by applying hierarchical clustering. They created a network of small battery-powered sensing nodes. These nodes report to a central node called base station after collecting information from its environment of deployment.

Through proper collaboration, these nodes fulfill their task. Since the energy source is constrained in WSNs, it should be used properly. Clustering has been used by the author to minimize energy dissipation in WSNs.

Michael R. Loken et al. in [11] proposed a system of applying hierarchical clustering to investigate the relationship between the presenting immunophenotype. In a large, controlled study of pediatric acute myeloid leukemia (AML) patients, this system will respond to therapy. On the basis of mathematical analysis of unsupervised hierarchical clustering, patients with similar diagnostic immunophenotypic expression profile (IEP) are grouped. An appropriate number of clusters were accomplished by minimizing within-cluster variation.

Dac-Tu Ho et al. in [12] proposed a method to find the optimal clusters by using an optimization method, i.e., particle swarm optimization (PSO). Bit error rate (BER), energy consumption, and unmanned aerial vehicle (UAV) travel time are reduced by the proposed method. To conserve energy in conventional wireless sensor networks (WSNs), low-energy adaptive clustering hierarchy (LEACH) is generally used. For large-scale deployments, conservation of energy is highly challenging than many other things.

Andy Podgurski and Charles Yang in [13] presented a new approach to reducing the manual labor required to estimate software reliability. To reduce the sample size necessary to estimate reliability, partition testing methods along with those of stratified sampling are combined with a given degree of precision. To stratify program executions, automatic cluster analysis is used and finally grouped those with similar features.

## 1.3 Reasons for less Disaster Regarding COVID-19 in South Asian Countries

The reason that makes COVID-19 [40, 41] a big threat is its spread rate. However, the conversion rate of affected cases to death cases varies in every country despite the high transmission rate. Quite a significant amount of margin has been noticed for the SAARC countries compared to the other nations with the correspondence of confirmed cases to death. Table 1.1 presents a marked difference between the death count of the top 4 counties and the SAARC nations with respect to the statistical data of COVID-19.

Figure 1.1 shows the death count's statistical visualization in eight different countries, which include four SAARC countries represented with dashed lines. The

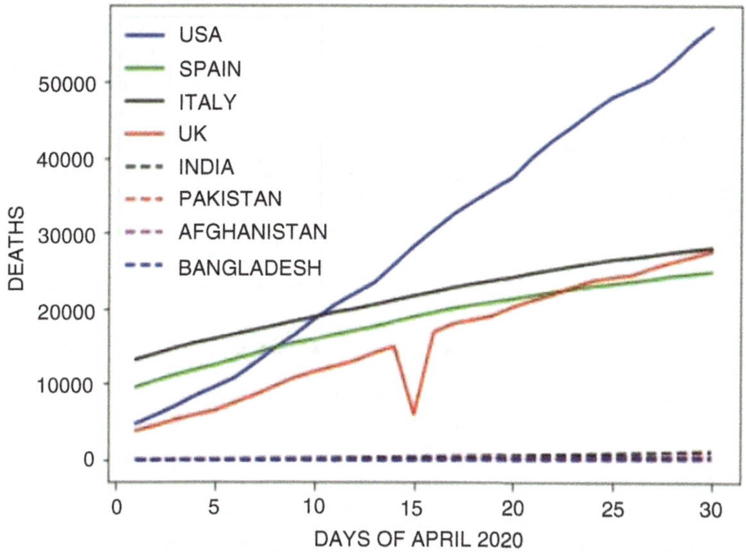


**Fig. 1.1** Death count of the top 4 counties and the SAARC nations due to COVID-19 in April 2020

four dashed different lines are clustered in the same space as the death count is very low in the SAARC countries.

**Crucial Factors Responsible for Low Death Rate in South Asian Countries**
All the fundamental factors that have been mentioned in Sect. 1.1 include (I) *Bacillus* Calmette-Guerin (BCG) vaccine, (II) average temperature, (III) average age, (IV) critical days, and (V) herd immunity which are described below elaborately.

I. *Bacillus* Calmette-Guerin (BCG) Vaccine: The objective of the BCG vaccine is to protect against tuberculosis [14]. Even though there has not been any direct link stating that this vaccine protects against COVID-19, however, it builds up the immune strength. Studies [15, 16] have proved that people with a strong immune system have better recovery chances from COVID-19 (see Table 1.2). Every SAARC nation takes the vaccine, whereas none of the countries with high death count takes it (Table 1.7).

II. *Average Temperature*: Zurich, London, Berlin, and Paris are the major cities that have recorded the highest death rate so far from COVID-19. During the months of February, March, and April, all these cities' average temperatures vary from 5.6 to 6.1 degrees Celsius [17]. In contrast, the temperature is quite high for the SAARC nations, which lies in 21.3 to 29.8 degrees Celsius. Studies have shown that the cumulative number of cases decreases by 0.86 [18] with every 1-degree Celsius increase in average temperature.

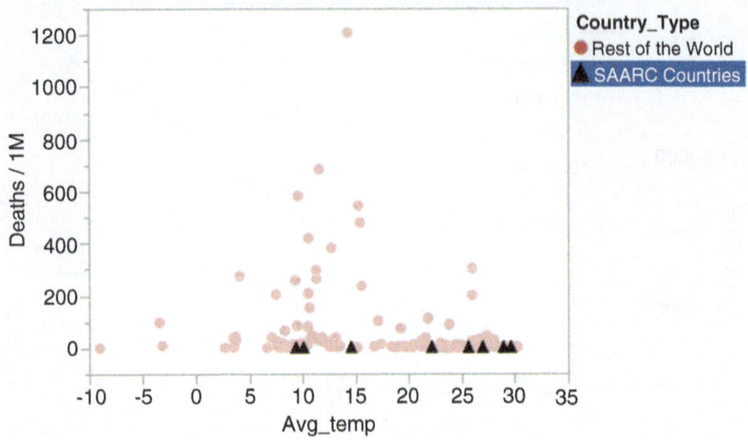


**Fig. 1.2** Death per million vs average temperature

The dependency of death per million corresponding to the average temperature is depicted in Fig. 1.2. Based on the data collected from 165 countries till 31 April, the graph is plotted. As a possible reason for this pandemic's fatalness, authors consider the average temperature of a country in this paper. The figure also depicts that three SAARC countries fall in the average temperature range of 7 to 15 degrees Celsius, which differs from the average temperature of other SAARC nations. For this reason, in order to make our prediction more robust and scalable, the weight given to average temperature during the calculation of risk factor (RF) in Eq. (1.1) carries the least value.

III. *Critical Days*: The critical days define the difference between the first day of occurrence of COVID-19 in that country and the day on which the government took action, i.e., localized recommendation, national recommendation, localized lockdown, and national lockdown [19]. Certain countries like Sri Lanka have been very proactive in their preparation against this virus and had taken action even before the country had its first confirmed case. On 25 March 2020, India declared the lockdown even when the overall death count of the country was below 50. In comparison, no proper lockdown was imposed in heavily affected places like the states in the United States and European countries like Sweden.

The SAARC nations have shown better results in the containment of the spread of COVID-19 on the scale of population density. Considering COVID-19, the impact of the critical days is relatively high compared to other infectious diseases. In Fig. 1.3, all the countries in the left section are the SAARC nations with low critical days compared to those countries with high critical days and high death rates in the right section.

**Table 1.2** Distribution of BCG vaccine taken by (a) countries with the highest deaths and (b) SAARC countries [14]

| (a) | | | | (b) | | | |
|---|---|---|---|---|---|---|---|
| Countries | Confirmed | Deaths | BCG Taken | Countries | Confirmed | Deaths | BCG Taken |
| USA | 14,97,244 | 89,420 | No | India | 90,927 | 2872 | Yes |
| Russia | 2,81,752 | 2631 | No | Pakistan | 40,151 | 873 | Yes |
| Spain | 2,77,719 | 27,650 | No | Bangladesh | 22,268 | 328 | Yes |
| UK | 2,40,161 | 34,466 | No | Afghanistan | 6664 | 169 | Yes |
| Brazil | 2,33,511 | 15,662 | Yes | Sri Lanka | 960 | 9 | Yes |
| Germany | 2,24,760 | 31,763 | No | Maldives | 1078 | 4 | Yes |
| Turkey | 1,48,067 | 4096 | Yes | Nepal | 292 | 2 | Yes |
| France | 1,42,291 | 27,625 | No | Bhutan | 21 | 0 | Yes |

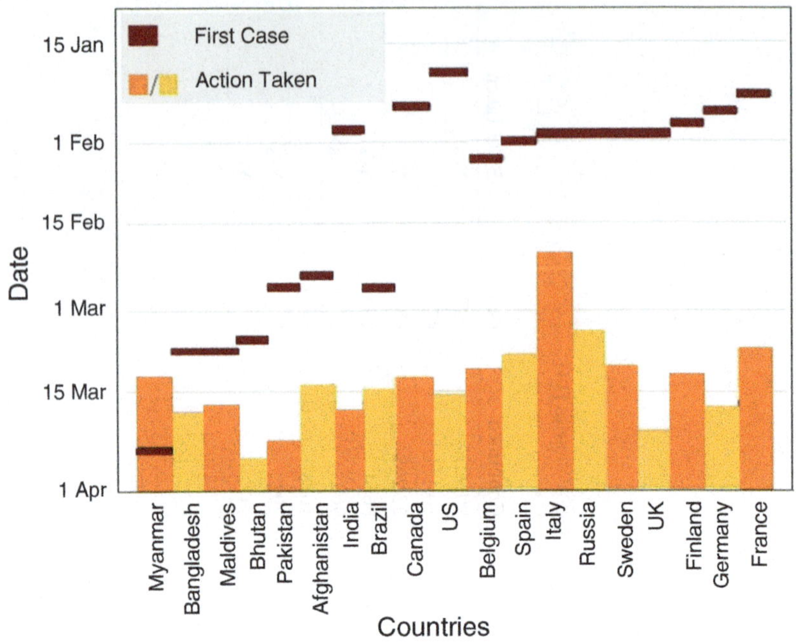


**Fig. 1.3** Duration between the first step taken and first COVID-19 confirmed case [20]

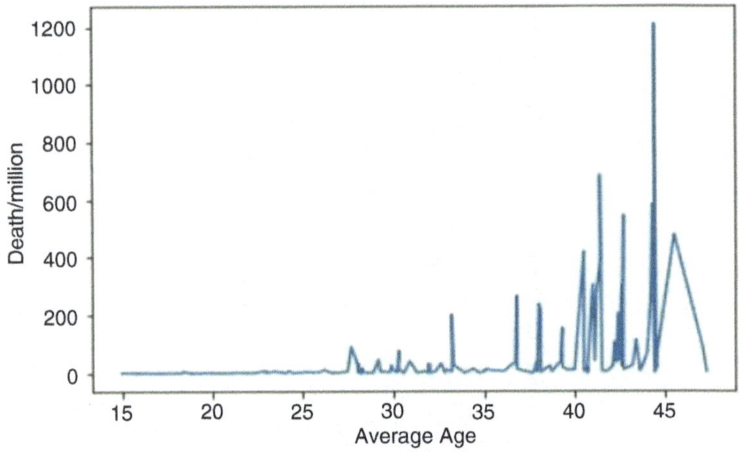


**Fig. 1.4** Death per million vs average age of a country

IV. *Average Age*: The immune system of the aged population is relatively weak against COVID-19 compared to the youth of the nation (see Fig. 1.4). The strong immune system of the younger people gives them the edge to fight against the virus. Moreover, the older people are surrounded by various diseases like heart disease, lung problems, etc., making them more vulnerable to getting COVID-19 infection. The age range of 18–44 years has been accounted for a low death rate of 3.9%. Whereas, the rate increases to 24.9% for 65–74 years old and to 48.7% for above 75 years of age [21]. The SAARC nations enjoy a low average age, in which India was the highest with an average age of 26.8. In contrast, the European countries like Italy, Germany, France, and the United Kingdom [22], all with high death counts, have an average age of over 40.

V. *Herd Immunity*: People from South Asian countries have experienced more exposure to highly infectious diseases as compared to the developed and leading nations of the world. With more exposure to pathogens, the white blood cells gain more power to recognize a virus by developing a broader memory that can trigger an immune response. The people of the SAARC countries tend to possess a wider variation in the leukocyte antigen genes, responsible for the immune response given the fact that their past history [23] has encounters with different infectious diseases like cholera, malaria, dengue, SARS-CoV-1 [24, 25], etc. As a result, the immune system becomes more proactive in producing antibodies that fight against viruses in the best way possible. This factor creates a severe impact in our study. When compared to the confirmed cases in SAARC countries, the number of death counts is relatively low, which solidifies the fact that a severe number of antibodies are generated by the immune system of the people in these countries, giving them the upper hand to fight against COVID-19. Not only the SAARC nations but also the African countries have a significantly low death count given the fact that they too enjoy a robust immune system that has been developed due to their previous encounters with diseases like Ebola and Zika. Compared to the European countries and American countries, people of all these underdeveloped nations have developed genetic diversity which has offered them better protection against COVID-19.

In this paper, the authors highlight five main factors, which are the prime cause for such a low death toll in SAARC nations. Few other points are also possible for this low death toll in SAARC nations, like the living style and public gathering habits of South Asian countries that are different from the rest of the world, i.e., South Asian people are living in big and wide houses, and there is very less culture of cluster living like high-roof multi-story building of Europe and America, food habits and hygiene, etc.

The authors have very carefully chosen the five key factors, as apart from five factors, all other factors are not uniformly applicable to all the SAARC countries. SAARC countries indeed have low testing and less capability to perform COVID PCR tests and insufficient epidemiological data, but one thing we must admit is that despite all difficulties, SAARC countries are showing the low death toll compared to the other nations.

The facts stated above showcase their impact and importance on the COVID-19 death count. With the help of these factors, we have analyzed each country corresponding to their death count. The outcome of this analysis has generated three clusters, namely, low risk, moderate risk, and high risk. To determine and generate the weights of these five factors with correspondence to their individual impact toward COVID-19 deaths, we have applied the multiple analytical hierarchy process. Then, we formulate an equation to calculate the risk of COVID-19 for each of the 165 countries with the help of the interdependency among each of these factors and the death rate. After the preprocessing of the data, we plot the three clusters on the basis of their risk index and death per million counts by applying hierarchical clustering. This entire methodology has been showcased in Fig. 1.8.

**Calculation of Risk Factor (RF)**

The authors have tried to estimate the "risk factor (RF)" associated with the individual country by investigating the situation with respect to the above attributes. The factors which are inversely proportional to the death count include high average temperature, usage of BCG, and immunity earned or herd immunity, whereas the factors which are directly proportional to the death count comprise of the high value of critical days and high average age. Hence, RF is calculated as mentioned below:

$$\begin{aligned} \mathrm{RF} = {} & 0.275 \times (\mathrm{Avg.Age}) + 0.243 \times (1/\mathrm{BCG}) \\ & + 0.215 \times (1/\mathrm{Herd\,Immunity}) \\ & + 0.116 \times (\mathrm{Critical\,Days}) \\ & + 0.083 \times (1/\mathrm{Avg.Temperature}) \end{aligned} \tag{1.1}$$

where the local weights of the five factors, i.e., avg. age, BCG given in % of the total population, immunity earned, critical days, and avg. temperature of the country, are obtained through M-AHP-based MCDM [32–36], i.e., multiple criteria decision-making technique [42–53]. In this chapter, the authors are considered four specialists' experience and mentioned as the four conditions to finally compute the weights of the factors.

1. *Condition 1.1*: Here, we recognize the average age is the most significant deciding factor, BCG given in % of the total population is the second, immunity earned is the third, critical days is the fourth, and average temperature of the country is the fifth vital deciding factor. Equation 1.2 shows the relative weight of the deciding factors.

$$Y = \begin{array}{c} \\ x1 \\ x2 \\ x3 \\ x4 \\ x5 \end{array} \begin{array}{c} \begin{array}{ccccc} x1 & x2 & x3 & x4 & x5 \end{array} \\ \begin{pmatrix} 1 & 2 & 3 & 4 & 5 \\ 1/2 & 1 & 2 & 3 & 4 \\ 1/3 & 1/2 & 1 & 2 & 3 \\ 1/4 & 1/3 & 1/2 & 1 & 2 \\ 1/5 & 1/4 & 1/3 & 1/2 & 1 \end{pmatrix} \end{array} \tag{1.2}$$

The normalized criteria weights of the five factors are calculated as W = {0.419, 0.263, 0.16, 0.097, 0.062}.

2. *Condition 1.2*: Here, for this condition, the expert assumes that all the factors have the same weight (see Eq. 1.3).

$$Y = \begin{array}{c} \\ x1 \\ x2 \\ x3 \\ x4 \\ x5 \end{array} \begin{array}{c} \begin{array}{ccccc} x1 & x2 & x3 & x4 & x5 \end{array} \\ \begin{pmatrix} 1 & 1 & 1 & 1 & 1 \\ 1 & 1 & 1 & 1 & 1 \\ 1 & 1 & 1 & 1 & 1 \\ 1 & 1 & 1 & 1 & 1 \\ 1 & 1 & 1 & 1 & 1 \end{pmatrix} \end{array} \tag{1.3}$$

The normalized criteria weights of the five factors are calculated as W = {0.2, 0.2, 0.2, 0.2, 0.2}.

3. *Condition 1.3*: Here, we consider the immunity earned is the most significant deciding factor, average age is the second, BCG given in % of the total population is the third, critical days is the fourth, and average temperature of the country is the fifth vital deciding factor. Equation 1.4 presents the relative weight of the deciding factors.

$$Y = \begin{array}{c} \\ x1 \\ x2 \\ x3 \\ x4 \\ x5 \end{array} \begin{array}{c} \begin{array}{ccccc} x1 & x2 & x3 & x4 & x5 \end{array} \\ \begin{pmatrix} 1 & 2 & 1/2 & 3 & 4 \\ 1/2 & 1 & 1/3 & 2 & 3 \\ 2 & 3 & 1 & 4 & 5 \\ 1/3 & 1/2 & 1/4 & 1 & 2 \\ 1/4 & 1/3 & 1/5 & 1/2 & 1 \end{pmatrix} \end{array} \tag{1.4}$$

The normalized criteria weights of the five factors are calculated as W = {0.263, 0.16, 0.419, 0.097, 0.062}.

4. *Condition 1.4*: Here, we consider the BCG given in % of the total population is the most significant deciding factor, average age is the second, immunity earned is the third, critical days is the fourth, and average temperature of the country is

the fifth vital deciding factor. Equation 1.5 presents the relative weight of the deciding factors.

$$Y = \begin{array}{c} \\ x1 \\ x2 \\ x3 \\ x4 \\ x5 \end{array} \begin{array}{c} \begin{array}{ccccc} x1 & x2 & x3 & x4 & x5 \end{array} \\ \begin{pmatrix} 1 & 1/2 & 2 & 3 & 4 \\ 2 & 1 & 3 & 4 & 5 \\ 1/2 & 1/3 & 1 & 2 & 3 \\ 1/3 & 1/4 & 1/2 & 1 & 2 \\ 1/4 & 1/5 & 1/3 & 1/2 & 1 \end{pmatrix} \end{array} \quad (1.5)$$

The normalized criteria weights of the five factors are calculated as W = {0.263, 0.419, 0.16, 0.097, 0.062}.

The normalized weights of the factors for different conditions are calculated by using an online computing software as mentioned below:

The normalized weights of the factors are calculated by using the formula of M-AHP (see Appendix A6), and the values are W = {0.275, 0.243, 0.215, 0.116, 0.083}, which shows weights of the average age, BCG given in % of the total population, immunity earned, critical days, and average temperature of the country, consecutively. The average temperature of the country is the least significant, and the average age is the most important criterion, which is cleared from Fig. 1.5.

To calculate the risk factor, we have generated a formula based on the weights calculated and the one-to-one relationship between each of the factors and the death rate. High average temperature, usage of BCG, and immunity earned or herd immunity are all inversely proportional to the death count. High average age and high value of critical days are directly proportional to the death count.

**Clustering Countries into Various Risk Regions via Hierarchical Clustering Process**

On the basis of the results of RF calculated with the help of Eq. 1.1, the countries have been grouped into three clusters like high risk, low risk, and moderate risk. *Hierarchical clustering algorithm* has been used to group the countries into different hazardous zones.

Hierarchical clustering is a powerful machine learning [31, 54–57] tool widely implemented in clustering techniques [30]. Based on the similarity between the nodes, they are being compared to produce a hierarchy of clusters. According to their relationship and similarity, the nodes are joined to build larger groups. Hierarchical clustering can be categorized into two different approaches, namely, *the agglomerative approach* and *the divisive approach*. The second one has been implemented in this study. The divisive approach is a top-down approach, while the agglomerative method is a bottom-up approach. Initially, all nodes belong to the same cluster in the divisive method, and gradually, they join based on their similarity to form its own cluster. A tree-like structure, known as dendrogram, is used to visualize the hierarchical clustering technique through the sequences of merges or splits (see Fig. 1.6).

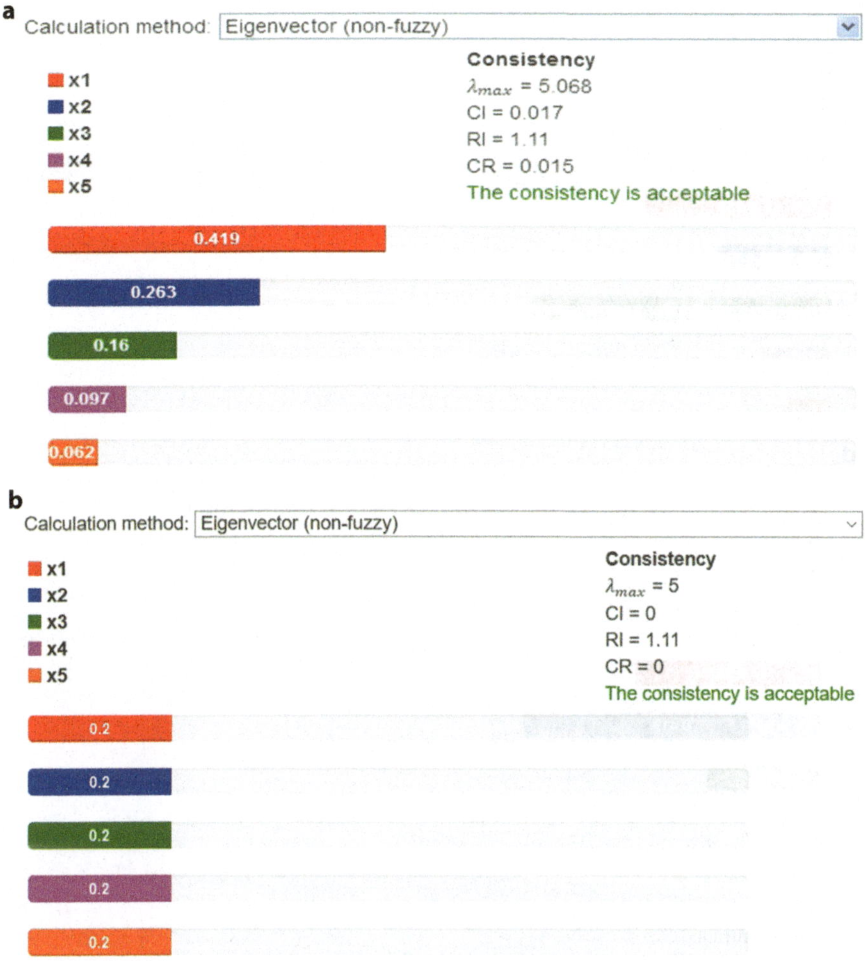


**Fig. 1.5** (**a–d**) Weights of the deciding factors using Saaty's AHP

c

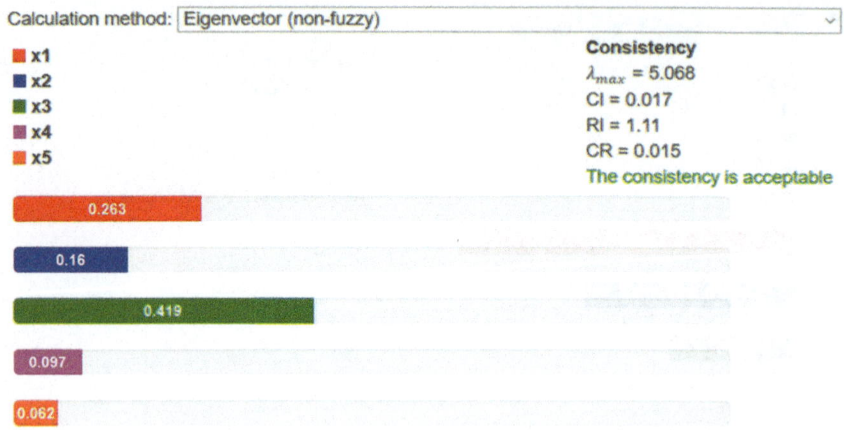


d

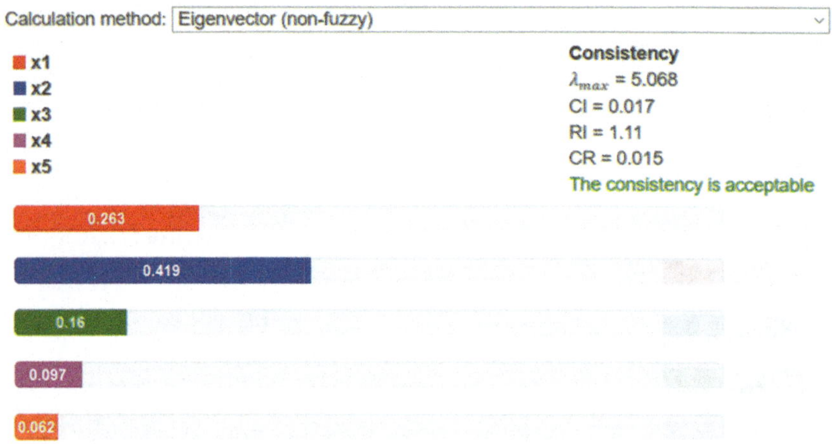


**Fig. .1.5** (continued)

**Stagewise Description of the Proposed Methodology**

This paper aims to establish the fact that South Asian countries have shown a less fatality rate concerning COVID-19. Figure 1.7 depicts the detailed sequence of the proposed approach. Firstly, authors have chosen the prime factors responsible for low death rates in South Asian countries, i.e., BCG, average temperature, critical days, average age, and herd immunity. Secondly, each of these attributes is to be weighed with the help of M-AHP. Thirdly, individual weights are to be designated corresponding to each of these attributes. Fourthly, combining the labeled attributes and the dataset for every individual country, the risk factor needs to be expressed. The countries are then to be clustered into low risk, moderate risk, and high risk through the hierarchical clustering technique. The clustering will provide the means necessary to analyze the SAARC countries with other countries.

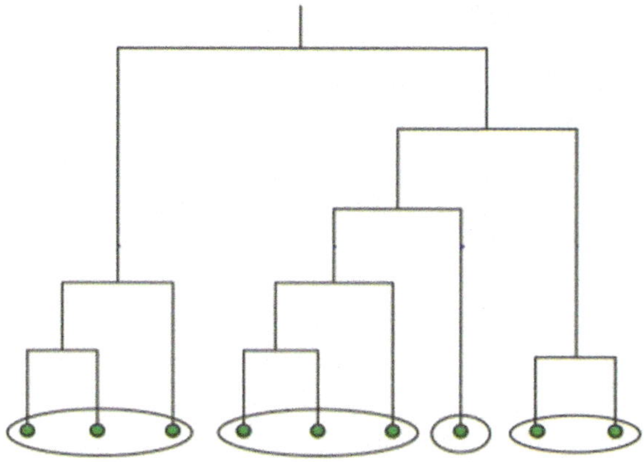

**Fig. 1.6** Dendrogram: an illustration of hierarchical clustering method

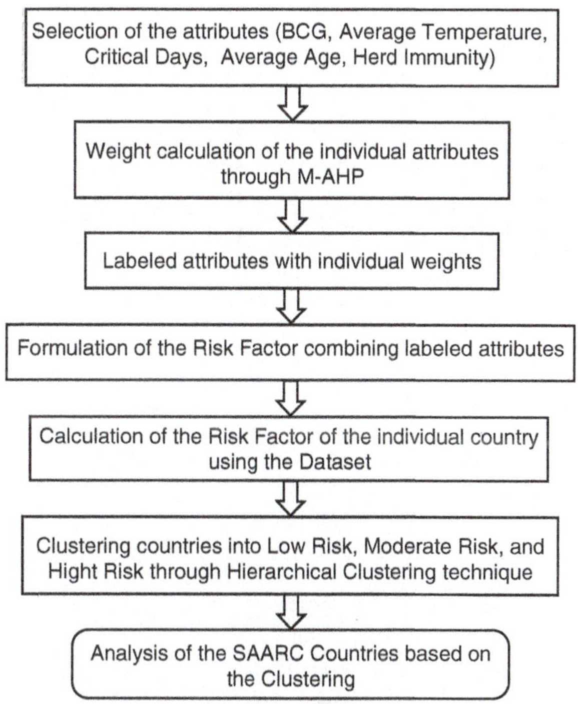


**Fig. 1.7** Step-by-step procedure of the proposed methodology

## 1.4 Experimental Result and Discussion

The purpose of our study is based on the fact that densely inhabited SAARC countries have accounted for a low death rate compared to the highly developed nations. The authors have arranged the dataset containing different attributes – death/million, the population density of each country (per km$^2$), and if the country is a member of SAARC or not (see Table 1.3). The dataset that has been used by the authors

**Table 1.3** Dataset-1 snapshot

| Country | Density (km$^2$) | Deaths /1 M | SAARC |
|---|---|---|---|
| Maldives | 1802 | 2.0 | Yes |
| Bangladesh | 1265 | 1.0 | Yes |
| Sint Maarten | 1261 | 303.0 | No |
| Bermuda | 1246 | 112.0 | No |
| Channel Islands | 907 | 236.0 | No |
| San Marino | 566 | 1208.0 | No |
| S. Korea | 527 | 5.0 | No |
| India | 464 | 1.0 | Yes |

**Table 1.4** Dataset-2 snapshot

| Country | BCG | Avg_temp | Critical Stage | Avg_Age | Immunity Earned | Deaths/1 M |
|---|---|---|---|---|---|---|
| San Marino | No | 14.33 | 17.0 | 44.4 | No | 1208.0 |
| Belgium | No | 11.55 | 11.55 | 41.4 | No | 684.0 |
| Andorra | No | 9.6 | 8.0 | 44.3 | No | 582.0 |
| Spain | No | 15.3 | 38.0 | 42.7 | Yes | 544.0 |
| Italy | No | 15.45 | 20.0 | 45.5 | Yes | 478.0 |
| UK | No | 10.55 | 51.0 | 40.5 | Yes | 419.0 |
| France | No | 12.7 | 44.0 | 41.4 | Yes | 381.0 |
| Sint Maarten | No | 26.0 | 18.0 | 41.0 | No | 303.0 |

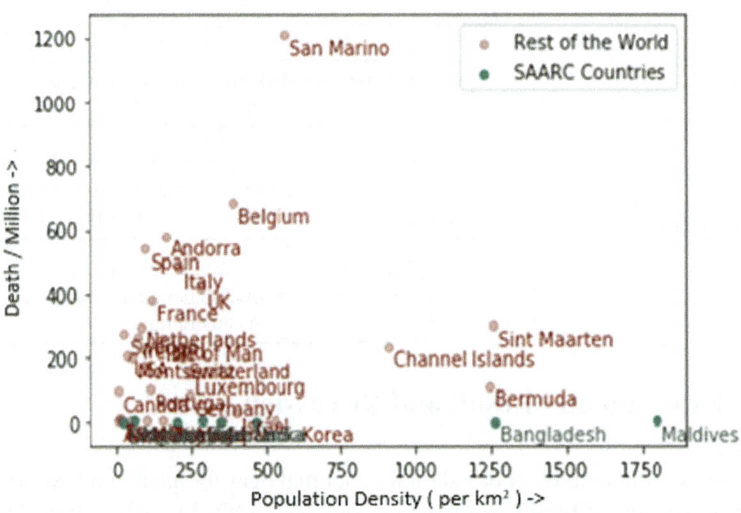


**Fig. 1.8** Distribution of countries on the basic of death/million vs population density

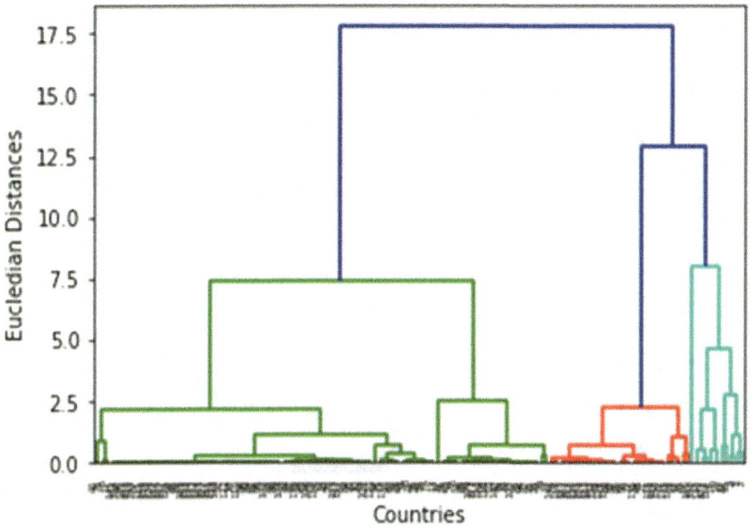


**Fig. 1.9** Dendrogram

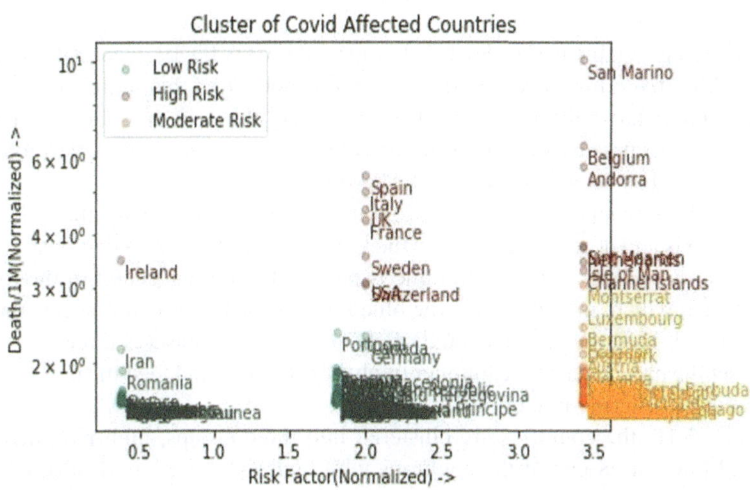


**Fig. 1.10** Cluster of COVID-19-affected countries (death/million vs risk factor)

for this report has been gathered from different sources from the Internet [14, 20, 25–28]. The dataset contains eight SAARC countries, countries with a high number of deceased, and developed countries along with South Korea and Singapore whose early check to COVID-19 strategy encourages the world.

Figure 1.8 portrays that SAARC countries like Bangladesh and Maldives, even with very high population density, still have a low deceased count of COVID-19-infected persons. The authors present an experimental outcome to showcase how

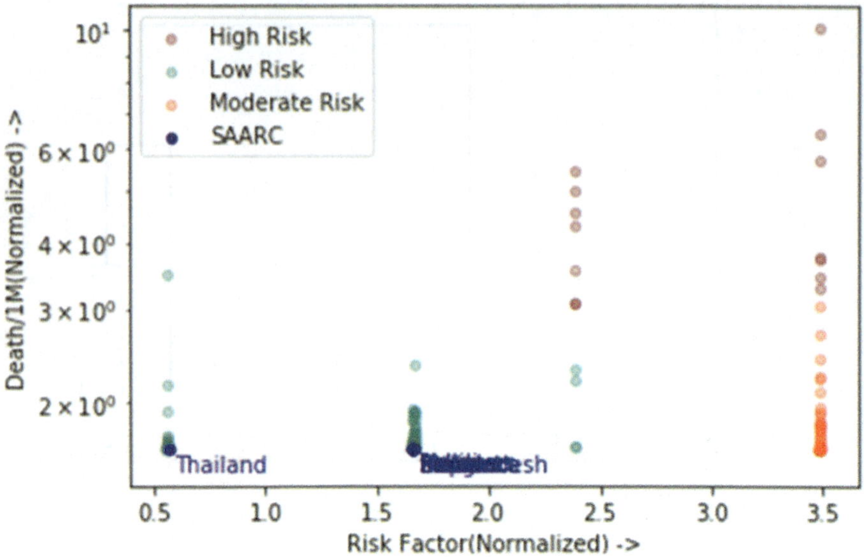


**Fig. 1.11** Cluster of affected SAARC countries (death/million vs risk factor)

the five factors established in Sect. 1.3 control the COVID-19 deceased count and why SAARC has a low deceased rate in the next portion of this segment.

The dataset has been constructed to study the effect of risk factors, and the deceased count contains the figures of 165 countries with 6 attributes (see Table 1.4). Here, the data has been considered till 31 April 2020.

The authors mapped out the dendrogram (see Fig. 1.9), taking the risk factor (RF) as x-axis and death per million as the y-axis. The dendrogram demonstrates the clusters' arrangement. A horizontal line is passed through the center of the longest vertical line, which, in this case, is the blue line. As the horizontal line cuts through three vertical lines, the optimal count of clusters for this dataset is three.

We set the parameter of the number of clusters to three and feed the dataset to our hierarchical clustering model [29].

In Fig. 1.10, the countries are clustered into three groups, high risk, moderate risk, and low risk. Some of the countries with high risk have low deaths, which is mainly due to their low population. The United States, the United Kingdom, France, and Italy are all clustered together in the high-risk zone and also have a higher death count. The figure clearly demonstrates that the countries with the lower risk factor also have lower death rates. In Fig. 1.10, we applied an extra filter to label the SAARC countries only to show the cluster in which these countries belong.

The position of the SAARC countries (colored and labeled blue) is shown in Fig. 1.11. The outcome proves the impact of the factors that we have taken into cognition. It is clearly demonstrated that the SAARC countries have a lower risk factor; as a result, the death rate is also low. Apart from the SAARC countries, the nations that satisfy the ideal conditions of the five factors we have considered also display a low deceased count, as shown in Fig. 1.10.

## 1.5 Concluding Remarks

COVID-19 virus is evolving day by day through mutations, as a result of which, the number of infected cases has shown an exponential rate of increase. Many of the countries, like the United States, France, and Italy, have reached the stage of community spread. Countries like India, Pakistan, and Bangladesh, with such high population density, still have some control over the death count due to COVID-19. In a similar likelihood, other SAARC countries have accounted for even very low infected cases. This paper has authenticated the factors that segregate the SAARC countries from the other nations with high infected cases and high death counts. Each of the factors has been considered with correspondence to their impact on 165 different countries. After a proper study of the interrelation between these factors with death count, they have been weighted. The risk index calculated displays accurate outcomes when matched with real-time data. Our study's aim and objective have been well-grounded with the help of cluster graphs, which give us a visualization of where the SAARC countries stand with regard to the COVID-19 death count when they are being compared to the other top nations with highly developed medical facilities.

## Appendix: Multiple Analytical Hierarchy Process (M-AHP)

For decision-making, AHP is a popularly used method, but the key disadvantage of AHP is that it follows a single expert's experience to build the evolutionary matrix, which sometimes does not match with real-time scenarios. Hence, the extension of AHP to cover the said disadvantage is also suggested, i.e., multiple AHP, where instead of a single expert's view, a couple of expert views can be considered.

The algorithm of basic AHP mainly has four steps as follows [36–39]:

*Step 1*: Based on the given problem, the decision hierarchy needs to be formed with the sub-problems or the independent factors.

*Step 2*: Decision-maker needs to calculate and decide the weights to the judgment factors. Pairwise comparison is executed on each decision factor.

**Table 1.5** 1 to 9 AHP scale (Saaty proposed)

| Saaty's rating | Description |
|---|---|
| 1 | Equal significance |
| 3 | Moderate significance |
| 5 | Essential or strong significance |
| 7 | Very strong significance |
| 9 | Extreme significance |
| 2, 4, 6, 8 | Intermediate values of the two adjacent judgments |

*Step 3*: It is very essential to confirm that the consistency ratio is maintained based on the calculation.

*Step 4*: The final ranking of each alternative is obtained considering the synthesized overall result.

Considering the pairwise comparison of each judgment factor, an evaluation matrix Y is to be formed. Experts will choose the value of the weight factors from the Saaty's 1 to 9 fundamental scale (Table 1.5). Now, square matrix Y can be written as:

$$Y = \left(y_{pq}\right)_{a\times a} = \begin{pmatrix} y_{11} & y_{12} & y_{13} \\ y_{21} & y_{22} & y_{23} \\ y_{31} & y_{32} & y_{33} \end{pmatrix} \quad (1.6)$$

pth and the qth judgment factor is expressed by $y_{pq}$, and here, a number of decision factors are considered. Each entry of the matrix can be written as the pairwise ratio, i.e., $y_{pq} = w_p/w_q$ where $p$, q = 1, 2, …, a. In AHP, each entry of the matrix maintains the reciprocal property $y_{pq} = 1/y_{qp}$.

The following condition needs to be met for becoming matrix Y as a consistent matrix:

$$y_{pr}\,y_{rq} = y_{pq}\ , \qquad p,q,r = 1,2,\ldots\ldots\ldots\ldots,a \quad (1.7)$$

The equation $Yw_{\mathrm{AHP}} = \lambda_{\max} w_{\mathrm{AHP}}$ provides the eigenvalue $\lambda_{\max}$ and eigenvector $w_{\mathrm{AHP}}$. Priority vector $w_{\mathrm{AHP}} = \{w_1, w_2, \ldots\ldots w_a\}$ expresses the local weights of the criteria. Due to the inconsistency of the matrices, it $w_{\mathrm{AHP}}$ is necessary to find out the decision error, which can be measured by the consistency ratio (C.R.). C.R. is simply a ratio of consistency index (C.I.) to random index (R.I.), viz., *C. R.* = C. I. : R. I. Table 1.6 shows all the R.I. values corresponding to the various number of decision factors. Again, C.I. can be described as $\mathrm{C.I.} = \frac{\left(\lambda_{\max} - \mathrm{a}\right)}{\left(\mathrm{a}-1\right)}$.

$$\text{where} \quad \lambda_{\max} = \left(\frac{1}{a}\right)\sum_{p=1}^{a} \frac{\left(Yw_{\mathrm{AHP}}\right)_p}{w_{\mathrm{AHP}p}} \quad (1.8)$$

Normally, $C.\,I. = 0$ is expected for consistent matrix and the accepted value of the $C.\,R. \leq 0.1$; otherwise when $C.\,R. > 0.1$, adjustment is required pairwise

**Table 1.6** Values of R.I

| Average Random Index (RI) | | | | | | | | | | |
|---|---|---|---|---|---|---|---|---|---|---|
| a | 1 | 2 | 3 | 4 | 5 | 6 | 7 | 8 | 9 | 10 |
| RI | 0 | 0 | 0.58 | 0.90 | 1.12 | 1.24 | 1.32 | 1.41 | 1.45 | 1.49 |

**Table 1.7** Distribution of BCG vaccine taken worldwide

| Country | BCG | Country | BCG |
|---|---|---|---|
| USA | No | Japan | Yes |
| Spain | No | UAE | Yes |
| Italy | No | Poland | Yes |
| UK | No | Romania | Yes |
| France | No | Ukraine | Yes |
| Germany | No | Indonesia | Yes |
| Russia | Yes | S. Korea | Yes |
| Turkey | Yes | Bangladesh | Yes |
| Brazil | Yes | Denmark | No |
| Iran | Yes | Serbia | No |
| China | Yes | Philippines | Yes |
| Canada | No | Dominican Republic | Yes |
| Belgium | No | Norway | No |
| Peru | Yes | Czechia | No |
| India | Yes | Colombia | Yes |
| Netherlands | No | Panama | Yes |
| Switzerland | No | Australia | No |
| Ecuador | No | South Africa | Yes |
| Saudi Arabia | Yes | Egypt | Yes |
| Portugal | Yes | Malaysia | Yes |
| Mexico | Yes | Finland | No |
| Sweden | No | Kuwait | Yes |
| Ireland | Yes | Morocco | Yes |
| Pakistan | Yes | Argentina | Yes |
| Chile | Yes | Algeria | Yes |
| Singapore | Yes | Moldova | Yes |
| Belarus | Yes | Kazakhstan | Yes |
| Israel | No | Luxembourg | No |
| Qatar | Yes | Bahrain | No |
| Austria | No | Hungary | Yes |
| Thailand | Yes | Tunisia | Yes |
| Afghanistan | Yes | Latvia | No |
| Oman | Yes | Cyprus | No |
| Greece | Yes | Kyrgyzstan | Yes |
| Nigeria | Yes | Albania | Yes |
| Armenia | Yes | Niger | Yes |
| Iraq | Yes | Andorra | No |
| Uzbekistan | Yes | Lebanon | No |
| Ghana | Yes | Costa Rica | Yes |
| Croatia | Yes | Sri Lanka | Yes |
| Azerbaijan | Yes | Guatemala | Yes |
| Bosnia and Herzegovina | Yes | Uruguay | Yes |
| | | Georgia | Yes |

(continued)

**Table 1.7** (continued)

| Country | BCG | Country | BCG |
|---|---|---|---|
| Iceland | No | San Marino | No |
| Estonia | Yes | Mali | Yes |
| Bulgaria | Yes | El Salvador | Yes |
| Cuba | Yes | Channel Islands | No |
| Bolivia | Yes | Maldives | Yes |
| North Macedonia | Yes | Kenya | Yes |
| New Zealand | No | Malta | Yes |
| Slovenia | No | Jamaica | Yes |
| Lithuania | Yes | Jordan | Yes |
| Slovakia | No | Taiwan | Yes |
| Ivory Coast | Yes | Paraguay | Yes |
| Senegal | Yes | Venezuela | Yes |
| Djibouti | Yes | Palestine | No |
| Honduras | Yes | Mauritius | Yes |
| Hong Kong | Yes | Montenegro | No |
| Isle of Man | No | Nepal | Yes |
| Equatorial Guinea | Yes | Cayman Islands | No |
| Vietnam | Yes | Libya | Yes |
| Guinea-Bissau | Yes | French Polynesia | No |
| Faeroe Islands | No | South Sudan | No |
| Cabo Verde | Yes | Malawi | Yes |
| Myanmar | Yes | Mongolia | Yes |
| Madagascar | Yes | Angola | Yes |
| Gibraltar | No | Zimbabwe | Yes |
| Ethiopia | Yes | Antigua and Barbuda | No |
| Brunei | No | | |
| Zambia | Yes | Timor-Leste | Yes |
| Togo | Yes | Botswana | Yes |
| Trinidad and Tobago | No | Belize | Yes |
| Bermuda | No | New Caledonia | No |
| Eswatini | No | Gambia | Yes |
| Aruba | No | Curaçao | No |
| Uganda | Yes | Sao Tome and Principe | Yes |
| Haiti | Yes | Burundi | Yes |
| CAR | Yes | Turks and Caicos | No |
| Bahamas | No | Montserrat | No |
| Guyana | Yes | Greenland | Yes |
| Barbados | Yes | Suriname | No |
| Liechtenstei | No | Mauritania | Yes |
| Mozambique | Yes | Bhutan | Yes |
| Sint Maarten | No | | |

comparison. Using Saaty's AHP, the final rankings of the alternatives are expressed by global ranking $w_{\mathrm{AHP}_{\mathrm{Global}}}$ where $\mathrm{w}_{\mathrm{AHP}\ q}$ are the local weights:

$$w_{\mathrm{AHP}_{\mathrm{Global}}} = w_{\mathrm{AHP}_{\mathrm{intermediate}}\ q} . \mathrm{w}_{\mathrm{AHP}\ q} \tag{1.9}$$

Instead of a single expert's view, a couple of expert views can be considered in the M-AHP process. Four expert views are considered using the M-AHP method in this chapter.

Using the experience of one specialist $p$, AHP weights, i.e., $w_{\mathrm{AHP}}$, are shown below:

$$w_{\mathrm{AHPp}} = \left[\mathrm{m}_{p1}, \mathrm{m}_{p2}, \ldots\ldots \mathrm{m}_{pa}\right] \quad \text{for} \quad \sum_{q=1}^{a} \mathrm{m}_{pq} = 1 \quad \text{where} \quad p = 1,2,\ldots,4 \tag{1.10}$$

Using M-AHP, the weight vector $w_{\mathrm{M-AHP}}$ is formulated by applying geometric mean method as shown below:

$$w_{\mathrm{M-AHP}} = \left[\mathrm{n}_1, \mathrm{n}_2, \ldots\ldots \mathrm{n}_{\mathrm{a}}\right], n_q = \sqrt[4]{\prod_{\mathrm{p=1}}^{4} \mathrm{m}_{\mathrm{pq}}} \quad \text{where} \quad q = 1,2,\ldots.\mathrm{a} \tag{1.11}$$

## References


1. WHO-China Joint Mission, Report of the WHO-China Joint Mission on Coronavirus Disease 2019 (COVID-19). (2020). https://www.who.int/docs/default-source/coronaviruse/who-china-joint-mission-on-covid-19-final-report.pdf. Accessed May 1, 2020.
2. https://en.wikipedia.org/wiki/Covid-19. accessed May 1, 2020.
3. https://theprint.in/health/why-south-asia-has-20-of-worlds-population-but-less-than-2-of-covid-19-cases/408471/. Accessed May 2, 2020.
4. Zhao, Y., Karypis, G., & Fayyad, U. (2005). Hierarchical clustering algorithms for document datasets. *Data Mining and Knowledge Discovery, 10*(2), 141–168.
5. Bar-Joseph, Z., Gifford, D. K., & Jaakkola, T. S. (2001). Fast optimal leaf ordering for hierarchical clustering. *Bioinformatics, 17*(suppl_1), S22–S29.
6. Luo, F., Tang, K., & Khan, L. (2003, March). Hierarchical clustering of gene expression data. In *Third IEEE Symposium on Bioinformatics and Bioengineering, 2003. Proceedings.* (pp. 328–335). IEEE.
7. Cai, D., He, X., Li, Z., Ma, W. Y., & Wen, J. R. (2004, October). Hierarchical clustering of WWW image search results using visual, textual and link information. In *Proceedings of the 12th annual ACM international conference on Multimedia* (pp. 952–959).
8. Bandyopadhyay, S., & Coyle, E. J. (2003, March). An energy efficient hierarchical clustering algorithm for wireless sensor networks. In *IEEE INFOCOM 2003. Twenty-second Annual Joint Conference of the IEEE Computer and Communications Societies* (IEEE Cat. No. 03CH37428) (Vol. 3, pp. 1713–1723). IEEE.
9. Cheng, R., & Milligan, G. W. (1995). Mapping influence regions in hierarchical clustering. *Multivariate Behavioral Research, 30*(4), 547–576.

10. Tiwari, T., & Roy, N. R. (2015, May). Hierarchical clustering in heterogeneous wireless sensor networks: a survey. In *International Conference on Computing, Communication & Automation* (pp. 1385–1390). IEEE.
11. Loken, M. R., Voigt, A. P., Gerbing, R. B., Brodersen, L. E., Menssen, A. J., Pardo, L., & Meshinchi, S. (2015). Hierarchical clustering of immunophenotypic cell surface antigen expression identifies clinically meaningful cohorts in childhood AML: A report from the Children's Oncology Group protocol AAML0531.
12. Ho, D. T., Grøtli, E. I., Sujit, P. B., Johansen, T. A., & Sousa, J. B. (2013, May). Cluster-based communication topology selection and UAV path planning in wireless sensor networks. In *2013 International Conference on Unmanned Aircraft Systems (ICUAS)* (pp. 59–68). IEEE.
13. Podgurski, A., & Yang, C. (1993). Partition testing, stratified sampling, and cluster analysis. *ACM SIGSOFT Software Engineering Notes, 18*(5), 169–181.
14. http://www.bcgatlas.org/. Accessed May 6, 2020.
15. https://www.bloomberg.com/news/articles/2020-04-02/fewer-coronavirus-deaths-seen-in-countries-that-mandate-tb-vaccine. Accessed May 6, 2020.
16. https://www.newindianexpress.com/opinions/2020/apr/29/coronavirus-and-the-bcg-vaccine-2136722.html. Accessed May 6, 2020.
17. Wang, J., Tang, K., Feng, K., & Lv, W. (2020). High temperature and high humidity reduce the transmission of COVID-19. Available at SSRN 3551767.
18. Wang, M., Jiang, A., Gong, L., Luo, L., Guo, W., Li, C., & Chen, Y. (2020). Temperature significant change COVID-19 Transmission in 429 cities. MedRxiv.
19. https://academic.oup.com/jtm/article/27/3/taaa037/5808003. Accessed May 10, 2020.
20. https://www.bbc.com/news/world-52103747. Accessed May 10, 2020.
21. https://www.worldometers.info/coronavirus/coronavirus-age-sex-demographics/. Accessed May 12, 2020.
22. https://www.vox.com/2020/3/12/21173783/coronavirus-death-age-covid-19-elderly-seniors. Accessed May 12, 2020.
23. https://www.jhsph.edu/covid-19/articles/achieving-herd-immunity-with-covid19.html. Accessed May 13, 2020.
24. https://en.wikipedia.org/wiki/2002%E2%80%932004_SARS_outbreak. Accessed May, 13, 2020.
25. https://www.worldometers.info/coronavirus/. Accessed May 15, 2020.
26. https://en.wikipedia.org/wiki/List_of_countries_by_median_age. Accessed May 15, 2020.
27. https://www.weather-atlas.com/en/climate, (accessed May 15, 2020).
28. https://en.wikipedia.org/wiki/Pandemic (accessed May 15, 2020).
29. https://en.wikipedia.org/wiki/Hierarchical_clustering
30. Banerjee, J., Maiti, S., Chakraborty, S., Dutta, S., Chakraborty, A., & Banerjee, J. S. (2019, March) Impact of machine learning in various network security applications. In *2019 3rd International Conference on Computing Methodologies and Communication (ICCMC)* (pp. 276–281). IEEE.
31. Pandey, I., Dutta, H. S., & Banerjee, J. S. (2019, March). WBAN: A Smart Approach to Next Generation e-healthcare System. In *2019 3rd International Conference on Computing Methodologies and Communication (ICCMC)* (pp. 344–349). IEEE.
32. Paul, S., Chakraborty, A., & Banerjee, J. S. (2019). The extent analysis based fuzzy AHP approach for relay selection in WBAN. In *Cognitive Informatics and Soft Computing* (pp. 331–341). Singapore: Springer.
33. Paul, S., Chakraborty, A., & Banerjee, J. S. (2017, November). A fuzzy AHP-based relay node selection protocol for wireless body area networks (WBAN). In *2017 4th International Conference on Opto-Electronics and Applied Optics (Optronix)* (pp. 1–6). IEEE.
34. Chattopadhyay, J., Kundu, S., Chakraborty, A., Banerjee, J.S. (2020) Facial expression recognition for human computer interaction, in *Proceedings of International Conference On Computational Vision and Bio Inspired Computing* (pp. 1181–1192). Springer, Cham.

35. Banerjee, J. S., Chakraborty, A., & Chattopadhyay, A. (2018). Relay node selection using analytical hierarchy process (AHP) for secondary transmission in multi-user cooperative cognitive radio systems. In *Advances in electronics, communication and computing* (pp. 745–754). Singapore: Springer.
36. Saha, O., Chakraborty, A., & Banerjee, J. S. (2017, November). A decision framework of IT-based stream selection using analytical hierarchy process (AHP) for admission in technical institutions. In *2017 4th International Conference on Opto-Electronics and Applied Optics (Optronix)* (pp. 1–6). IEEE.
37. Saha, O., Chakraborty, A., & Banerjee, J. S. (2019). A fuzzy AHP approach to IT-based stream selection for admission in technical institutions in India. In *Emerging technologies in data mining and information security* (pp. 847–858). Singapore: Springer.
38. Banerjee, J. S., Chakraborty, A., & Chattopadhyay, A. (2018). Reliable best-relay selection for secondary transmission in co-operation based cognitive radio systems: a multi-criteria approach. *Journal of Mechanics of Continua and Mathematical Sciences, 13*(2), 24–42.
39. Banerjee, J. S., Chakraborty, A., & Chattopadhyay, A. (2018). A novel best relay selection protocol for cooperative cognitive radio systems using fuzzy AHP. *Journal of Mechanics of Continua and Mathematical Sciences, 13*(2), 72–87.
40. Guhathakurata, S., Kundu, S., Chakraborty, A., Banerjee, J. S. (2021). A Novel Approach to Predict COVID-19 Using Support Vector Machine. In *Data Science for COVID-19*, Elsevier (press).
41. Biswas, S., Sharma, L. K., Ranjan, R., & Banerjee, J. S. (2020). Go-COVID: An Interactive Cross-platform Based Dashboard for Real-time Tracking of COVID-19 using Data Analytics. *Journal of Mechanics of Continua and Mathematical Sciences, 15*(6), 1–15.
42. Banerjee, J. S., Chakraborty, A., & Chattopadhyay, A. (2017). Fuzzy based relay selection for secondary transmission in cooperative cognitive radio networks. In *Advances in optical science and engineering* (pp. 279–287). Singapore: Springer.
43. Chakraborty, A., Banerjee, J. S., & Chattopadhyay, A. (2020). Malicious node restricted quantized data fusion scheme for trustworthy spectrum sensing in cognitive radio networks. *Journal of Mechanics of Continua and Mathematical Sciences, 15*(1), 39–56.
44. Chakraborty, A., Banerjee, J. S., & Chattopadhyay, A. (2019). Non-uniform quantized data fusion rule for data rate saving and reducing control channel overhead for cooperative spectrum sensing in cognitive radio networks. *Wireless Personal Communications, 104*(2), 837–851.
45. Chakraborty, A., Banerjee, J. S., & Chattopadhyay, A. (2017). Non-uniform quantized data fusion rule alleviating control channel overhead for cooperative spectrum sensing in cognitive radio networks". In *2017 IEEE 7th International Advance Computing Conference (IACC)* (pp. 210–215). IEEE, 2017.
46. Roy, R., Dutta, S., Biswas, S., & Banerjee, J. S. (2020). Android things: A comprehensive solution from things to smart display and speaker. In *Proceedings of International Conference on IoT Inclusive Life (ICIIL 2019), NITTTR Chandigarh, India* (pp. 339–352). Singapore: Springer.
47. Das, D., Pandey, I., Chakraborty, A., & Banerjee, J. S. (2017). Analysis of Implementation Factors of 3D Printer: The Key Enabling Technology for making Prototypes of the Engineering Design and Manufacturing. *International Journal of Computer Applications, 1*, 8–14.
48. Das, D., Pandey, I., & Banerjee, J. S. (2016). An in-depth study of implementation issues of 3D Printer. In: *Proc. MICRO 2016 Conference on Microelectronics, Circuits and Systems*, pp. 45–49.
49. Banerjee, J.S., Goswami, D. & Nandi, S. (2014). OPNET: A new paradigm for simulation of advanced communication systems. In: *Proc. International Conference on Contemporary Challenges in Management, Technology & Social Sciences, SEMS*, pp. 319–328, Lucknow, India.
50. Banerjee, J. S., & Chakraborty, A. (2015). Fundamentals of software defined radio and cooperative spectrum sensing: A step ahead of cognitive radio networks. In N. Kaabouch & W. Hu (Eds.), *Handbook of research on software-defined and cognitive radio technologies for dynamic spectrum management* (pp. 499–543). Hershey: IGI Global.

51. Banerjee, J. S., & Chakraborty, A. (2014). Modeling of software defined radio architecture & cognitive radio, the next generation dynamic and smart spectrum access technology. In M. H. Rehmani & Y. Faheem (Eds.), *Cognitive radio sensor networks: Applications, architectures, and challenges* (pp. 127–158). Hershey: IGI Global.
52. Banerjee, J. S., Chakraborty, A., & Karmakar, K. (2013). Architecture of cognitive radio networks. In N. Meghanathan & Y. B. Reddy (Eds.), *Cognitive radio technology applications for wireless and mobile ad hoc networks* (pp. 125–152). Hershey: IGI Global.
53. Banerjee, J. S., & Karmakar, K. (2012). A Comparative study on cognitive radio implementation issues. *International Journal of Computer Applications, 45*(15), 44–51.
54. Guhathakurata, S., Saha, S., Kundu, S., Chakraborty, A., & Banerjee, J. S. (2021). A new approach to predict COVID-19 using artificial neural networks. In *Cyber-Physical Systems: AI and COVID-19*, Elsevier (press).
55. Saha, P., Guhathakurata, S., Saha, S., Chakraborty, A., & Banerjee, J. S. (2021). Application of machine learning in app-based cab booking system: A survey on Indian scenario. *In 2020 1st Global Conference on Artificial Intelligence and Applications (GCAIA)*, Springer (press).
56. Chakraborty, A., & Banerjee, J. S. (2013). An advance Q learning (AQL) approach for path planning and obstacle avoidance of a mobile robot. *International Journal of Intelligent Mechatronics and Robotics (IJIMR), 3*(1), 53–73.
57. Biswas, S., Sharma, L.K., Ranjan, R., Saha, S., Banerjee, J. S. (2021). Smart farming & water saving based intelligent irrigation system implementation using IoT. In Recent trends in computational intelligence enabled research. Elsevier (press).

# Chapter 2
# Application of Deep Learning Strategies to Assess COVID-19 Patients

**V. Ramasamy, Chhabi Rani Panigrahi, Joy Lal Sarkar, Bibudhendu Pati, Abhishek Majumder, Mamata Rath, and Sheng-Lung Peng**

## 2.1 Introduction

Coronavirus 2019 (COVID-19) is a particularly infectious illness leading to severe acute coronavirus syndrome. In December 2019, the epidemic originated in Wuhan, a city in China, and has then spread to more than 212 countries worldwide [27]. If an infect person sneezed and/or coughed, the COVID-19 virus mostly spreads by droplets of saliva or discharge from the nose. The structure of a coronavirus looks like as shown in Fig. 2.1. The effect is such that the World Health Organization (WHO) declared the on-going COVID-19 pandemic of international significance as a public health emergency. No unique vaccinations or therapies are presently available for COVID-19. Nonetheless, several research trials are underway to evaluate possible therapies. As long as clinical results are accessible, WHO can continue to have updated details about the statistics of the affected patients. The basic procedure for COVID-19 is considered as polymerase chain reaction (PCR) monitoring to identify antibodies with a specific infection. But, it was found that the check has a lot of issues. The diagnostic gold standard is the pathogenic laboratory check; this

V. Ramasamy (✉)
Park College of Engineering and Technology, Coimbatore, Tamil Nadu, India

C. R. Panigrahi · B. Pati
Rama Devi Women's University, Bhubaneswar, India

J. L. Sarkar · A. Majumder
Tripura University (A Central University), Tripura, India

M. Rath
Birla Global University, Bhubaneswar, India

S.-L. Peng
Taoyuan Campus, National Taipei University of Business, Taoyuan, Taiwan
e-mail: slpeng@ndhu.edu.tw



S. Kautish et al. (eds.), *Computational Intelligence Techniques for Combating COVID-19*, EAI/Springer Innovations in Communication and Computing,
https://doi.org/10.1007/978-3-030-68936-0_2

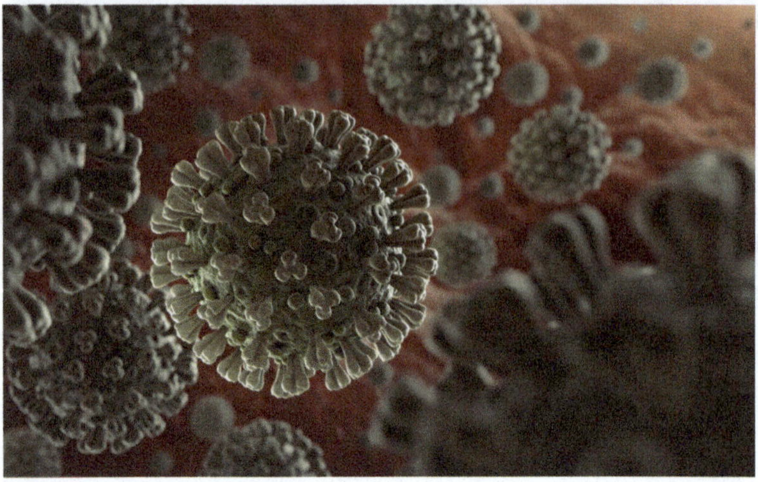

**Fig. 2.1** Novel coronavirus 2019 [28]

needs time for significant false negatives. A wide-ranging application of COVID-19 experiments which are incredibly costly will not be rendered possible in both developing and underdeveloped countries. Therefore, we can use artificial intelligence (AI) and machine learning (ML) techniques to exploit historical evidence for a concurrent diagnosis or testing process.

In the extraction of image features, including shape and spatial relationship features, AI involving medical imaging deep learning (DL) systems have been developed. In fact, feature selection and learning has demonstrated the convolutional neural network (CNN). CNN was introduced to classify the origin of pulmonary nodules via computed tomography (CT) scans, paediatric pneumonia diagnosis through X-ray chest pictures, automatic polyp precision and polyp mark and cystoscopy picture identification from videos during colonoscopic examination [8, 9].

### *2.1.1 Deep Learning*

"Deep learning is one specific form of machine learning which gains tremendous strength and versatility by learning to view the environment as an elongated spectrum of theories with every theory described in contrast to basic and less abstract theories [3]".

DL is an artificial neural network subset of ML that imitates the human brain and is a type of emulation of the humans as well. We do not have to plan anything directly in DL. For a few years since, it has been widely used and is now trending as humans did not have so much computing resources before. As, over the last 20 years, the computing capacity has expanded rapidly, the DL and ML become popular day by day.

The chapter is organized as follows. Section 2.2 presents the deep learning strategies with image processing to classify COVID-19 patients. Section 2.3 provides a proposed hybrid model for COVID-19 classification. In Sect. 2.4, we have identified certain possible future research directions which will be helpful for the other researchers working in this area to carry forward their research. Finally, the chapter is concluded in Sect. 2.5.

## 2.2 Deep Learning with Image Processing to Classify COVID-19 Patients

In this section, we have described the methods of DL which are applied to both CT scan images and X-ray scans to identify coronavirus along with their results. CT process is quite precise and accurate than the standard radiograph. CT images can be used to detect penetration, ground-glass opacity, and bottom section convergence [26].

### *2.2.1 Using CT Scan Images*

Radioactivity imagery is a popular COVID-19 detection device. Most of the COVID-19 instances provide common characteristics with CT images along with ground-glass opacity and later become respiratory assembly. A circular form and external pulmonary spread are often seen occasionally [4, 5]. While standard CT photos can help to detect suspicious instances in earlier stage, photographs of distinct viral pneumonia become identical as well as correlate with many other contagious and allergic lung disorders. Radiologists also seem to have difficulty in distinguishing between COVID-19 and some other viral pneumonia diseases. AI through clinical imagery DL models is also established in the field of image processing, which include the structure and geographical connection. In specific, the convolutional neural network (CNN) was demonstrated in the detection and processing of characteristics. CNN has been utilized to boost low-light video endoscopy with restricted training data consisting of only 55 videos [6]. The CNN has also been used to detect pulmonary nodular characteristics using CT scans to diagnose paediatric pneumonia from the heart X-ray photos, to automate the process of polyp precision and marking during colonoscopy videos and images and to detect cystoscopic scan from videos [7–10].

Many characteristics are correlated mostly with particular pathogenesis for the detection of viral pathogens on the support of imagery patterns [12]. COVID-19 characteristics include mutual shadowy spread and ground-glass opacity [11]. On this basis, it is felt that CNN can support to recognize special features that could not be readily identifiable. To check the concept, 453 CT photos of COVID-19 pathogen-reported incidents and historically normal viral pneumonia have been documented in retrospect. To create the model, 217 pictures have trained with the help of inception migration-learning model. With 80.5% specificity and 84% sensitivity for testing, overall accuracy of 83% was obtained. Total precision with specificities of 67% and specificity of 74% is demonstrated in the outside experiments. The evidence-of-principle is demonstrated by such findings utilizing the DL approach to derive radiological attributes in diagnosing COVID-19.

#### 2.2.1.1 Methods and Materials

**Retrospective Collection of Datasets**
CT samples of 99 individuals are retrospectively obtained [1]. The cohort contains 55 instances of common viral pneumonia and 44 additional instances of SARS-COV-2-verified nucleic acid tests from 3 separate clinics. Xi'an Jiaotong University's Medical College is one such clinic that sponsors such photos. All CT images are de-identified in the initial stage of the analysis process.

**Overview of the Deep Learning Architecture**
Figure 2.2 shows the structural network for the design of predictions [1]. There are three key stages throughout the design, i.e. (1) randomized set of region of interests (ROIs), (2) CNN method of training in extracting attributes and (3) complete system categorization algorithm training and multi-classifier predictions. The ROIs are selected randomly and utilized an inception network to derive characteristics of every person to measure tomography test and forecast them.

**Intercept ROIs from CT Images**
CT pictures, with roughly 1 * 1 in-plane pixel density, have been captured by video recorder. ROIs were derived in CT scans to minimize the difficulty in measurement and dependent upon the symptoms of pneumonia. It is between 395*223 and 636 * 533 pixels for every ROI. We had selected 195 ROIs from 44 COVID-19 victims who were positive pneumonia and 258 ROIs from 50 COVID-19 victims who were doubtful, and an Inception-based neural transfer learning network was created. The whole neural network is then split into approximately double sections: the first portion utilizes a well-trained inception network for translation of picture data into

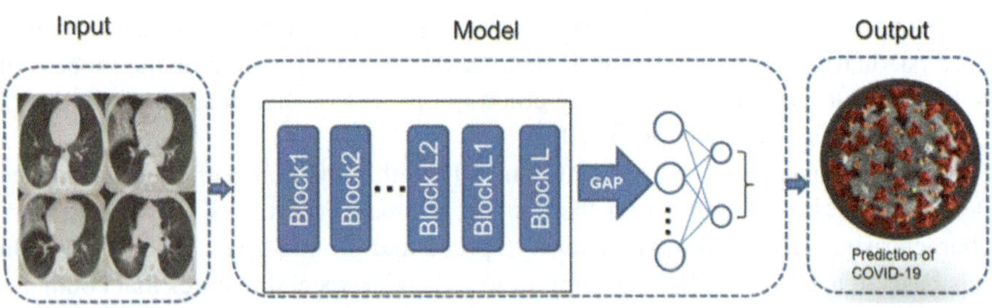


**Fig. 2.2** System with deep learning algorithms

standard vectors, and the second section utilizes a complete network, which is primarily built for categorization. There are two to three photographs of the specific cases arbitrarily taken to construct a learning dataset. There are roughly equivalent numbers of different forms of images in the training sample, with a minimum of 236. For testing, the leftover CT images were included. The process is iterated 15,000 times in 0.01 phase scale. A total of 236 computational ROIs have been utilized and 217 ROIs for testing have been collected.

**Feature Extraction Using Transfer Learning**

The regular Inception network is updated and the Modified Inception (M-Inception) with pre-trained weights is strengthened. The initial Inception portion is not educated across the training process, and only a changed component was equipped. The M-Inception framework is outlined in Table 2.1. The disparity in distinction among the Inception and M-Inception remains over the final completely linked layers. Until being submitted to the final classifying layer, the scale of the functionality is decreased. All of the above listed changes comprise the training dataset.

**Prediction**

The last phase would be to categorize pneumonia focused on certain attributes after the attributes are produced. The categorization quality was enhanced via the assembly of the classifiers. In this work, decision tree and AdaBoost classifiers are merged and used to find the results.

**Performance Evaluation Metrics**

The efficiency of classification is computed by sensitivity, accuracy, specificity, positive predictive value (PPV), area under curve (AUC), F1 score, negative predictive value (NPV) and Youden index. The true positive (TP) and true negative (TN) are the real number of positive and negative tests. The amount of false positive and negative samples is the FP and FN value, respectively. Sensitivity calculates the accurately segregated affirmative percentage. Specificity is used to test the

**Table 2.1** The M-Inception framework.

| Inception section | Layer | Patch size/stride or remarks |
|---|---|---|
| | conv | 3*3/2 |
| | conv | 3*3/1 |
| | conv padded | 3*3/1 |
| | pool | 3*3/2 |
| | onv | 3*3/1 |
| | conv | 3*3/2 |
| | conv | 3*3/1 |
| | Inception | “3x5x2x” |
| | pool | 8x8 |
| | linear | Logits |
| | softmax | Classifier |
| Changed section | Fc1 | [batchnorm dropout(0.5) 512d Linear] |
| | Fc2 | [batchnorm dropout(0.5) 2d Linear] |

percentage of appropriately marginalized negatives. AUC is an index for calculating the classifier's efficiency. NPV has been utilized to test the screening algorithm, and PPV is expected to get disease if the diagnostic index is accurate. The Youden index defines the optimum relation. F1 score is a metric to measure binary model performance. Furthermore, F-measure (F1) efficiency was analysed in order to assess similitude and output variability.

**Results and Discussion**

In this section, the results obtained by using DL on CT scan images are presented and are given as in Table 2.2. From the results obtained, it indicates that DL approach yields significant performance in classifying CT scan images.

Person under investigations (PUIs) are vital to prompt detection and triage for the management of evolving inflammatory conditions like the present COVID-19. As nucleic acid-oriented laboratory research is minimal, it is imperative to consider speedy alternatives for simple and precise diagnosis of the infection by ground force clinical staff. In this work, an AI system via a profound analysis method is established for processing symbolic CT pictures. It is a descriptive analysis, with multi-cohort, diagnostic research. A migration neuro network Inception has been developed which has an acquired accuracy of 82.9%. In contrast, the designed DL model was validated using the external test and the accuracy obtained was found to be 73%. The results indicate that DL can retrieve CT picture characteristics from COVID-19 for diagnosis applications. This device may be further established to greatly reduce the testing period to monitor infection. It may also lower the burden of doctors on the ground for diagnostics. This work focuses on the use of AI for effective COVID-19 scanning in CT pictures.

Nucleic acid-based identification of unique SARS-COV-2 gene sequences became the golden norm for diagnostic COVID-19. When diagnosing the disease, it also emphasizes the role of nucleic acid identification. Nevertheless, there are still considerations such as technical drawbacks, disease phases and species selection procedures that could hinder diagnosis and management of disease due to the extremely large numbers of false negatives. The quality of nuclear acid processing is only about 30–50%, according to recent reports. Through the retrieval of CT images, it will obtain more than 83% accuracy and outplay nucleic acid experiments substantially. Furthermore, this technique has low cost and is not aggressive. It gives

**Table 2.2** The output of DL approach.

| Performance Metric | Internal | External |
|---|---|---|
| AUC95%CI | 0.90(0.86 to 0.94) | 0.78(0.71 to 0.84) |
| Accuracy,% | 82.9 | 73.1 |
| Sensitivity | 0.81 | 0.67 |
| Specificity | 0.84 | 0.76 |
| PPV | 0.73 | 0.61 |
| NPV | 0.88 | 0.81 |
| FI score | 0.77 | 0.63 |
| Yoden index | 0.69 | 0.44 |

confidence with the original outcome, but assumes that it can gain greater precision including more CT pictures used in the preparation. This device is developed and checked properly. However, this work involves certain restrictions. Because of the massive amount of parameters, particularly the pictures beyond the lungs that are non-concerned for pneumonia, CT pictures pose a complicated categorization task [11]. The ROI region has been identified within analysis by only a single radiologist. Moreover, the dataset for training is fairly thin. The method is anticipated to improve its productivity by growing the amount of instruction. The CT images of the fully developed stage of the lung lesions were considered for analysis. In order to refine the treatment method, an analysis is required to relate this to the development of all pathological phases of COVID-19.

### *2.2.2 X-Ray Scans Using CNN and Class Activation Maps*

Both advanced and emerging countries are struggling to introduce wide-scale experiments on COVID-19, which are incredibly costly, although it can use AI and ML in any concurrent diagnosis or screening processes and exploit empirical evidence. This will aid to pick those who are predominantly tested. A quick, reliable form of treatment for battling the infection is essential. The current work used transfer learning on 1119 CT images using CNN. The validation accuracy for the model both internally and externally is reported at 89.5% and 79.3%, respectively. A related research in this review is primarily based on heart X-ray pictures to render CXRs which is more available in urban and remote locations than to obtain CT scans.

**CNN Approach to Detect the Presence of COVID-19 from X-Rays**
The CNN has been used on three classification problems:

1. Classification of normal vs. COVID-19 cases.
2. Classification of pneumonia vs. COVID-19 cases.
3. Classification of normal vs. COVID-19 vs. pneumonia cases.

The transfer learning via VGG-16 is utilized, and some of the end layers are getting fine-tuned. The number of parameters of this model is as follows.

1. Total parameters: 14,747,650.
2. Trainable parameters: 2,392,770.
3. Non-trainable parameters: 12,354,880.

The model has been trained using Kaggle GPU. The pattern can be differentiated within the dual instances of approximately 100% precision. In addition to achieve better comprehension, gradient-based class maps as given in Fig. 2.3 have been utilized to identify which part of the picture has been the most significant that allows the system to correctly categorize. The Grad CAM heatmaps for regular cases, COVID-19 cases and pneumonia cases are shown in Figs. 2.4, 2.5 and 2.6, respectively. The model indicates that the focused portion relies mostly on the detection and diagnosis of ordinary healthy cases. Likewise, the segment outlined would go to the right end of the chart, suggesting that this portion may be a significant factor in deciding whether or not the patients had COVID-19 or COVID-19 in the portion. The clinical reports can confirm this in this scenario.

Yet this solution has a tremendous capability, and it might be a perfect means of providing an effective, quick and time-consuming diagnostic method. The benefits of this source are listed as follows.

1. The check or test distribution is still a primary drawback in PCR technology, although the issue may be solved by X-ray machines.
2. AI will render a tentative evaluation and determine whether a patient is affected or not and can also augment the role of radiologists and doctors without replacing them.

So if they are utilizing X-ray pictures in the archive of the impacted COVID-19 patients, it is necessary to support the registry because it would be helpful at this crucial period.

### 2.2.3 *COVID-19 Detection Using X-Ray Images and CNN*

**Deep Transfer Learning**

DL is an exciting subset of the brain function in the ML area. The DL strategies employed in past years demonstrate an outstanding efficiency in the field of medical image processing just like in other domains. It is attempted to derive useful findings from medical data by the use of DL techniques. In several sectors including diagnosis, segmentation and lesion recognition in medical details, DL method is being widely adopted. DL methods in medical imaging such as MRI, CT, and X-ray help to analyze the image and signal data. Such measures offer ease for identifying and diagnosing diseases such as diabetes mellitus, brain tumour, skin cancer and breast cancer [13–18].

The key challenge confronting scientists in the study of medical data is the insufficient amount of datasets that are accessible. DL models also require a lot of information. This information is therefore expensive and time-intensive to mark by researchers. It makes data processing with less datasets and requires fewer computing costs as the greatest benefit of utilizing the transfer learning process. The data obtained from the pre-trained method in a broad dataset may be passed to the model

$$\alpha_k^c = \overbrace{\frac{1}{Z}\sum_i\sum_j}^{\text{global average pooling}} \underbrace{\frac{\partial y^c}{\partial A_{ij}^k}}_{\text{gradients via backprop}}$$

**Fig. 2.3** Action maps in gradient-based class

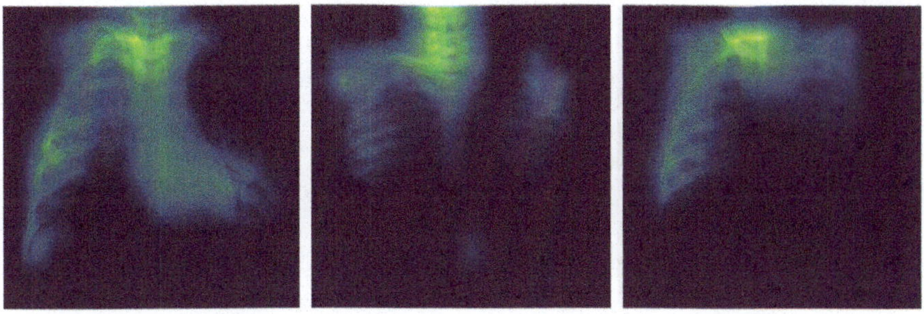

**Fig. 2.4** Grad CAM heatmap for regular cases

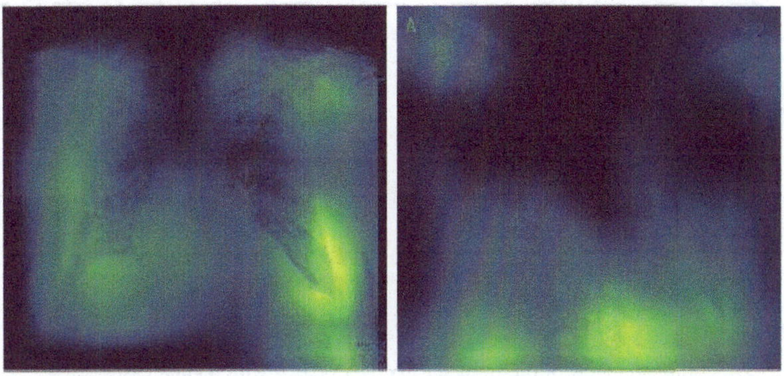

**Fig. 2.5** Grad CAM heatmap for COVID-19 cases

to be trained using the transfer learning approach that is commonly utilized in the field of DL.

The research is focused on ResNet50, InceptionV3 and Inception-ResNetV2 for classifying COVID-19 heart X-ray photographs to regular groups as well as COVID-19 groups by creating CNN. Furthermore, the transfer learning methods were used to address inadequate knowledge and training time by the use of ImageNet. The graphical depiction of conventional CNN, along with the ResNet50 and the ResNetV2 predictive models for COVID-19 and ordinary patient predictions, is shown as in Fig. 2.7 [2].

The residual neural network (ResNet) template is also an updated variant of the CNN. ResNet provides shortcuts to fix issues across layers. It avoids interference, which happens with the depth and complexity of the network. Bottleneck frames are often included to render ResNet system activities faster [19]. ResNet50 is an ImageNet application qualified 50-layer platform. ImageNet is an image archive developed for image recognition contests, with over 14 million pictures in over 20,000 categories [20]. InceptionV3 is based on the CNN model. There are several phases and the fastest rate of pooling. It comprises a neural network during the latter stage totally linked [21]. Like the ResNet50 method, ImageNet trains the network.

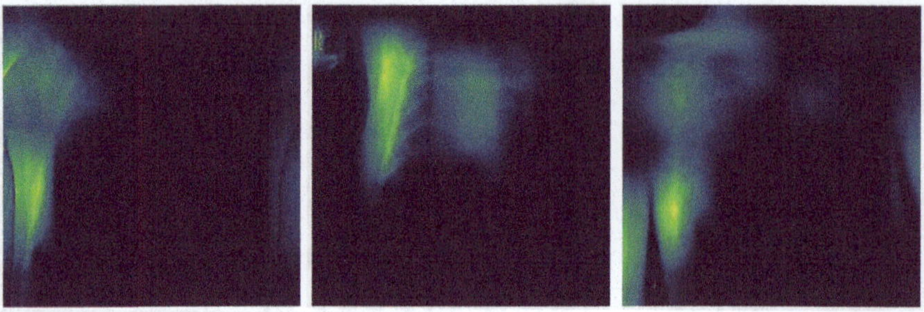

**Fig. 2.6** Grad CAM heatmap for cases with pneumonia

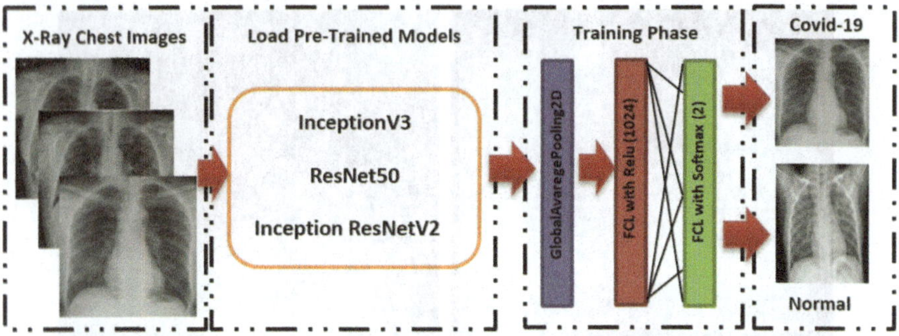


**Fig. 2.7** Diagrammatic view of pre-trained COVID-19 cases with regular cases

The model consists of a deep convolutionary network with the ResNetV2 Inception design, trained on the ImageNet-2012 data collection. The model entry represents a picture of 299*299, and the output is an approximate class probability [22].

**Discussions**

The key benefits of this research are summed up as follows in comparison to other findings in the literature:

1. Chest X-ray photographs were included in the research. X-ray pictures can be collected from any hospital easily and fastly with no complexity.
2. This process is the whole end-to-end framework. Thus, no extracting or selecting functionality is available.
3. Three popular pre-trained versions, such as ResNet50, InceptionV3 and Inception-ResNetV2, are correlated.
4. However, this is an incredibly recent topic with a small amount of details, but the findings are very good.

The key concern of this research is the insufficient amount of X-ray photographs included in the preparation of DL frameworks of COVID-19. Deep transfer learning methods are employed to solve this issue. When more data can be obtained over the upcoming days, various versions will boost the operating model.

### 2.2.4 *DL System to Screen COVID-19 Pneumonia*

#### 2.2.4.1 Process

The entire COVID-19 diagnosis report development cycle is illustrated in Fig. 2.8 of this analysis [3]. First, pre-processed CT photographs were utilized for extracting effective pulmonary areas. Second, several picture cubes were separated using a 3D CNN interface. For more phases, the central picture was collected along with the two neighbourhoods of each block. Third, all the picture patches were categorized as three forms in the picture classification model displayed in Fig. 2.9: COVID-19, influenza A viral pneumonia and unrelated infection. Photo patches of the same cube were voted for the candidate's general form and durability. The overall result was then estimated with the noisy or Bayesian method for one CT study.

#### 2.2.4.2 Dataset Pre-processing and Candidate Region Segmentation

The research has been driven by the same approach and method as in the preceding pulmonary tuberculosis analysis at the data and applicant clustering phases [23]. The emphasis of tuberculosis infections has been on many systems and forms, including the military, infiltrative, gaseous, tuberculosis and cavitary disease. The clustering patterns were checked using VNET [24] and VNET-IR-RPN in such a way to distinguish the candidate patches from viral pneumonia to pulmonary tuberculosis. In addition, both segregation and grouping were utilized in the analysis of pulmonary tuberculosis, using the VNET-IR-RPN method. Only the clustering boundary regression portion was retained, irrespective of the classified outcomes, since at this point in this analysis only the previous task was needed.

#### 2.2.4.3 Image Data Processing and Augmentation

Numerous regions which are not important to this analysis, along with fibrotic form of lung, calcification patches or safe areas that were poorly defined, were also split using the 3D model of clustering. A new type, in comparison to COVID-19 and influenza A viral pneumonia, was introduced as unrelated to disease.

There were 618 CT samples in the analysis (219 COVID-19, 224 flu A viral pneumonia and 175 stable cases). The 3D clustering method then creates a number of 3957 candidate cubes. Only the region near the centre of this cube held full details on this disease focal point. Thus, for potential classification measures, only the picture of the middle along with both neighbourhoods of every cube is obtained. Furthermore, two qualified radiologists personally graded every picture patch into two forms of meaningless pneumonia and infection. The second type photographs were immediately known as COVID-19 or as influenza A viral pneumonia depending on the findings of medical diagnosis.

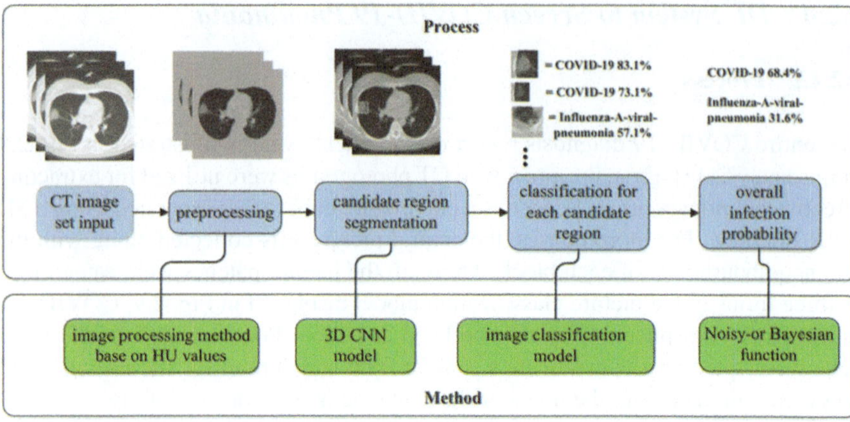


**Fig. 2.8** COVID-19 diagnosis report development cycle

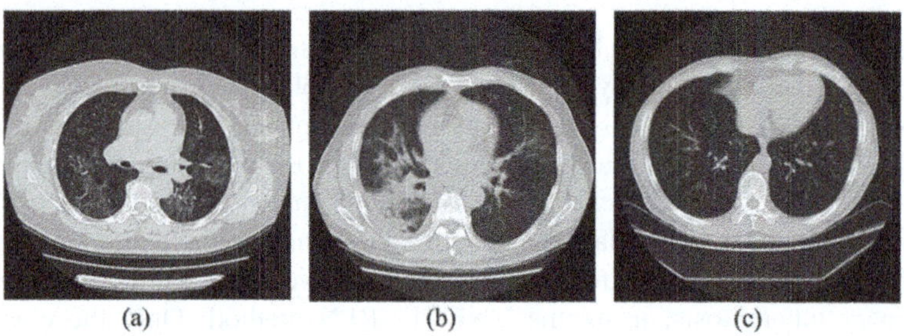


**Fig. 2.9** CT photos in traditional cross-section: (**a**) COVID-19. (**b**) Influenza a viral pneumonia. (**c**) No signs of pneumonia

The above measures contained 11,871 image pieces, of which 2634 were COVID-19, 2661 were obtained with the influenza A viral pneumonia and 6576 were unrelated to infections. Based on the earlier assessment of results, the training and validation sets consisted of 529 CT tests, which equates to 10,161 (85.6%) pictures, which included 2301 COVID-19, 2244 flu A viral pneumonia and 5616 non-reporting pictures. Reservation for the study dataset is rendered for the leftover 1710 (14.4%) images. COVID-19 and influenza A viral pneumonia cases' sampling possibilities have been extended three times to equilibrate the test volume for unrelated diseases, thereby minimizing effects on the current data collection from the unequal allocation of the various picture forms. The same move was taken in order to maximize the amount of testing samples and avoid duplication of data in common data enlargement processes such as RCC, left-right, up-down and mirroring activities.

#### 2.2.4.4 DL Model for Classification

**Location-Attention Classification**

Three distinctive attributes of COVID-19 namely ground glass, hitting peripherals together with pleura were identified in Jeffrey Kanne's work (21) and Chung M et al. (22) work and is shown as in Fig. 2.10. Based on these results, the frameworks have been configured. The picture recognition cock is built to differentiate between the presence of various diseases and the shape. In order to obtain relative position details on the pulmonary picture, comparatively distance-from-end as excess weight was also utilized for the layout. The subject of diseases around the pleura has been more generally known as COVID-19.

Every patch's relative length of the edge was determined as follows:

1. Calculate the total gap between the mask and the middle of this patch (double-headed arrow as seen in Fig. 2.10c).
2. Achieve diagonal of the pulmonary image minimal circumscribed triangle (Fig. 2.10d).
3. Otherwise, divide the relative gap between phase 1 and stage 2.

**Network Structure**

The research tested two CNN 3D classification types as seen in Fig. 2.11. It was a comparatively conventional ResNet23 network, and another model was built by integrating the emphasis method with the full link layer to increase the overall accuracy performance based on the first network topology. For picture retrieval, the classical network framework ResNet18 was utilized. In addition, pooling activities were employed to reduce data dimension to avoid overfitting and to boost the generalization issue. The performance of the convolution layer was reduced to a 256-dimensional vector and then transformed by a full-connector network into a 16-dimensional functional vector. The meaning of the relative distance from the edge was first averaged in the same order of magnitude in the location-care network and then connected to the complete network structure. Then the overall classified result and the trust score were obtained in three layers full-linked.

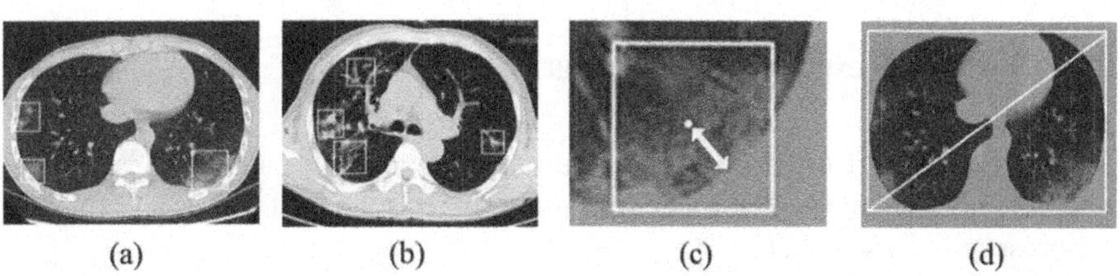


**Fig. 2.10** (**a**) A focused COVID-19 photo of 3 ground glass of infection. (**b**) Picture of influenza A virus pneumonia including 4 focus of infections. (**c**) The total gap between the mask and the middle of this patch (arrow with double heading) and (**d**) minimal level diagonally circumcised pulmonary feature rectangle

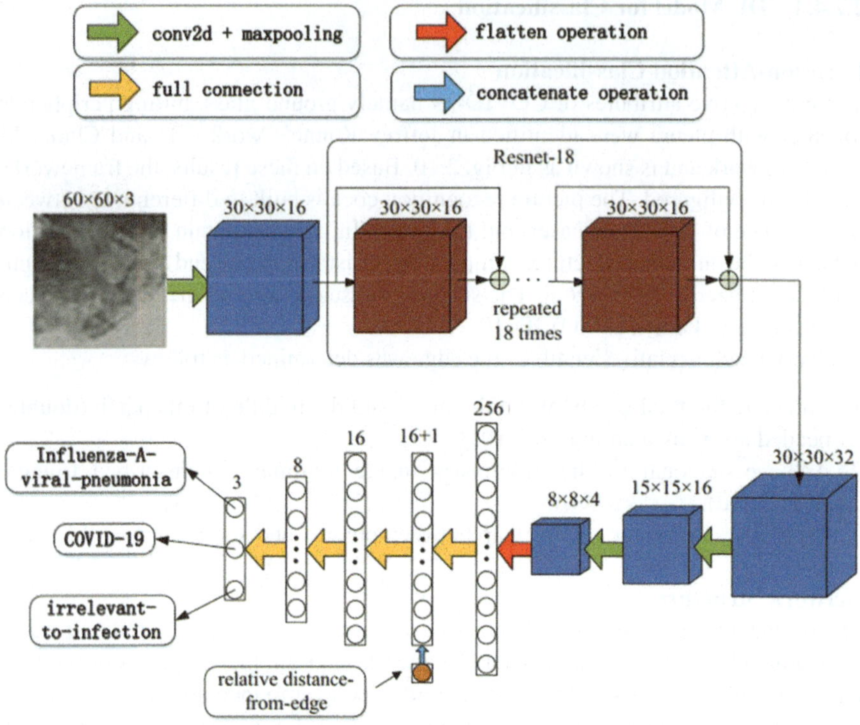


**Fig. 2.11** Area-oriented design of network layout

## 2.3 Hybrid Model for COVID-19 Classification

In this section, we propose a hybrid model for COVID-19 classification as shown in Fig. 2.12 which is the combinations of CNN and LSTM models using DL concepts. In this method, CNN is used for feature extraction, and LSTM is used for successful classification of COVID-19 instances.

## 2.4 Future Research Directions

In the context of COVID-19, there are a variety of fields in which ambitious researchers can explore. The accessible study subjects are explored as a framework for prospective researchers.

- Hybrid DL frameworks provide further scope in the dataset of clinical photos to classify COVID-19 cases.
- A field of study with specific CNN model may be evaluated by growing the amount of photos in the dataset to enhance classification efficiency.

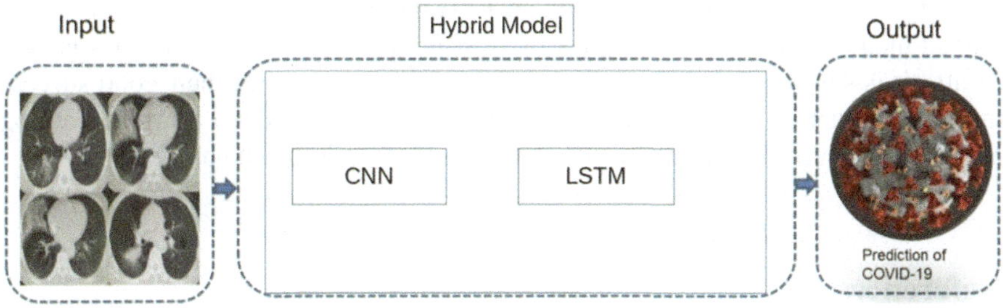


**Fig. 2.12** Hybrid model for COVID-19 classification

- In order to enhance the exactness of COVID-19 clinical evaluation, patients have to be paired with a better preparation and the numbers of tests of their contact past, travel experience, original signs and clinical research.
- Several multicentre research experiments to resolve the complicated health condition will be performed.
- A stronger model can be established through testing and evaluation of output generality utilizing a wider dataset to enhance clustering and classification performance.
- Future work needs to relate centralized characteristics of CT photos to attributes of others, for example, genomic, epidemiological and clinical evidence in multi-omic and multifaceted applications, to improve infection diagnostics.
- The key research goal of reinforcement learning is to improve more efficiently and utilize the existing resources and enhance patient satisfaction where the rooms, personnel and other services available are minimal.
- In turn, the usage of such models in comparison to historic data (and related hospitals) will ideally support the hospital detect shortfalls, especially when paired with the above epidemic frameworks, for improved control in the future [25].
- Prospective work needs to address significant holes in cause awareness, epidemiology, patient transmission period and the medical infection continuum.
- Deep learning drug discovery technologies will be a significant element in the creation of medicines for the regulation of such coronaviruses.
- CT images are paired with computational features such as genetic, epidemiotic, non-omic and non-modelling work to help identify pathogens and epidemiological and medical information.

## 2.5 Conclusions

In order to avoid transmission of the infection to others, the earlier diagnosis of COVID-19 victims is important. In this work, we suggest a deep transfer learning method by utilizing heart X-ray photographs taken from COVID-19 victims and ordinary for the automated detection of COVID-19 victims. The ResNet50 pre-trained method reveals best accuracy of 98% among its three versions. Despite the results, it is suspected that doctors are motivated to assess with their good success in clinical practice. This research offers insights into how deep transfer learning approaches can be utilized to identify COVID-19 at an initial stage.

## References

1. Wang, S., Kang, B., Ma, J., Zeng, X., Xiao, M., Guo, J., Cai, M., Yang, J., Li, Y., Meng, X., & Xu, B. (2020). A deep learning algorithm using ct images to screen for corona virus disease (covid-19). *medRxiv*.
2. Narin, A., Kaya, C., & Pamuk, Z. (2020). Automatic detection of coronavirus disease (COVID-19) using X-ray images and deep convolutional neural networks. *ArXiv*, abs/2003.10849.
3. Xu, X., et al. (2020). A deep learning system to screen novel coronavirus disease 2019 pneumonia. *Engineering, 6*(10), 1122–1129.
4. Huang, C., Wang, Y., Li, X., Ren, L., Zhao, J., Hu, Y., et al. (2020). Clinical features of patients infected with 2019 novel coronavirus in Wuhan, China. *The Lancet, 395*, 497–506.
5. Chung, M., Bernheim, A., Mei, X., Zhang, N., Huang, M., Zeng, X., et al. (2020). CT imaging features of 2019 novel coronavirus (2019-nCoV). *Radiology, 295*, 200230.
6. Gomez, P., Semmler, M., Schutzenberger, A., Bohr, C., & Dollinger, M. (2019). Low-light image enhancement of high-speed endoscopic videos using a convolutional neural network. *Medical & Biological Engineering & Computing, 57*, 1451–1463.
7. Choe, J., Lee, S. M., Do, K. H., Lee, G., Lee, J. G., Lee, S. M., et al. (2019). Deep learning-based image conversion of CT reconstruction kernels improves Radiomics reproducibility for pulmonary nodules or masses. *Radiology, 292*, 365–373.
8. Kermany, D. S., Goldbaum, M., Cai, W., Valentim, C. C. S., Liang, H., Baxter, S. L., et al. (2018). Identifying medical diagnoses and treatable diseases by image-based deep learning. *Cell, 172*, 1122–31.e9.
9. Negassi, M., Suarez-Ibarrola, R., Hein, S., Miernik, A., & Reiterer, A. (2020). Application of artificial neural networks for automated analysis of cystoscopic images: A review of the current status and future prospects. *World Journal of Urology, 38*(10), 2349–2358.
10. Wang, P., Xiao, X., Glissen Brown, J. R., Berzin, T. M., Tu, M., Xiong, F., et al. (2018). Development and validation of a deep-learning algorithm for the detection of polyps during colonoscopy. *Nature Biomedical Engineering, 2*, 741–748.
11. Wang, D., Hu, B., Hu, C., Zhu, F., Liu, X., Zhang, J., et al. (2020). Clinical characteristics of 138 hospitalized patients with 2019 novel coronavirus-infected pneumonia in Wuhan, China. *JAMA, 323*(11), 1061–1069.
12. Koo, H. J., Lim, S., Choe, J., Choi, S. H., Sung, H., & Do, K. H. (2018). Radiographic and CT features of viral pneumonia. *Radiographics, 38*, 719–739.
13. Yildirim, O., Talo, M., Ay, B., Baloglu, U. B., Aydin, G., & Acharya, U. R. (2019). Automated detection of diabetic subject using pre-trained 2D-CNN models with frequency spectrum images extracted from heart rate signals. *Computers in Biology and Medicine, 113*, 103387.
14. Saba, T., Mohamed, A. S., El-Affendi, M., Amin, J., & Sharif, M. (2020). Brain tumour detection using fusion of hand crafted and deep learning features. *Cognitive Systems Research, 59*, 221–230.
15. Dorj, U. O., Lee, K. K., Choi, J. Y., & Lee, M. (2018). The skin cancer classification using deep convolutional neural network. *Multimedia Tools and Applications, 77*(8), 9909–9924.
16. Kassani, S. H., & Kassani, P. H. (2019). A comparative study of deep learning architectures on melanoma detection. *Tissue and Cell, 58*, 76–83.

17. Ribli, D., Horvth, A., Unger, Z., Pollner, P., & Csabai, I. (2018). Detecting and classifying lesions in mammograms with deep learning. *Scientific Reports, 8*(1), 1–7.
18. Celik, Y., Talo, M., Yildirim, O., Karabatak, M., & Acharya, U. R. (2020). Automated invasive ductal carcinoma detection based using deep transfer learning with whole-slide images. *Pattern Recognition Letters, 133*, 232–239.
19. Wu, Z., Shen, C., & Van Den Hengel, A. (2019). Wider or deeper: Revisiting the ResNet model for visual recognition. *Pattern Recognition, 90*, 119–133.
20. Russakovsky, O., Deng, J., Su, H., Krause, J., Satheesh, S., Ma, S., Huang, Z., Karpathy, A., Khosla, A., Bernstein, M., Berg, A. C., & Fei-Fei, L. (2015). ImageNet large scale visual recognition challenge. *International Journal of Computer Vision, 115*, 211–252.
21. Ahn, J. M., Kim, S., Ahn, K. S., Cho, S. H., Lee, K. B., & Kim, U. S. (2018). A deep learning model for the detection of both advanced and early glaucoma using fundus photography. *PLoS One, 13*(11), e0207982.
22. Byra, M., Styczynski, G., Szmigielski, C., Kalinowski, P., Michalowski, L., Paluszkiewicz, R., Ziarkiewicz-Wrblewska, B., Zieniewicz, K., Sobieraj, P., & Nowicki, A. (2018). Transfer learning with deep convolutional neural network for liver steatosis assessment in ultrasound images. *International Journal of Computer Assisted Radiology and Surgery, 13*(12), 1895–1903.
23. Wu, W., Li, X., Du, P., et al. (2019). A deep learning system that generates quantitative CT reports for diagnosing pulmonary tuberculosis. *arXiv preprint arXiv*, 1910.02285.
24. Milletari, F., Navab, N., & Ahmadi, S. A. (2016). V-net: Fully convolutional neural networks for volumetric medical image segmentation. *arXiv preprint arXiv*, 1606.04797.
25. Sarkar, J. L., Majumder, A., Panigrahi, C. R., & Roy, S. (2020). MULTITOUR: A multiple itinerary tourists recommendation engine. *Electronic Commerce Research and Applications, 40*, 100943.
26. Kooraki, S., Hosseiny, M., Myers, L., & Gholamrezanezhad, A. (2020). Coronavirus (COVID-19) outbreak: What the Department of Radiology Should Know. *Journal of the American College of Radiology, 17*(4), 447–451. https://doi.org/10.1016/j.jacr.2020.02.008.
27. Wang, C. (2020). A novel coronavirus outbreak of global health concern. *Lancet, 395*, 470–473. https://doi.org/10.1016/S0140-6736(20)30185-9.
28. "[Online]. Available:." https://www.who.int/images/default-source/health-topics/coronavirus/corona-virus-getty.tmb-1200v.jpg.

# Chapter 3
# Applications of Artificial Intelligence (AI) Protecting from COVID-19 Pandemic: A Clinical and Socioeconomic Perspective

**Ritwik Patra, Nabarun Chandra Das, Manojit Bhattacharya, Pravat Kumar Shit, Bidhan Chandra Patra, and Suprabhat Mukherjee**

## 3.1 Introduction

The novel coronavirus disease 2019 (COVID-19) is an ongoing pandemic emergency, caused by the severe acute respiratory syndrome coronavirus 2 (SARS-CoV-2). The World Health Organization (WHO) reported on 6 July 2020 that there are about 215 countries with 11,327,790 confirmed cases of coronavirus disease and around 532,340 deaths [1]. The pathological and physiological consequences lead to difficulties in breathing, inflammation in the lungs leading to fluid accumulation, fever, and multi-organ failure, which occurs due to overexpression of inflammatory cytokines resulting in cytokine storm [2]. The unavailability of appropriate therapy with effective drugs or vaccines, a tremendous effect on human health, property, well-being, as well as the global economic condition, is elevating and worsening regularly. Even though RT-PCR testing is used and marked as the worldwide standard for the detection of the COVID-19 [3], however, in these fast-spreading pandemic situations, it becomes considerate as major threats and challenges to the healthcare welfare of human civilization.

R. Patra · N. C. Das · S. Mukherjee (✉)
Integrative Biochemistry & Immunology Laboratory, Department of Animal Science, Kazi Nazrul University, Asansol, West Bengal, India
e-mail: suprabhat.mukherjee@knu.ac.in

M. Bhattacharya
Department of Zoology, Fakir Mohan University, Balasore, Odisha, India

P. K. Shit
Department of Geography, Faculty of Science, Raja N.L. Khan Women's College, Medinipur, West Bengal, India

B. C. Patra
Department of Zoology, Vidyasagar University, Midnapore, West Bengal, India



S. Kautish et al. (eds.), *Computational Intelligence Techniques for Combating COVID-19*, EAI/Springer Innovations in Communication and Computing,
https://doi.org/10.1007/978-3-030-68936-0_3

To get rid of such a worldwide health crisis, the use of an artificial intelligence (AI) algorithm-based and data-based trained model may be serving as a promising tool. AI works on machine learning technology and advanced bio-computational techniques that are purposefully used in medical science for fast diagnosis, rapid treatment, and well-prepared advancements for any future crisis allied with the healthcare system. A computer-based healthcare system uses data from various sources in different machine languages to train the model, forming a logical network topology, and works through a digital framework and automated library [4]. In this present emergency of the worldwide SARS-CoV-2 outbreak, artificial intelligence-based detection, diagnosis, and responses are very operative in the clinical approach and, subsequently, help to manage its therapeutics impacts and socio-economic constraints. The main objective of this chapter is to discuss the various applications and development of an AI-based model for the fight against the global pandemic of COVID-19. The advancement in the technologies of AI-based algorithm leads to multiple functions of AI in the fight against COVID-19 and is depicted in Fig. 3.1. The data related to coronavirus disease available across various sources is collected and analyzed, and output is generated using the AI-based model. It can provide early warning and alert for the worldwide spread and pandemic of COVID-19. The use of AI-based radiological technologies for the fast detection and diagnosis of COVID-19 increases the efficiency of disease diagnosis and treatment

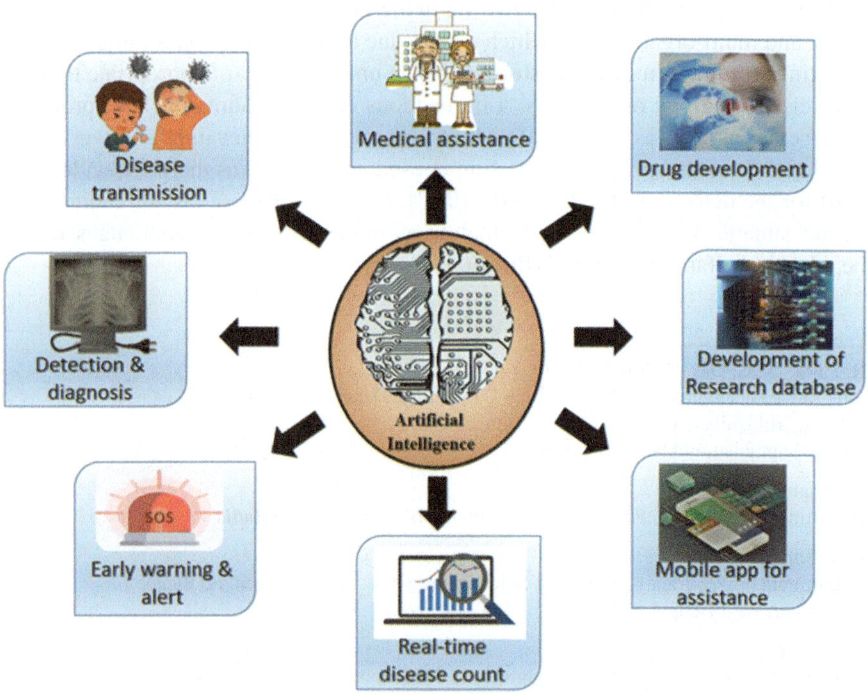


**Fig. 3.1** Application of artificial intelligence in COVID-19

and also helps the healthcare worker to deliver contactless healthcare facilities. The use of smartphones and web server based on AI algorithm for managing the crisis in every industrial sector. The enhancement in the use of an AI algorithm-based pre-trained model for the development and repurposing of drug and discovery of a vaccine. Nevertheless, the management of worldwide lockdown, isolation, and home quarantine across various countries is monitored and managed through the use of AI-based devices and algorithms. Collectively, it can be concluded that the use of AI in this pandemic situation of COVID-19 effectively manages the crisis and promotes advancement in the healthcare facilities, drug and vaccine development, and socioeconomic management.

## 3.2 Artificial Intelligence-Based COVID-19 Early Warning and Management

On 9 January 2020, the World Health Organization (WHO) declares the outbreak of coronavirus disease, COVID-19 officially, after getting confirmation reports from China [5]. Although the virus has already been detected and confirmed on earlier December 2019 at Wuhan hospital, China [6]. The use of AI-driven algorithms can provide early notices of this pandemic globally and its potential aid for better preparedness in the future. BlueDot is an AI-based algorithm that provided the warning and detection of COVID-19, 7 days before the official statement by WHO [7]. It uses various natural language processing algorithms to collect data from news reports, official and unofficial statements, airline ticketing, infectious disease alert system, climatic conditions, and also vector-borne disease reservoirs and outbreak cases. It predicted the possibilities of spreading the disease to other regions from the originating place of China [8]. The Boston Children's Hospital in the USA used an innovative AI-based model HealthMap for warning even earlier than that of BlueDot; however, its level of significance is very low for the SARS-CoV-2 outbreak [9].

An epidemic monitoring company called Metabiota, based on data analysis, machine language function, and natural language processing (NLP) algorithms, alerted South Korea, Japan, Thailand, and Taiwan about this devastating viral disease outbreak [8]. Moritz Kraemer, an epidemiologist from the University of Oxford, UK, developed a web-based platform, for visually representing and tracking the outbreak, based on real location and time [10]. Consequently, the LSTM-GRU architecture modeling technique is applied for time series analysis and prediction of confirmed cases on a daily basis [11].

The Government of India developed an AI-based mobile app known as Aarogya Setu, built on a web access platform that can use GPS tracking, Bluetooth, and proximity sensors to provide an application programming interface (API) [12]. It augments the initiatives of the health department to share best practices and assured advisories. Bluetooth and proximity sensors determine the risk if one has been near within 6 feet of a COVID-19-infected person, by scanning through a developed database of known cases across India [13]. Similarly, the Chinese government developed a monitoring system, Health Code. The user has to register to it with their Alipay or WeChat account and was assigned color codes like red for 14 days of self-quarantine, yellow for 7 days of self-quarantine, and green for no quarantine based on their travel history and exposure to contamination hotspots [14]. These innovative initiatives have forecast all possibilities and consequences to and from the available governmental report, media platforms, and social media to minimize the risk chances of the COVID-19 spread and infection.

## 3.3 Clinical Perspective of AI in COVID-19

### *3.3.1 Detection and Diagnosis*

Reverse transcription-PCR (RT-PCR) is the primary and globally standardized test for the detection and confirmation of COVID-19-positive patients [3]. However, it has various limitations, like sample collection, inadequacy throughout all region, and prolonged analysis process, and is not sufficient in this thriving emergency [15]. On the other hand, the artificial intelligence-based deep learning models, Internet of Things (IoT), and machine learning are very useful in the detection, diagnosis, and analysis of medical data of coronavirus-infected patients, and their comparison is represented in Fig. 3.2. Upon comparing the conventional method of diagnosis and treatment of COVID-19 with the advanced AI-based technology, it is found to be more fast and precise and also have fewer chances of being contagious. The conventional methods of swab testing using RT-PCR require a prolonged process of sample collection and testing, which is time-effective and also has huge probabilities of contamination. Furthermore, these results are manually analyzed by the healthcare workers that require much more manpower during this worldwide situation of crisis, and treatment based on symptomatic treatment, resulting in prolonged treatment procedures. On the other hand, the application of advanced AI algorithm-based pre-trained model precisely can detect and diagnose the COVID-19 patients and further assisted the healthcare workers to prototype the treatment procedure to speed up the process of cure. AI algorithm prototype-based automated radiology techniques including computed tomography (CT) scan, magnetic resonance imaging (MRI), and digital X-ray are efficient for the detection and diagnosis of several diseases [16]. It works based on contactless scanning, benefiting the health workers from contamination and also in faster ways. Shanghai United Imaging Intelligence (UII) utilizes this method for visualization techniques to test the changes in size, volume, biomass density, and other clinical consequences toward providing data-driven guidance to medical experts, to further use this information in determining the suitable strategy for treatment action plans [17]. In China, an automated diagnosis tool is developed by Alibaba Group's research and innovation institute, DAMO Academy, to form a deep learning AI-enabled system trained by CT scan records of 5000

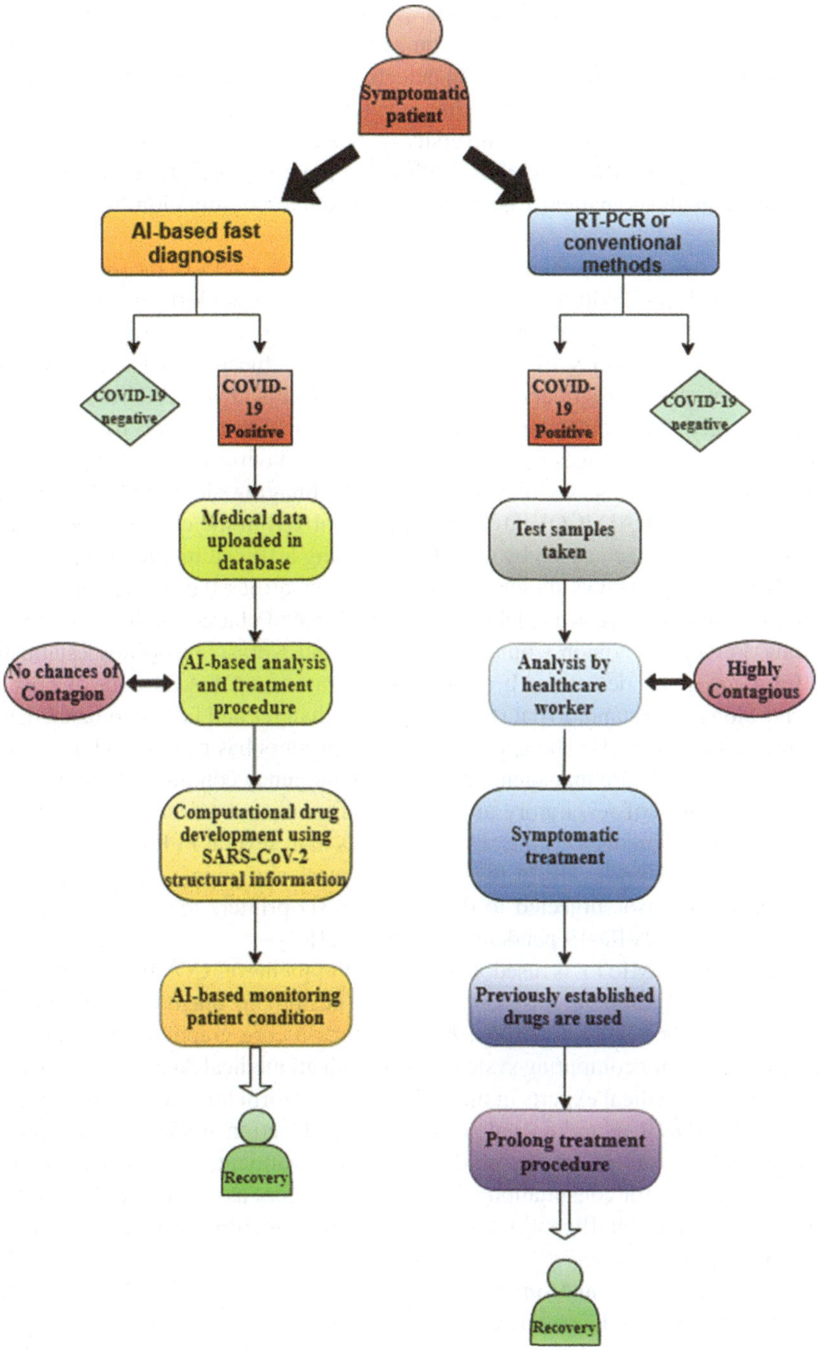


**Fig. 3.2** Comparison between the AI-based and conventional mode of COVID-19 treatment

patients for diagnosis within 20 seconds with 96% accuracy [18]. Another company named Infervision (www.infervision.com) developed a coronavirus AI solution to help the first-line healthcare worker in detecting and monitoring the patients [19]. It was first used at the epicenter of the outbreak in Tongji Hospital in Wuhan (Tongji Medical College of Huazhong University of Science and Technology) and is efficiently assisting healthcare workers with pneumonia segmentation, abnormal and severe case analysis, patient triage, medical resource coordination, and treatment assessments.

Narin et al. developed a pre-trained model, ResNet50, InceptionV3, and Inception-ResNetV2 with using convolutional neural network (ConvNet/CNN) for prediction and accuracy of COVID-19 through the patients' X-ray dataset. The results show an accuracy of 97% and 87% for the InceptionV3 and Inception-ResNetV2 model, respectively [20]. The COVID-Net is also a CNN-designed prototype merged with machine-driven design forming a network framework, to analyze chest X-ray images for the diagnosis of coronavirus disease [21].

CAD4COVID software is developed by Delft Imaging along with their partner Thirona to create CAD4COVID-CT [22]. It is utilized in the clinical investigation for extents of damage caused by COVID-19. Using artificial intelligence, the heatmap data of lungs shows its abnormalities and quantifies the percentage of viral infection. This software is available globally and free of charge for these emergency periods. Perception Vision Company (PVmed) and Keras/TensorFlow establish a platform for quick detection. It aligned the X-ray and CT scan data of positive patients along with standard data to correlate the changes and fast, automated detection techniques [17, 23]. The application of 3D printers has been found very much beneficial in healthcare management amid the emergency condition. Hospitals with a shortage supply of respiratory aids and venturi valves are found to be benefited after the application of 3D printers [24]. Besides that, several PPE kits such as copper 3D NanoHack mask, HEPA mask, Creality mask and goggle, Lowell mask, and face shields are also subjected to design using 3D printers to support healthcare workers in this COVID-19 pandemic situation [24].

Medical IoT (MIoT) is used for the development of COVID-19 Intelligent Diagnosis and Treatment Assistant Program (nCapp) to diagnose and clinically assist in the fight against COVID-19 [25]. It uses a core graphics processing unit (GPU)-based cloud computing system linked with all medical data along with assistance from top medical experts in this field. It can perform up to ten major functions against COVID-19 including online monitoring, location tracking, three-linkage response alarm function for graded diagnosis and treatment, command and control plan management for consultation of patients, intelligent assisted severity stratification, precise and intelligent treatment, and also security privacy of data of patients [25].

XGBoost algorithm and support vector machines developed by Chen et al. were trained to use various diagnostic data of patients like the amount of lactate dehydrogenase, blood pressure, C-reactive protein (CRP) level, monocyte ratio, and body temperature to monitor the severity and to predict mortality risk of patients admitted to hospitals [26, 27]. The crisis of availability of healthcare workers and social distancing in this pandemic condition created worldwide mismanagement in the health facility. Regarding these, the advancement of AI-based devices overtakes this condition and replaces human experts, for health assessments and disease predictions. Maghdid et al. recently developed a smartphone-based framework, which includes smartphones, algorithms, and embedded sensors, like cameras, inertial sensors, microphones, and temperature sensors, to use as a symptom checker for coronavirus diseases. It is also designed to capture CT scan images of lung and tally with the established databases [28]. Researcher from King's College, health science company ZOE, in collaboration with Massachusetts General Hospital and the University of Nottingham, developed an AI-based smartphone app called COVID Symptom Study app [29]. Using the data shared by the user, it can predict the COVID-19 infection without any testing based on the symptoms. It is used by over 3.3 million peoples globally and is very much efficient [29]. The list of several AI-based software developed for the fast detection and diagnosis of COVID-19 is discussed in Table 3.1.

**Table 3.1** List of various AI software used for clinical manifestation in COVID-19

| AI-based software | Mode of action | Consequence | Reference/ developer |
|---|---|---|---|
| Keras, TensorFlow, and deep learning | Chest X-ray plate detection and comparison | Fast and automated detection | PyImageSearch community |
| ResNet50, InceptionV3, and inception-ResNetV2 software | Chest X-ray radiographs | 97% accuracy for InceptionV3 and 87% accuracy for inception-ResNetV2 | [20] |
| CAD4COVID; CAD4COVID-CT software | Chest X-ray images and CT scans | Indicates the affected lung tissue and the severity of the infection | Delft imaging; Thirona |
| COVID-net | Chest X-ray images | CNN designed detection of COVID-19 | [21] |
| XGBoost algorithm | Clinical data of the patient | The severity of patients and mortality risk | [26, 27] |
| AI-enabled smartphone-embedded sensors | Chest CT scan images and body touch | Symptoms checker low-cost disease detection | [28] |
| nCapp | Medical data cloud using IoT | Medical assistance, diagnosis, monitoring, and management | [25] |
| COVID symptom study app | COVID-19 database | Predict infection without testing | [29] |

### 3.3.2 *Structural and Molecular Analysis*

AI has been used for a better understanding of the structure of proteins associated with the SARS-CoV-2 virus targeted for potential treatments and the development of drugs or vaccines. Computational models are used to predict protein structure using the template-based sequence and also by template-free sequence modeling aspects [11]. Cleemput et al. developed a web-based software application called Genome Detective Coronavirus Typing Tool for assembling the virus genome from next-generation sequencing datasets. It can identify the phylogenetic clusters and genotype of the SARS-CoV-2 genome and also can submit and analyze 2000 sequences within a 1-minute duration [30].

DeepMind is an AI program developed by Google adapted to get the computationally derived structure of the viral protein and associated structure of SARS-CoV-2. It uses AlphaFold System relying upon the amino acid sequences by contrasting the features with a similar type. Multiple sequence alignment (MSA) is employed for collecting the information regarding distance and the bond angle between amino acid residues and also for designing protein's shape [31]. Heo and Feig developed a pipeline using a machine learning-based method from trRosetta to predict the structural model. It was further updated by implementing molecular dynamics simulation-based refinement and AlphaFold models to analyze and correlate with the C-I-TASSER models [32].

### 3.3.3 *Drug Development*

Artificial intelligence-aided computational drug designing is the key to progress in the process of producing drugs and vaccines for coronavirus disease in this situation of a fast-spreading pandemic [33]. Molecule Transformer-Drug Target Interaction (MT-DTI), a pre-trained deep learning model, analyzes the various previously available drugs for different viruses, like HIV, Ebola, and Zika, to check its effectiveness against SARS-CoV-2 [34]. BenevolentAI and Imperial College London, using deep learning database, approved the drug baricitinib, previously used in the treatment of rheumatoid arthritis, which might be effective against the SARS-CoV-2. In Hong Kong, in silico medicine-based AI reported that their algorithm had designed new molecules that could stop the viral replication [10].

Atazanavir, an antiretroviral drug for HIV, functions against the 3C-like proteinase of SARS-CoV-2 with inhibitory potency of Kd value = 94.94 nM [35]. Baricitinib, a NAK inhibitor having a higher affinity to AAK1, regulates the clathrin-mediated endocytosis, thereby inhibiting viral infection [36]. Selective JAK-STAT inhibitors, like fedratinib and ruxolitinib, are generally used for the treatment of rheumatoid arthritis and myelofibrosis disease. It suppresses expression of IL17, IL22, and IL23 with no effect on IL22, thus reducing cytokine storm associated with COVID-19 infection [37]. Abacavir is a reverse transcriptase inhibitor generally used in the treatment of HIV and, on testing against SARS-CoV-2, showed a high binding affinity to its various proteins [38]. The list of various drugs developed using AI-based pre-trained model is listed in Table 3.2.

Molecular docking simulations are the modern approach for drug re-designing and discovery [39]. It uses a wide range of ligands that interact with the protein in different orientations and conformations, illustrating various binding modes to predict the ligand's binding affinity. Development of a Deep Docking (DD) platform that works on a neural network to predict the outcomes of docking simulations [40]. It has the potential to identify a set of 3 million of 3C-like protease inhibitors from a set of over 1 billion compounds extracted from the ZINC database [41]. Using the bioinformatics platform, researchers predict the epitopic regions of the SARS-CoV-2 for computer-aided peptide-based vaccine designing [42]; along with that, it is also being used for the analysis of the phylogenetic relationship of SARS-CoV-2 across different animals, origin of virus, and transmission to the human host and the mechanism of pathogenesis within the host body [43].

## 3.4 AI-Based Robotic Technologies

The above section describes the use of AI for detection, diagnosis, and health assessment and also the various applications of AI in structural and molecular analysis and drug development against SARS-CoV-2. The highly contagious disease leads to social distancing and isolation all across the world which reduces the availability of manpower, and the advancement of AI-based robotic technologies came forward as extremely useful and efficient in this COVID-19 pandemic. The replacement of the workers associated with cleaning and management across various hospitals for providing essential services with AI-based robots efficiently overcome the situation of contamination and spreading of disease [44]. The deployment of robots in China by Pudu Technology to facilitate food catering, cleaning, and sterilizing within the hospital complex [45]. UVD robots from Blue Ocean Robotics were designed to kill the virus and sterilize using UV light [44]. The collaboration of various universities in Europe to develop a humanoid serving robot named Amigo Prototype under the RoboEarth project can provide nursing and patient handling [46]. Automated Venipuncture Device (AVD) robot developed in the joint collaboration of Rutgers

**Table 3.2** AI-based drugs developed against COVID-19

| Drug | Target | Mode of action | Reference |
|---|---|---|---|
| Atazanavir | Protease inhibitor | Inhibit 3C-like proteinase of virus | [35] |
| Baricitinib | NAK inhibitor | Regulate clathrin-mediated endocytosis | [36] |
| Fedratinib and ruxolitinib | JAK-STAT signalling inhibitors | Suppress expression of IL17, IL22, and L23 with no effect on IL22 | [37] |
| Abacavir | Nucleoside analogue reverse transcriptase inhibitor | High binding affinity with several proteins of SARS-CoV-2 | [38] |

University and Robert Wood Johnson University Hospital assists in fast blood sample collecting from patients with high accuracy [47]. Flying drones for logistic support are being used in this situation of home quarantine and nationwide lockdown. Further, it is also used for the surveillance of the peoples violating the lockdown, social distancing, and precautionary measures.

## 3.5 Socioeconomic Perspectives

In an attempt to fight against the COVID-19 pandemic, many countries have started public policy interventions, such as social distancing and quarantining of individuals showing symptoms of COVID-19 along with nationwide lockdown [48]. The consequences of these can be modeled using AI-based models for managing and monitoring people, public places, railway, and airport checkpoints, by scanning for potential threats and contamination. Vivacity Labs installed 200 sensors in surveillance cameras across 10 cities of the UK, focused on traffic surveillance systems, to monitor whether people were staying at home [49]. Social distancing measuring software, Cameo, installed along with the security cameras for automatically calibrating the rate and development of social distancing data [50]. SenseTime, an AI-based company in China, created "Smart AI Epidemic Prevention Solutions" for fast monitoring crowd to detect fever and invigilating the violation of quarantine rules by peoples based on facial recognition and thermal screening [14].

WHO data reports are used to train various models like Modified AutoEncoder (MAE) and Topological AutoEncoder (TA) to predict the number of confirmed cases, deceased, and recovery daily across 240 countries [38]. Development of time-varying Bayesian auto-regressive model for counts (TVBARC) with a linear link function for better temporal modeling of the virus spread with using time-dependent coefficient [51]. The AI-based drones and robotic technology are shown to be very much effective during the worldwide pandemic and lockdown situation. The use of human in essential service is being reduced to avoid contagion. Terra drone is used for the supply of medical delivery to the disease control center of Xinchang County from other places of supply [52].

National and international organizations are now using the online platform like the Internet blog and social media for sharing the information and to communicate with the public regarding this pandemic [11]. But it is seen that propagation of misinformation, fake news, and rumors is increasingly prevalent, resulting in panic and disturbance within the community. In this current situation of lockdown across many places around the globe, functional human staffs have been reduced. To overcome this problem, social media platforms like YouTube and Facebook including WhatsApp and Twitter have advanced their AI more intensively for monitoring and moderating its contents uploaded by the user for checking rumors, fake news, and misconceptions regarding the disease [53]. Infodemic Risk Index (IRI) is developed to quantify the rate a generic user is exposed to such unreliable posts from different classes of unverified humans and also verified or unverified bots [54]. In Taiwan,

Google Trends is used to monitor public activity across the Internet platform. It analyzes the increased search keywords like "COVID-19" and "face masks" across the Internet after the first infection to determine the public risk awareness and communication strategy [55]. The outbreak of COVID-19 leads to global economic crises all across the world resulting in unemployment, share market downfall, and unprecedented debt levels. The United Nations' report for 2020–2021 states that the repayment on the debt by the developing countries may lead to ascending across a value of $2.6 trillion and $3.4 trillion. The World Bank estimated that the global pandemic of COVID-19 surges 40–60 million peoples to poverty [56]. The use of AI to monitor the world economy can promote the growth and management of global economics. The increase in the growth of AI-based technologies in the healthcare and medical industries provides a huge market and dependency in the near future. The COVID-19 pandemic situation offers an opportunity to AI-based industries to flourish and proliferate to contribute to mankind and socioeconomic progression.

## 3.6 Limitations and Future Perspectives

Artificial intelligence (AI) has the potential to help us in tackling the current issues raised by the COVID-19 pandemic. It uses the knowledge and creativity of the human developer and user. The application of AI-based model during the COVID-19 worldwide crisis brings back advantageous changes in the healthcare industries; fastens the process and reduces the chances of contamination; helps in the management of social status emerging due to the worldwide lockdown, self-isolation, and social distancing; and also proves to be a powerful tool in managing the world economic crisis. However, the wide application and dependency on AI-based model may result in certain limitations [58]. The radiology data used for the diagnosis of COVID-19 is insufficient, is imprecise, and is not enough for the complete training of the AI-based model to form a precise segmentation and diagnostic framework network [17]. The dataset available for COVID-19 is limited so the training and development of AI-dependent treatment are still underdeveloped. Impoverished deep learning networks could result in poor segmentation and abnormality classification. Overriding consent and privacy rights used for disease surveillance may cause distrust and misuse of personal data and sooner become inconvenient for peoples [57]. The complete dependency on the AI-based technologies for the diagnosis and treatment of COVID-19 is beneficial but some time may result in data falsification and inaccurate result. The use of network servers may lead to technical problems and glitches that can hinder the healthcare system. Furthermore, the experience and basic instinct to handle an emergency situation by an expert healthcare worker cannot be replaced by the AI-based model. The use of AI-based model in the management of socioeconomic parameters requires expert knowledge and training, which is still under development and evolving.

In the upcoming days, more advanced training and the dataset are especially desired on COVID-19 including collaborative and multidisciplinary research for improving the ability of AI. There is favorable progress in the importance of advancement in building a proper database regarding this disease and also sharing its information globally with free and quick access. The World Health Organization's (WHO) Global Research on Coronavirus Disease database is a good example of this progress. For the futuristic use of AI, the joint initiative between various research database publishers, different Institutes of Artificial Intelligence, global digital companies like of digitization of the economy and growing digital market.

## 3.7 Conclusion

The development of the AI-based model is very much efficient and effectively brings up the advancement of technologies from healthcare to industrial sectors. The use of AI algorithm-based radiological techniques promotes fast and smooth detection of COVID-19. Further, the use of robotic technologies and drones based on the AI algorithm replaces the human intervention for managing and providing services in this pandemic situation of COVID-19 to prevent contamination. This chapter summarizes the various applications of AI in the worldwide emergency of coronavirus disease, to counteract the problem and to promote better management. The use in early warning and alert of the pandemic helps in preparing for the consequences of the disease. The application of AI shows a broad sense domain, and this study is to highlight its emerging applications in early detection, monitoring, diagnosis, treatment, drug or vaccine discovery and development, various social managements, monitoring epidemiology, and also economic tracking. The advancement in the healthcare facilities based on AI promotes fast detection, diagnosis, and even assisting of the healthcare worker for health management. Deep learning technology has shown great performance in extracting segmentation data, and features in radiology reports may hold the promise to alleviate this outbreak. Early diagnosis and quarantine of suspected patients are the most important ways to prevent the further spread of coronavirus disease. The use of robotic technologies and drone replaces human labor to prevent contagion. The use of AI enhances and can manage the global economic crisis and social misanthropic. It can provide worldwide connectivity and database for the fight against COVID-19. Collectively, the use of AI-based technologies over the conventional method of healthcare and social management shows much more efficiency and is better during this pandemic condition. However, its use is confined by an insufficient dataset and mishandling. International initiatives regarding this should be encouraged for the development and advancement of AI models operational for regulating this pandemic and reducing its severity in terms of mortality, livelihood, and economic loss.

**Acknowledgments** Ritwik Patra thanks the Department of Higher Education, Govt. of West Bengal, for awarding Swami Vivekananda Merit Cum Means Fellowship. We acknowledge the efforts of all the doctors, health workers, scientists, researchers, and society management workers for their endless contribution against COVID-19 pandemic.

**Conflict of Interest** The author declares no conflict of interest relevant to this article.

**Ethical Approval** This article does not require any ethical approval.

## References

1. WHO (2020) Coronavirus Disease (COVID-19) Situation Reports. https://www.who.int/emergencies/diseases/novel-coronavirus-2019/situation-reports. Accessed 16 Jul 2020.
2. Cao, W., & Li, T. (2020). COVID-19: Towards understanding of pathogenesis. *Cell Research, 30*, 367–369. https://doi.org/10.1038/s41422-020-0327-4.
3. Ai, T., Yang, Z., Hou, H., Zhan, C., Chen, C., Lv, W., Tao, Q., Sun, Z., & Xia, L. (2020). Correlation of chest CT and RT-PCR testing in coronavirus disease 2019 (COVID-19) in China: A report of 1014 cases. *Radiology, 296*(2), E32–E40. 200642.
4. Bhattacharya, M., Kar, A., Malick, R. C., Chakraborty, C., Das, B. K., & Patra, B. C. (2020). Application of internet assistance computation for disease prediction and bio-modeling: Modern trends in medical science. In *Principles of Internet of Things (IoT) ecosystem: Insight paradigm* (pp. 327–346). Springer.
5. Li, Q., Guan, X., Wu, P., Wang, X., Zhou, L., Tong, Y., Ren, R., Leung, K. S. M., Lau, E. H. Y., Wong, J. Y., Xing, X., Xiang, N., Wu, Y., Li, C., Chen, Q., Li, D., Liu, T., Zhao, J., Liu, M., Tu, W., Chen, C., Jin, L., Yang, R., Wang, Q., Zhou, S., Wang, R., Liu, H., Luo, Y., Liu, Y., Shao, G., Li, H., Tao, Z., Yang, Y., Deng, Z., Liu, B., Ma, Z., Zhang, Y., Shi, G., Lam, T. T. Y., Wu, J. T., Gao, G. F., Cowling, B. J., Yang, B., Leung, G. M., & Feng, Z. (2020). Early transmission dynamics in Wuhan, China, of novel coronavirus–infected pneumonia. *The New England Journal of Medicine, 382*, 1199–1207. https://doi.org/10.1056/NEJMoa2001316.
6. Peng, P. W. H., Ho, P.-L., & Hota, S. S. (2020). Outbreak of a new coronavirus: What anaesthetists should know. *British Journal of Anaesthesia, 124*, 497.
7. Dananjayan, S., & Raj, G. M. (2020). Artificial intelligence during a pandemic: The COVID-19 example. *International Journal of Health Planning and Management*. https://doi.org/10.1002/hpm.2987.
8. Allam, Z., Dey, G., & Jones, D. S. (2020). Artificial intelligence (AI) provided early detection of the coronavirus (COVID-19) in China and will influence future urban health policy internationally. *AI, 1*, 156–165.
9. Naudé, W. (2020). Artificial intelligence vs COVID-19: Limitations, constraints and pitfalls. *AI and Society*. https://doi.org/10.1007/s00146-020-00978-0.
10. McCall, B. (2020). COVID-19 and artificial intelligence: Protecting health-care workers and curbing the spread. *Lancet Digital Health, 2*, e166–e167.
11. Bullock, J., Pham, K. H., Lam, C. S. N., & Luengo-Oroz, M. (2020). Mapping the landscape of artificial intelligence applications against COVID-19. arXiv Prepr arXiv200311336.
12. India G of Aarogya Setu Mobile App | MyGov.in. In: 2020. https://www.mygov.in/aarogya-setu-app/. Accessed 16 Jul 2020.
13. Garg, S., Bhatnagar, N., & Gangadharan, N. (2020). A case for participatory disease surveillance of the COVID-19 pandemic in India. *JMIR Public Health & Surveillance, 6*, e18795.
14. Chawla, S., & Saxena, S. K. (2020). Preparing for the perpetual challenges of pandemics of coronavirus infections with special focus on SARS-CoV-2. In *Coronavirus disease 2019 (COVID-19)* (pp. 165–186). Springer.
15. Kanne, J. P., Little, B. P., Chung, J. H., Elicker, B. M., & Ketai, L. H. (2020). Essentials for radiologists on COVID-19: An update—radiology scientific expert panel. *Radiology, 296*(2), E113–E114.

16. Hosny, A., Parmar, C., Quackenbush, J., Schwartz, L. H., & Aerts, H. J. W. L. (2018). Artificial intelligence in radiology. *Nature Reviews. Cancer, 18*, 500–510. https://doi.org/10.1038/s41568-018-0016-5.
17. Shi, F., Wang, J., Shi, J., Wu, Z., Wang, Q., Tang, Z., He, K., Shi, Y., & Shen, D. (2020). Review of artificial intelligence techniques in imaging data acquisition, segmentation and diagnosis for covid-19. *IEEE Rev Biomed Eng, 4*, 4–15.
18. Pham, Q.-V., Nguyen, D. C., Hwang, W.-J., & Pathirana, P. N. (2020). Artificial Intelligence (AI) and big data for coronavirus (COVID-19) pandemic: A survey on the state-of-the-arts. *IEEE Access, 8*, 130820–130839.
19. Infervision in the Frontlines Against the Coronavirus I Imaging Technology News. https://www.itnonline.com/content/infervision-frontlines-against-coronavirus. Accessed 16 Jul 2020.
20. Narin, A., Kaya, C., & Pamuk, Z. (2020). Automatic detection of coronavirus disease (COVID-19) using x-ray images and deep convolutional neural networks. arXiv Prepr arXiv200310849.
21. Wang, L., & Wong, A. (2020). COVID-Net: A tailored deep convolutional neural network design for detection of COVID-19 cases from Chest X-Ray Images. arXiv Prepr arXiv200309871.
22. Murphy, K., Smits, H., Knoops, A. J. G., Korst, M. B. J. M., Samson, T., Scholten, E. T., Schalekamp, S., Schaefer-Prokop, C. M., Philipsen, R. H. H. M., & Meijers, A. (2020). COVID-19 on the chest radiograph: A multi-reader evaluation of an AI system. *Radiology, 296*(3), E166–E172. 201874.
23. Arora, K., Bist, A. S., Chaurasia, S., & Prakash, R. Analysis of deep learning techniques for COVID-19 detection.
24. Tino, R., Moore, R., Antoline, S., Ravi, P., Wake, N., Ionita, C. N., Morris, J. M., Decker, S. J., Sheikh, A., & Rybicki, F. J. (2020). COVID-19 and the role of 3D printing in medicine. *3D Printing in Medicine, 6*(1), 11.
25. Bai, L., Yang, D., Wang, X., Tong, L., Zhu, X., Zhong, N., Bai, C., Powell, C. A., Chen, R., Zhou, J., Song, Y., Zhou, X., Zhu, H., Han, B., Li, Q., Shi, G., Li, S., Wang, C., Qiu, Z., Zhang, Y., Xu, Y., Liu, J., Zhang, D., Wu, C., Li, J., Yu, J., Wang, J., Dong, C., Wang, Y., Wang, Q., Zhang, L., Zhang, M., Ma, X., Zhao, L., Yu, W., Xu, T., Jin, Y., Wang, X., Wang, Y., Jiang, Y., Chen, H., Xiao, K., Zhang, X., Song, Z., Zhang, Z., Wu, X., Sun, J., Shen, Y., Ye, M., Tu, C., Jiang, J., Yu, H., & Tan, F. (2020). Chinese experts' consensus on the Internet of Things-aided diagnosis and treatment of coronavirus disease 2019 (COVID-19). *Clinical eHealth, 3*, 7–15. https://doi.org/10.1016/j.ceh.2020.03.001.
26. Chen, T., & Guestrin, C. (2016). Xgboost: A scalable tree boosting system. In: Proceedings of the 22nd ACM SIGKDD international conference on knowledge discovery and data mining. pp. 785–794.
27. Yan, L., Zhang, H.-T., Xiao, Y., Wang, M., Sun, C., Liang, J., Li, S., Zhang, M., Guo, Y., & Xiao, Y. (2020). Prediction of criticality in patients with severe Covid-19 infection using three clinical features: A machine learning-based prognostic model with clinical data in Wuhan. MedRxiv.
28. Maghdid, H. S., Ghafoor, K. Z., Sadiq, A. S., Curran, K., & Rabie, K. (2020). A novel Ai-enabled framework to diagnose coronavirus COVID 19 using smartphone embedded sensors: Design study. arXiv Prepr arXiv200307434.
29. Menni, C., Valdes, A. M., Freidin, M. B., Sudre, C. H., Nguyen, L. H., Drew, D. A., Ganesh, S., Varsavsky, T., Cardoso, M. J., & Moustafa, J. S. E.-S. (2020). Real-time tracking of self-reported symptoms to predict potential COVID-19. *Nature Medicine, 26*(7), 1037–1040.
30. Cleemput, S., Dumon, W., Fonseca, V., Abdool Karim, W., Giovanetti, M., Alcantara, L. C., Deforche, K., & De Oliveira, T. (2020). Genome detective coronavirus typing tool for rapid identification and characterization of novel coronavirus genomes. *Bioinformatics, 36*, 3552–3555.
31. Senior, A. W., Evans, R., Jumper, J., Kirkpatrick, J., Sifre, L., Green, T., Qin, C., Žídek, A., Nelson, A. W. R., & Bridgland, A. (2020). Improved protein structure prediction using potentials from deep learning. *Nature, 577*, 706–710.

32. Heo, L., & Feig, M. (2020). Modeling of Severe Acute Respiratory Syndrome Coronavirus 2 (SARS-CoV-2) proteins by machine learning and physics-based refinement. bioRxiv.
33. Salehi, A. W., Baglat, P., & Gupta, G. (2020). Review on machine and deep learning models for the detection and prediction of coronavirus. *Materials Today: Proceedings, 33*, 3896–3901.
34. Shin, B., Park, S., Kang, K., Ho, J. C. (2019). Self-attention based molecule representation for predicting drug-target interaction. arXiv Prepr arXiv190806760.
35. Beck, B. R., Shin, B., Choi, Y., Park, S., & Kang, K. (2020). Predicting commercially available antiviral drugs that may act on the novel coronavirus (SARS-CoV-2) through a drug-target interaction deep learning model. *Computational and Structural Biotechnology Journal, 18*, 784–790.
36. Richardson, P., Griffin, I., Tucker, C., Smith, D., Oechsle, O., Phelan, A., & Stebbing, J. (2020). Baricitinib as potential treatment for 2019-nCoV acute respiratory disease. *Lancet (London, England), 395*, e30.
37. Wu, D., & Yang, X. O. (2020). TH17 responses in cytokine storm of COVID-19: An emerging target of JAK2 inhibitor Fedratinib. *Journal of Microbiology, Immunology, and Infection, 53*(3), 368–370.
38. Hu, Z., Ge, Q., Li, S., Boerwincle, E., Jin, L., & Xiong, M. (2020). Forecasting and evaluating intervention of COVID-19 in the World. arXiv Prepr arXiv200309800.
39. Rahman, M. M., Karim, M. R., Ahsan, M. Q., Khalipha, A. B. R., Chowdhury, M. R., & Saifuzzaman, M. (2012). Use of computer in drug design and drug discovery: A review. *International Journal of Pharmacy and Life Sciences, 1*. https://doi.org/10.3329/ijpls.v1i2.12955.
40. Gentile, F., Agrawal, V., Hsing, M., Ton, A.-T., Ban, F., Norinder, U., Gleave, M. E., & Cherkasov, A. (2020). Deep docking: A deep learning platform for augmentation of structure based drug discovery. *ACS Central Science, 6*, 939–949.
41. Ton, A., Gentile, F., Hsing, M., Ban, F., & Cherkasov, A. (2020). Rapid identification of potential inhibitors of SARS-CoV-2 main protease by deep docking of 1.3 billion compounds. *Molecular Informatics, 39*(8), e2000028.
42. Bhattacharya, M., Sharma, A. R., Patra, P., Ghosh, P., Sharma, G., Patra, B. C., Lee, S.-S., & Chakraborty, C. (2020). Development of epitope-based peptide vaccine against novel coronavirus 2019 (SARS-COV-2): Immunoinformatics approach. *Journal of Medical Virology, 92*, 618–631. https://doi.org/10.1002/jmv.25736.
43. Choudhury, A., & Mukherjee, S. (2020). In silico studies on the comparative characterization of the interactions of SARS-CoV-2 spike glycoprotein with ACE-2 receptor homologs and human TLRs. *Journal of Medical Virology*. https://doi.org/10.1002/jmv.25987.
44. Bogue, R. (2020). Robots in a contagious world. *Industrial Robot*. https://doi.org/10.1108/IR-05-2020-0101.
45. In COVID-19, Pudu Robotics Provides Non-contact Delivery Service in Hundreds of Hospitals Worldwide | Business Wire. https://www.businesswire.com/news/home/20200605005095/en/COVID-19-Pudu-Robotics-Non-contact-Delivery-Service-Hundreds. Accessed 16 Jul 2020.
46. Fong, S. J., Dey, N., & Chaki, J. AI-enabled technologies that fight the coronavirus outbreak. In *Artificial intelligence for coronavirus outbreak* (pp. 23–45). Springer.
47. Leipheimer, J. M., Balter, M. L., Chen, A. I., Pantin, E. J., Davidovich, A. E., Labazzo, K. S., & Yarmush, M. L. (2019). First-in-human evaluation of a hand-held automated venipuncture device for rapid venous blood draws. *Technology, 7*, 98–107.
48. Dubey, S., Biswas, P., Ghosh, R., Chatterjee, S., Dubey, M. J., Chatterjee, S., Lahiri, D., & Lavie, C. J. (2020). Psychosocial impact of COVID-19. *Diabetes and Metabolic Syndrome: Clinical Research and Reviews, 14*, 779–788. https://doi.org/10.1016/j.dsx.2020.05.035.
49. AI exposed Brits ignoring advice to stay home and socially distance. https://artificialintelligence-news.com/2020/03/27/ai-exposed-brits-ignoring-advice-stay-home-socially-istance/. Accessed 16 Jul 2020.

50. Tummers, J., Catal, C., Tobi, H., Tekinerdogan, B., & Leusink, G. (2020). Coronaviruses and people with intellectual disability: An exploratory data analysis. *Journal of Intellectual Disability Research, 64*, 475–481.
51. Roy, A., & Karmakar, S. (2020) Bayesian semiparametric time varying model for count data to study the spread of the COVID-19 cases. arXiv Prepr arXiv200402281.
52. Terra Drone business partner Antwork helps fight coronavirus in China with medical delivery drones. https://www.terra-drone.net/global/2020/02/07/terra-drones-business-partner-antwork-helps-fighting-corona-virus-with-drones/. Accessed 16 Jul 2020.
53. Facebook, YouTube, and Twitter warn that AI systems could make mistakes – Vox. https://www.vox.com/recode/2020/3/17/21183557/coronavirus-youtube-facebook-twitter-social-media. Accessed 16 Jul 2020.
54. Gallotti, R., Valle, F., Castaldo, N., Sacco, P., & De Domenico, M. (2020). Assessing the risks of "infodemics" in response to COVID-19 epidemics. arXiv Prepr arXiv200403997.
55. Husnayain, A., Fuad, A., & Su, E. C.-Y. (2020). Applications of google search trends for risk communication in infectious disease management: A case study of COVID-19 outbreak in Taiwan. *International Journal of Infectious Diseases, 95*, 221–223.
56. Coronavirus and the rise of the AI Economy. https://www.forbes.com/sites/rainermichaelpreiss/2020/05/29/coronavirus-and-the-rise-of-the-ai-economy/#5240cd33446d. Accessed 16 Jul 2020.
57. Ienca, M., & Vayena, E. (2020). On the responsible use of digital data to tackle the COVID-19 pandemic. *Nature Medicine, 26*, 463–464.
58. Sampathkumar, A., Rastogi, R., Arukonda, S., Shankar, A., Kautish, S., & Sivaram, M. (2020). An efficient hybrid methodology for detection of cancer-causing gene using CSC for micro array data. *Journal of Ambient Intelligence and Humanized Computing*, 1–9.

# Chapter 4
# COVID-19 Risk Assessment Using the C4.5 Algorithm

**Sarmistha Nanda, Chhabi Rani Panigrahi, Bibudhendu Pati, Mamata Rath, and Tien-Hsiung Weng**

## 4.1 Introduction

COVID-19 is reported first in Wuhan, a city in the Hubei province of China [1]. In cattle and camel, coronavirus is common but now humans are also getting infected by the detected new strain. It affects the upper respiratory tract, such as the throat, nose, and sinus. The lower respiratory tract such as the lungs and windpipe is also infected [2]. It means it infects the whole respiratory system. Before COVID-19, six types of coronavirus were also identified that could harm humans [3]. Out of these, four are responsible for mild symptoms in respiratory organs and can be recovered without any special treatment.

In contrast, Middle East Respiratory Syndrome-coronavirus (MERS-CoV) and Severe Acute Respiratory Syndrome-coronavirus (SARS-CoV) was found to have critically high mortality rates. The seventh type of coronavirus disease was detected in December 2019 and hence the name COVID-19. After getting infected by the virus, it takes 5–6 days to show the symptoms on an average.

In some cases, it takes 14 days, and some are asymptotic. The most common symptoms found in this case are dry cough, fever, and tiredness, whereas there are some other symptoms such as sore throat, diarrhea, headache, discoloration of fingers and toes, loss of taste or smell, and rash on the skin, among others. When the

S. Nanda · C. R. Panigrahi (✉) · B. Pati
Department of Computer Science, Rama Devi Women's University, Bhubaneswar, Odisha, India

M. Rath
School of Management (IT), Birla Global University, Bhubaneswar, Odisha, India

T.-H. Weng
Department of Computer Science & Information Engineering, Providence University, Taichung, Taiwan
e-mail: thweng@gm.pu.edu.tw



S. Kautish et al. (eds.), *Computational Intelligence Techniques for Combating COVID-19*, EAI/Springer Innovations in Communication and Computing,
https://doi.org/10.1007/978-3-030-68936-0_4

disease reached the critical stage, breathing difficulty, chest pain, and speech loss, among others, are observed [4]. The mortality rate is high compared to other viral infections [5]. So, it is always advisable to consult with the doctor from the preliminary stage. Nose discharges and saliva droplets are responsible for spreading COVID-19 from the infected person to the healthy ones. Since there are no vaccines invented to date, the whole globe is struggling with this. America, Europe, Italy, Spain, and others [6] are the developed countries, but they also struggled to handle this pandemic. WHO suggests some guidelines that include regular frequent handwashing with soap and water, hand rub with an alcohol-based sanitizer, social distancing [7], staying at home, covering the nose and mouth while sneezing and coughing, avoiding lung-weakening activities like smoking, and unnecessary travel and social gathering [8].

In addition to some guidelines mentioned above, the chatbot may be used to avoid physical person-to-person interaction. The chatbot is a multidisciplinary, virtual tool that observes and records the human conversation in an automated way using AI [9, 10]. It can be implemented in many areas, such as education, medicine, social network, business, and organizations [11]. The whole system can be automated in education, including learning, teaching, student/teacher feedback, and many more. The chatbot in medicine includes patient diagnosis and medicine recommendation. Social interaction, business deals, and employee-level communication can also be achieved using this concept. Many researchers and organizations are busy developing chatbots nowadays, such as Meena, an open-domain chatbot developed by Google; ROSS, an AI-based legal advisor developed by IBM; and Ernest, an aggregator of bank and Facebook messenger [12]. During this COVID-19 crisis, a chatbot can be developed to collect the symptoms from the persons and that will help to analyze one's condition [13].

Section 4.2 describes the ML-assisted COVID-19 healthcare system, general ML process, the C4.5 algorithm, and ML challenges in COVID-19. Section 4.3 describes the global status of COVID-19 that includes dataset containing the COVID-19 information and visualization of COVID-19 confirmed cases across the globe. The C4.5 algorithm is also presented. We plotted a graph of confirmed, recovered, active, and death cases worldwide. The time series forecast for the next 30 days is also done. Section 4.4 presents the proposed work, and Sect. 4.5 concludes the work with specific future directions.

## 4.2 ML-Assisted COVID-19 Healthcare System

The COVID-19 health crisis causes an acute respiratory problem. Many researchers of versatile fields such as medical, chemical, technical, etc. are working on its betterment across the globe. ML researchers are also having a significant contribution to it. Patient diagnostic and drug suggestion, risk level prediction, and much more automation can help this critical situation using ML [14]. The use of ML algorithms results in faster execution with less human interaction.

The COVID-19 data can be analyzed using artificial intelligence (AI) and data science (DS) to resolve many problems. AI is a broad area of computer science. It refers to building machines by embedding programs in such a way that it is capable of simulating human intelligence. ML is a subset of AI where models are built to determine the future outcome by learning from its experience [15]. According to Tom Mitchell, "A computer program is said to learn from experience E concerning some class of tasks T and performance measure P, if its performance at tasks in T, as measured by P, improves with experience E.", and is called ML [16]. A computer program that automatically can improve its performance with experience is the primary goal of ML. Deep learning (DL) is a subset of ML, and it helps the machine trains itself from its inputs subsequently. The relationship between AI, ML, DL, and data science is shown in Fig. 4.1.

### *4.2.1 ML Process*

It is a predictive model and the main goal is to improve the prediction accuracy. Depending upon the addressed problem, different approaches such as supervised learning, unsupervised learning, and reinforcement learning are used [18, 19].

ML process goes through a number of steps that are shown as in Fig. 4.2.

***Data Collection:*** To build an accurate and efficient model, data collection plays a vital role [21]. The quality of the data determines the accuracy of the model. The output of this step is the raw data and is taken as the input to the data preparation step. There are many open data repositories such as UCI, Kaggle, etc., where pre-collected data are available. Some of these need preprocessing, and some datasets

**Fig. 4.1** Relationship between AI, ML, DL, and DS [17]

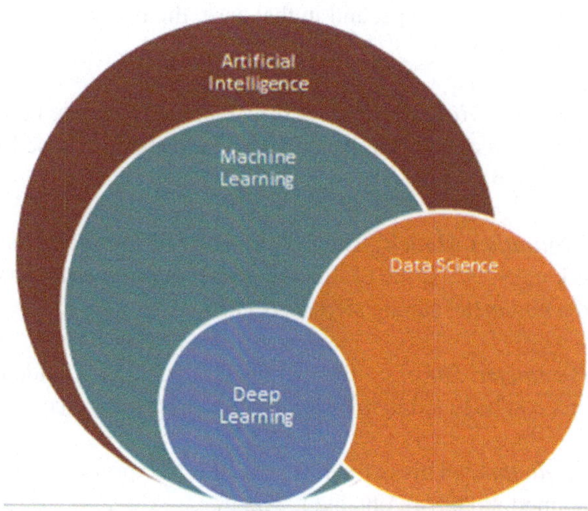

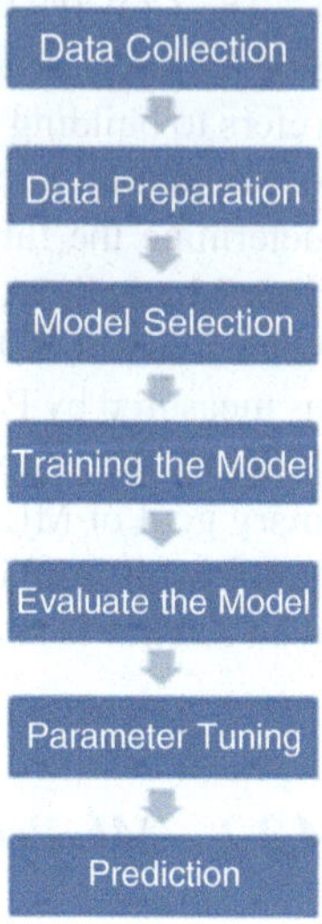


**Fig. 4.2** Steps of ML process [20]

can be used directly. The data can be collected by mounting sensors and other data collecting equipments or can be collected manually.

***Data Preparation:*** This step aims to prepare the data for training. It can go through many steps such as removing redundant values, data normalization, filling the missing values, data type conversion, etc. Also data randomization or arranging the data in the order of collection and others is done in this step. The splitting of data into training and testing data is also done if required.

***Model Selection:*** Versatile datasets are available, and depending upon the type, a correct approach needs to be chosen. There may be multiple numbers of algorithms that fit the data type, and in that case, the models are compared, and the best model is chosen.

***Train the Model:*** Training is given as input to the model for pattern or rule recognition. Once the rule is confirmed, test data is passed through it and the output is predicted.

***Evaluation Model:*** The performance of the model is evaluated in terms of time, accuracy, etc. If the evaluation model is not satisfactory, then previous mistakes or the parameter tuning step is checked.

***Parameter Tuning:*** The parameters such as confidence factor value, batch size, etc. can be tuned in this step for better performance.

***Prediction:*** This is the last step of a ML process, and the prediction results of an applied model are obtained.

### 4.2.2 *The C4.5 Algorithm*

The C4.5 is the most popular decision tree algorithm developed by a decision theory researcher of computer science named Ross Quinlan in 1993 [22, 23]. It is an extension of the ID3 algorithm developed by the same researcher. From a set of training data, the decision tree is formed by considering the information entropy [24]. The difference in entropy or information gain is used as the criteria of splitting, and this process occurs recursively. The test is done in each internal node of the decision tree, and the path to be followed is decided.

The *gain ratio* and split information denoted as *SplitInfo* for test *T* at position *p* are calculated as follows [25]:

$$\text{Gain ratio}\left(p,T\right)=\frac{\text{Gain}\left(p,T\right)}{\text{SplitInfo}\left(p,T\right)} \tag{4.1}$$

$$\text{SplitInfo}\left(p,\ \text{test}\right)=-\sum_{j=1}^{n}p'\left(\frac{j}{p}\right)\log\left(p'\left(\frac{j}{p}\right)\right) \tag{4.2}$$

Taking the value of *j*th test, $p'\left(\frac{j}{p}\right)$ is the proportion of elements present at the position *p*. Here in this decision tree, each end node is called leaf, and each non-final internal node is represented by test.

There are many advantages of this algorithm. Firstly, it is suitable for both continuous and discrete data. Secondly, it can manage the missing values very well by evaluating the gain ratio, and it also does the tree pruning after the creation of the decision tree.

### 4.2.3 *ML Challenges in COVID-19*

Many healthcare applications are developed by using ML [26] and the same can be done for COVID-19. To make the COVID-19 loss minimization, various activities associated with COVID-19 can be automated using ML techniques. Some of the application areas of COVID-19 where ML algorithms can be implemented are shown in Fig. 4.3.

***COVID-19 prediction:*** From the dataset of COVID-19 patient symptoms, the positive and negative information of a person can be calculated using ML classification algorithms. There are several classification algorithms available in ML, such as K-Nearest Neighbour (KNN), Random Forest (RF), Support Vector Machine (SVM), C4.5, etc.

***Social distance identification:*** COVID-19 is spreading very fast from person to person. To control the spreading several measures such as lockdown, shutdown, etc.

are implemented by both state as well as central governments in each country. The main intention behind this is to maintain social distancing. The social distancing can be identified and maintained using the Internet of Things (IoT) and can be done if a wrist band or any wearable can be designed with the integration of sensors which are capable of identifying the location, and then the distance of the nearest people can be calculated. Here alarm or buzzer can be set to inform the concerned person for the appropriate action.

***Case analysis and forecastination:*** The number of cases in terms of confirmed, recovered, active, and death is increasing day by day. The use of ML algorithms can help in analyzing such data. A time-series forecasting can also be done to find the number of cases in short intervals.

***Risk level analysis:*** To find the level of risk for COVID-19, a symptom dataset with a risk level is required. As the data grow, the algorithm will behave more efficiently. Based on the risk level, the person will decide whether it is necessary to consult with the doctor.

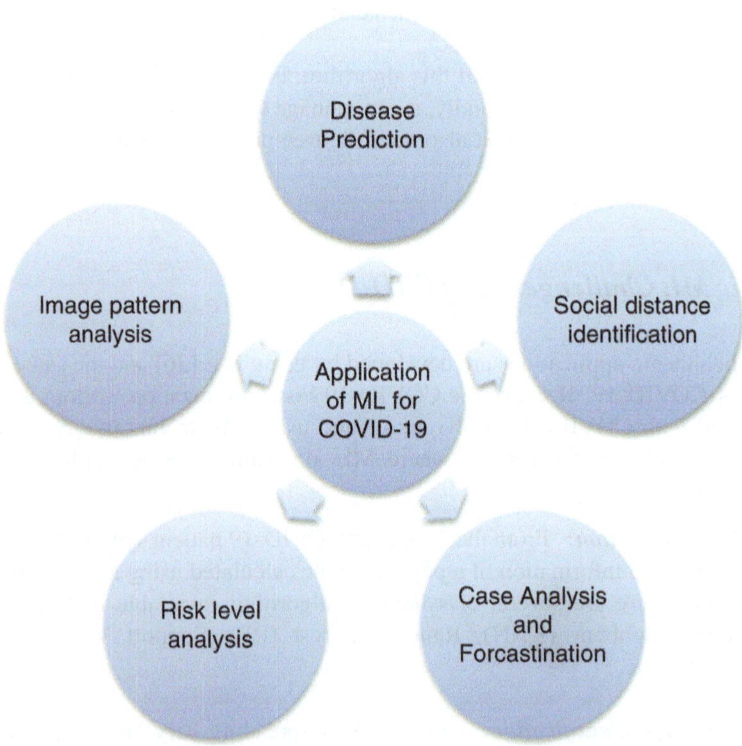


**Fig. 4.3** ML applications for COVID-19

***Image pattern analysis:*** COVID-19 is causing mainly problems in respiratory organs. If the automation of X-ray image analysis [27] can be done, then diagnosis and treatment can be made faster. The number of patient to doctor ratio is becoming very challenging gradually. So a faster treatment process can save many lives.

## 4.3 COVID-19 Global Status

In this section, we have presented a summary of the dataset used to create the confirmed case map and plot COVID-19 case status.

### *4.3.1 Dataset Description*

The considered COVID-19 dataset is publicly available in Kaggle [28]. It is an active dataset and is updated frequently with current data, containing the WHO region-wise confirmed, recovered, death, and active cases. This dataset contains data from 22 January 2020 to 20 June 2020. Table 4.1 summarizes the dataset.

The environmental setup required to show the pictorial representation of the COVID-19 dataset is given in Table 4.2.

### *4.3.2 COVID-19 Global Map*

Figure 4.4 shows the country-wise COVID-19 confirmed case map which is created from the COVID-19 dataset. The intensity of peach color in Fig. 4.4 indicates the number range of confirmed cases. The color intensity in Fig. 4.4 signifies that it is directly proportional to the range of confirmed cases.

### *4.3.3 COVID-19 Case Status*

The number of confirmed, death, active, and recovered cases concerning date is plotted from the considered dataset and shown in Fig. 4.5.

**Table 4.1** COVID-19 dataset description

| Dataset name | Dataset source | From | To | Data format |
|---|---|---|---|---|
| COVID-19 dataset | Kaggle | 22-Jan-2020 | 20-Jun-2020 | .csv |

**Table 4.2** Environmental setup for a pictorial representation of COVID-19 dataset

| | |
|---|---|
| Environment | Google Colab |
| Language | Python 3.6 |
| Libraries | Pandas, seaborn, matplotlib etc. |

### *4.3.4 Time-Series Forecast of Confirmed Cases*

The datestamp (ds) vs. numerically confirmed cases (y) data is plotted and is shown in Fig. 4.6. The actual data from January to June 2020 is taken, and the number of confirmed cases for the next 30 days is forecasted. The solid line indicates the forecast, and the shaded area refers to the possibility of deviation.

## 4.4 Proposed Work

In this work, we implemented a ML classification algorithm named C4.5 to identify the COVID-19 risk factor by taking the symptoms such as body temperature, dry cough, drowsiness, breathing problem, weakness, etc. into consideration. Age and gender are also important factors during disease identification and treatment. We have also considered the attributes of age, gender, and some previously identified diseases like diabetes, high blood pressure, lung disease, heart disease, etc. The remote treatment facility can be available by using this concept [29–31]. The audio and speech analysis is also required to make the system robust [32].

### *4.4.1 Dataset Description*

The considered dataset is collected from the Kaggle repository [33]. The dataset contains 21 columns, where the first column is serial number removed while classification is done. From the remaining 20 columns, 19 are symptoms and are treated as features of the classification problem. The last column indicates the target that includes low risk, medium risk, and high risk. This dataset has 127 instances. The dataset is summarized in Table 4.3.

### *4.4.2 Environmental Setup and the C4.5 Algorithm Implementation*

The considered dataset is classified using Python 3.6 in the Google colab environment. The dot CSV file contains both patient symptoms and the COVID-19 risk factor. The risk factors are high, medium, and low. The risk factor column is taken

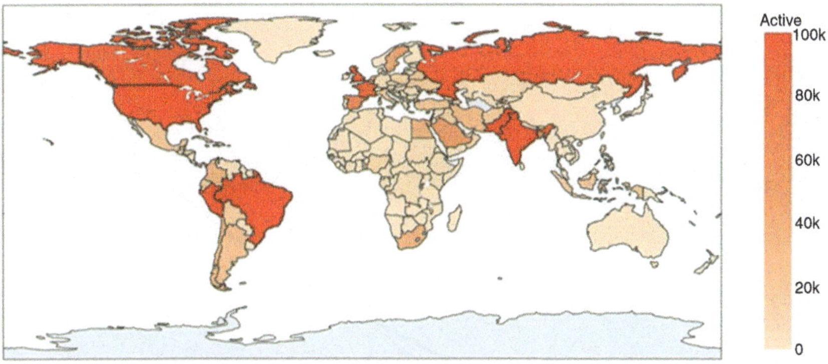


**Fig. 4.4** COVID-19 global map

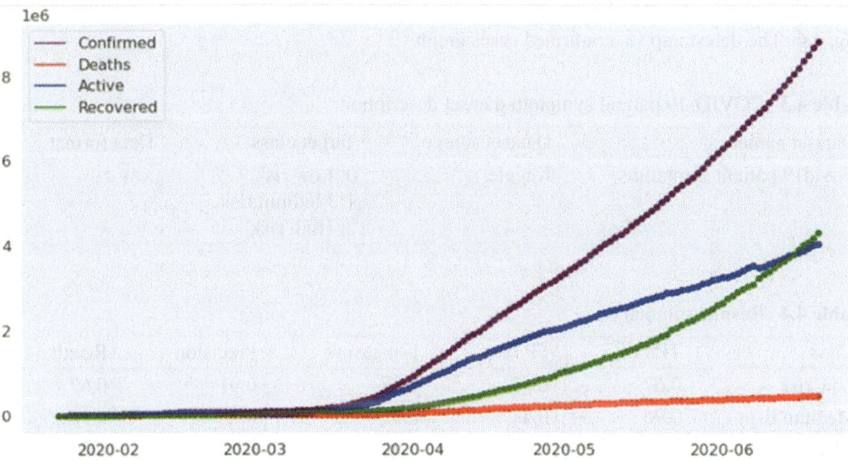


**Fig. 4.5** Different COVID-19 cases for date

as a target class that is to be classified. The body symptoms of the patient are treated as features based on which the classification can be done. There are many classification algorithms, such as Multilayer Perception (MLP), KNN, SVM, decision tree, C4.5, etc. [34–37]. In this work, we have used the C4.5 algorithm.

***C4.5 algorithm:*** Among the classification algorithms, the C4.5 algorithm is very popular and is used in many research areas. This is a fast and reliable classifier [22, 38]. The C4.5 algorithm verifies the information gain, that is, the difference in entropy, and decides splitting the data into different branches efficiently.

***Data split:*** The total data is divided into two sets: one is a training set and another is the test set. The model is built with the training set data. The test cases are used to check the accuracy of the built model.

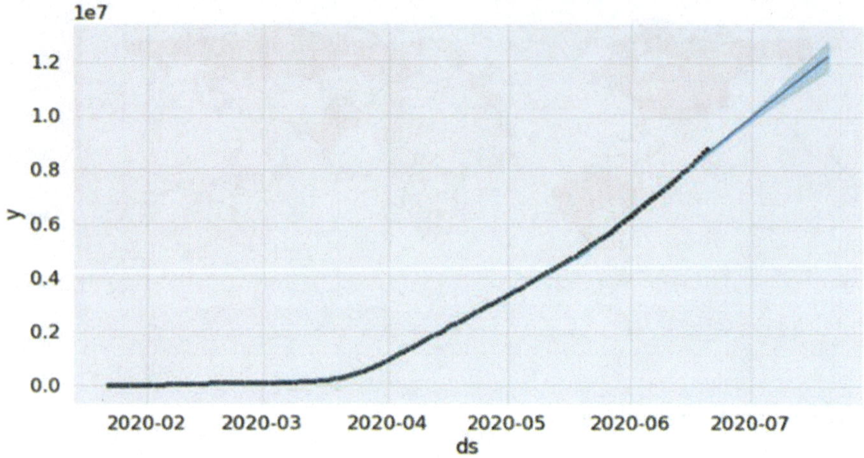


**Fig. 4.6** The datestamp vs. confirmed cases graph

**Table 4.3** COVID-19 patient symptom dataset description

| Dataset name | Dataset source | Target class | Data format |
|---|---|---|---|
| Covid19 patient symptoms | Kaggle | 0: Low risk,<br>1: Medium risk,<br>2: High risk | .csv |

**Table 4.4** Results summary

| Class | TP rate | FP rate | F-measure | Precision | Recall |
|---|---|---|---|---|---|
| Low risk | 0.67 | 0.03 | 0.77 | 0.91 | 0.67 |
| Medium list | 0.96 | 0.41 | 0.81 | 0.7 | 0.96 |
| *High risk* | 0.28 | 0.03 | 0.40 | 0.67 | 0.29 |

***Confidence factor:*** It is also known as the confidence interval. For statistical significance tests, it is preferably used.

***Batch size:*** In one iteration, how many training data will be utilized is indicated as batch size.

We have used the C4.5 as it results in better accuracy as compared to the other algorithms. The total data is split into training and test with a 65:35 ratio. The C4.5 tree construction algorithm [39] is applied with confidence factor 0.25 and batch size 100.

### 4.4.3 Results

We considered various parameters such as true-positive (TP) rate, false-positive (FP) rate, F-measure, precision, and recall for analyzing the obtained results.

***TP Rate:*** TP is correctly identified instances, and $P$ is the actual positive cases in the data. It can be computed as in Eq. (4.3).

$$\text{TP rate} = \text{TP} / P \tag{4.3}$$

***FP Rate:*** FP is the data that is incorrectly identified, and $N$ is the real negative case in the data. It can be computed as in Eq. (4.4).

$$\text{TP rate} = \text{FP} / N \tag{4.4}$$

***Precision:*** Precision is the ratio of correctly predicted positive observations of the total predicted positive observations [40]. The higher precision relates to the low false-positive rate. It can be computed as in Eq. (4.5).

$$\text{Precision} = \text{TP} / \left(\text{TP} + \text{FP}\right) \tag{4.5}$$

***F-Measure:*** It is the weighted harmonic mean of the precision and recall of the test.

The class, true-positive (TP) rate, false-positive (FP) rate, F-measure, precision, and recall after the classifier's implementation are given in Table 4.4.

The obtained results indicate that 75% of data are correctly classified and 25% are wrongly classified. The Kappa statistics, mean absolute error, and root mean square error are found to be 0.56, 0.22, and 0.38 respectively for the considered dataset.

The confusion matrix is used to describe a classification model's performance on a set of test data for which the correct values are known [41]. Columns of the matrix represent the prediction class result, whereas the actual class result is represented by rows [42]. The number of correct and incorrect predictions is summarized with count values and is separated by class. The confusion matrix of the data after applying the C4.5 algorithm is shown in Fig. 4.7. In Fig. 4.7, 0, 1, and 2 represent a low risk, medium risk, and high risk, respectively, for COVID-19 prediction.

The decision tree is somehow similar to flowchart. Each node except the leaf node represents a test condition that decides the branch to follow. The value of the cost function is calculated for each node, where a minimum is treated as a root of a tree. During the tree creation, the entropy decreases while splitting the tree downward, and the information gain decreases, or in other words, we can say the entropy and information gain are inversely proportional to each other [43]. The decision tree of the C4.5 algorithm for the considered dataset is presented in Fig. 4.8.

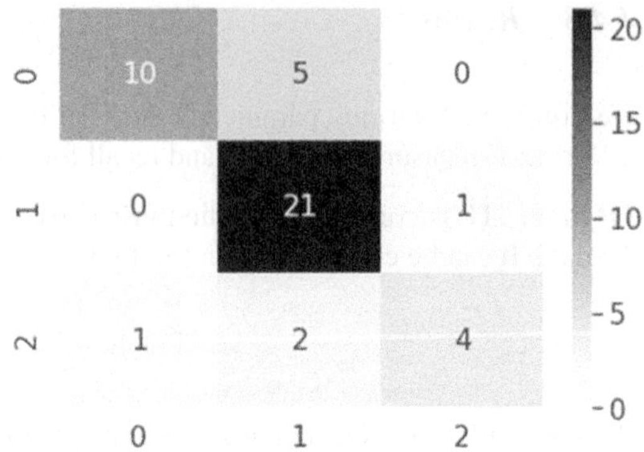


Fig. 4.7 Confusion matrix after the C4.5 algorithm implementation

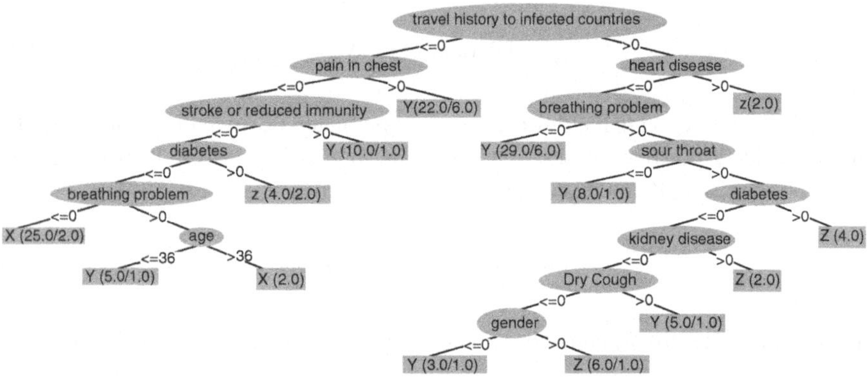


Fig. 4.8 Decision tree for the C4.5 algorithm on COVID-19 risk assessment

## 4.5 Conclusion and Future Work

In this work, we have taken the world case study for COVID-19 patients. The dataset is used for analyzing the present global scenario. We have implemented the C4.5 classifier on the COVID-19 patient symptom dataset to determine the person's risk level based on its recorded symptoms. The experimental results indicate that the C4.5 algorithm results in a classification accuracy of 75%.

As a future work, this model can be used in a chatbot in which a person can predict the risk and decide whether to consult the doctor or not. Since it is a highly contagious disease and unnecessary outdoor activities are to be avoided, a chatbot is a good option. The chatbot works on the cloud and hence while embedding the model into the chatbot, the network connectivity, service latency, symptom offloading time, cloud computation cost, etc. need to be considered. As the dataset will grow, deep learning can be applied to get higher accuracy. The optimization algorithms can also be integrated with ML algorithms to find the best fit for the application.

## References


1. https://www.medicalnewstoday.com/articles/coronavirus-causes#origin. Accessed 29 June 2020.
2. https://www.webmd.com/lung/coronavirus. Accessed 29 June 2020.
3. Kooraki, S., Hosseiny, M., Myers, L., & Gholamrezanezhad, A. (2020). Coronavirus (COVID-19) outbreak: What the department of radiology should know. *Journal of the American College of Radiology, 17*(4), 447–451.
4. Sohrabi, C., Alsafi, Z., O'Neill, N., Khan, M., Kerwan, A., Al-Jabir, A., & Agha, R. (2020). World Health Organization declares global emergency: A review of the 2019 novel coronavirus (COVID-19). *International Journal of Surgery, 76*, 71–76.
5. Ahuja, A. S., Reddy, V. P., & Marques, O. (2020). Artificial intelligence and COVID-19: A multidisciplinary approach. *Integrative Medicine Research, 9*(3), 100434.
6. Remuzzi, A., & Remuzzi, G. (2020). COVID-19 and Italy: What next? *The Lancet, 395*(10231), 1225–1228.
7. Singh, R., & Adhikari, R. (2020). Age-structured impact of social distancing on the COVID-19 epidemic in India. *arXiv preprint arXiv:2003.12055*.
8. https://www.who.int/emergencies/diseases/novel-coronavirus-2019. Accessed 29 June 2020.
9. Nguyen, T. T. (2020). Artificial intelligence in the battle against coronavirus (COVID-19): A survey and future research directions. *arXiv preprint arXiv:2008.07343*.
10. Ghosh, S., Bhatia, S., & Bhatia, A. (2018). Quro: Facilitating user symptom check using a personalized chatbot-oriented dialogue system. *Studies in Health Technology and Informatics, 252*, 51–56.
11. Madhu, D., Jain, C. N., Sebastain, E., Shaji, S., & Ajayakumar, A. (2017). A novel approach for medical assistance using trained chatbot. In *2017 international conference on inventive communication and computational technologies (ICICCT)* (pp. 243–246). Piscataway: IEEE.
12. https://chatbotslife.com/10-ai-bots-with-human-names-7efd7047be34. Accessed 29 June 2020.
13. https://www.analyticsinsight.net/chatbots-coronavirus-detecting-covid-19-symptoms-virtual-assessment-tool/. Accessed 29 June 2020.
14. Alimadadi, A., Aryal, S., Manandhar, I., Munroe, P. B., Joe, B., & Cheng, X. (2020). Artificial intelligence and machine learning to fight COVID-19. *Physiological Genomics, 52*(4), 200–202.
15. https://www.mygreatlearning.com/blog/what-is-machine-learning/. Accessed 29 June 2020.
16. https://machinelearningmastery.com/what-is-machine-learning/. Accessed 29 June 2020.
17. https://becominghuman.ai/ultimate-guide-and-resources-for-data-science-2019-f663f9384fc7. Accessed 29 June 2020.
18. https://www.geeksforgeeks.org/supervised-unsupervised-learning/. Accessed 29 June 2020.
19. Hastie, T., Tibshirani, R., & Friedman, J. (2009). Unsupervised learning. In *The elements of statistical learning* (pp. 485–585). New York: Springer.
20. https://www.kdnuggets.com/2018/05/general-approaches-machine-learning-process.html. Accessed 29 June 2020.
21. Sampathkumar, A., Rastogi, R., Arukonda, S., Shankar, A., Kautish, S., & Sivaram, M. (2020). An efficient hybrid methodology for detection of cancer-causing gene using CSC for micro array data. *Journal of Ambient Intelligence and Humanized Computing, 11*, 4743–4751.
22. Salzberg, S. L. (1994). *C4.5: Programs for machine learning* by J. Ross Quinlan. Morgankaufmann Publishers, Inc., 1993.
23. Kotsiantis, S. B., Zaharakis, I., & Pintelas, P. (2007). Supervised machine learning: A review of classification techniques. *Emerging Artificial Intelligence Applications in Computer Engineering, 160*(1), 3–24.
24. https://en.wikipedia.org/wiki/C4.5_algorithm. Accessed 29 June 2020.

25. Hssina, B., Merbouha, A., Ezzikouri, H., & Erritali, M. (2014). A comparative study of decision tree ID3 and C4.5. *International Journal of Advanced Computer Science and Applications, 4*(2), 13–19.
26. https://www.upgrad.com/blog/machine-learning-applications-in-healthcare/. Accessed 29 June 2020.
27. Zheng, C., Deng, X., Fu, Q., Zhou, Q., Feng, J., Ma, H., et al. (2020). Deep learning-based detection for COVID-19 from chest CT using weak label. *medRxiv*.
28. https://www.kaggle.com/imdevskp/corona-virus-report. Accessed 29 June 2020.
29. Wright, J. H., & Caudill, R. (2020). Remote treatment delivery in response to the COVID-19 pandemic. *Psychotherapy and Psychosomatics, 89*(3), 1.
30. Smith, A. C., Thomas, E., Snoswell, C. L., Haydon, H., Mehrotra, A., Clemensen, J., & Caffery, L. J. (2020). Telehealth for global emergencies: Implications for coronavirus disease 2019 (COVID-19). *Journal of Telemedicine and Telecare, 26*(5), 309–313.
31. Connors, J. M., & Levy, J. H. (2020). COVID-19 and its implications for thrombosis and anticoagulation. *Blood: The Journal of the American Society of Hematology, 135*(23), 2033–2040.
32. Deshpande, G., & Schuller, B. (2020). An overview on audio, signal, speech, & language processing for COVID-19. *arXiv preprint arXiv:2005.08579*.
33. https://www.kaggle.com/bitsofishan/covid19-patient-symptoms? Accessed 29 June 2020.
34. Kumar, R., & Verma, R. (2012). Classification algorithms for data mining: A survey. *International Journal of Innovations in Engineering and Technology (IJIET), 1*(2), 7–14.
35. Deng, Z., Zhu, X., Cheng, D., Zong, M., & Zhang, S. (2016). Efficient kNN classification algorithm for big data. *Neurocomputing, 195*, 143–148.
36. Saritas, M. M., & Yasar, A. (2019). Performance analysis of ANN and Naive Bayes classification algorithm for data classification. *International Journal of Intelligent Systems and Applications in Engineering, 7*(2), 88–91.
37. Wu, X., Kumar, V., Quinlan, J. R., Ghosh, J., Yang, Q., Motoda, H., et al. (2008). Top 10 algorithms in data mining. *Knowledge and Information Systems, 14*(1), 1–37.
38. Quinlan, J. R. (2014). *C4.5: Programs for machine learning*. Amsterdam: Elsevier.
39. Ruggieri, S. (2002). Efficient C4. 5 [classification algorithm]. *IEEE Transactions on Knowledge and Data Engineering, 14*(2), 438–444.
40. Miner, A. S., Laranjo, L., & Kocaballi, A. B. (2020). Chatbots in the fight against the COVID-19 pandemic. *NPJ Digital Medicine, 3*(1), 1–4.
41. World Health Organization. (2020). *Coronavirus disease 2019 (COVID-19): Situation report, 72*.
42. Xu, J., Zhang, Y., & Miao, D. (2020). Three-way confusion matrix for classification: A measure driven view. *Information Sciences, 507*, 772–794.
43. https://towardsdatascience.com/what-is-the-c4-5-algorithm-and-how-does-it-work-2b971a9e7db0. Accessed 29 June 2020.

# Chapter 5
# Recent Diagnostic Techniques for COVID-19

**Rajeshwar Kamal Kant Arya, Meena Kausar, Dheeraj Bisht, Deepak Kumar, Deepak Sati, and Govind Rajpal**

## 5.1 Introduction

Coronavirus disease 2019 was previously initiated as a bunch of cases from Wuhan, China, that has now covered over 135 countries worldwide [1]. Till 20 July 2020, about 14 million cases were reported with 0.6 million deaths worldwide [2]. This virus was named 2019-nCoV due to the similarity of the virus that caused the SARS outbreak (SARS-CoVs) [3]. Coronavirus belongs to a group of viruses ranging from regular flu to MERS (Middle East respiratory syndrome), coronavirus, and SARS coronavirus. The coronavirus RNA positioned in ORF1 (open reading frame 1a/b) [4] that converts polyproteins (pp1a and pp1ab) and also codify 16 non-structural proteins and structure-forming proteins. Coronavirus gene codifies the four necessary structural proteins, like spike (S) glycoprotein, matrix (M) protein, envelope (E) protein, and nucleocapsid (N) protein [4, 5], and also codifies various appended proteins, probably obstructing the inherent host immunity [6]. The lower respiratory tract of humans possesses SARS-COVID receptor [7] and regulates both the human-to-human and cross-species transmissions [5, 8]. Generally the incubation period is 1–14 days, but in most cases, it is 3–7 days, and the infection is manifested by fever, tiredness, and dry cough and in some cases blocked nose, runny nose, throat ache, and diarrhea. Severe patients show dyspnea and hypoxemia after 7 days and progressed to acute respiratory distress syndrome and finally multiple organ failure. Some patients carry mild symptoms such as low fever and tiredness [1]. Initially when the outbreak started, every country followed and implemented several action

R. K. K. Arya (✉) · M. Kausar · D. Bisht · D. Sati · G. Rajpal
Department of Pharmaceutical Sciences, Bhimtal Campus, Kumaun University Nainital, Bhimtal, Uttarakhand, India

D. Kumar
Department of Pharmaceutical Chemistry, School of Pharmaceutical Sciences, Shoolini University, Solan, Himachal Pradesh, India



S. Kautish et al. (eds.), *Computational Intelligence Techniques for Combating COVID-19*, EAI/Springer Innovations in Communication and Computing,
https://doi.org/10.1007/978-3-030-68936-0_5

plans for testing. WHO initiated a mission to ensure the availability of the diagnostic facilities for detecting, protecting, and treating for breaking the chain of transmission. Therefore preliminary testing and quick treatment can minimize the number of cases; thus, the diagnosis plays an important role in regulating and limiting the coronavirus infection [1]. For a preventive measure of coronavirus, there is only one method, i.e., tracing, tracing, and tracing the suspect; only this provides a real-time patient condition. The diagnosis can prevent the spreading of the viruses, hence protecting the life of other peoples. The entire world is making an effort for developing a new rapid diagnostic system which can provide quick and efficient diagnosis at an affordable price. Although there are several diagnostic kits available in the market, they are very expensive and take 2–5 days for diagnosis. Still, some rapid diagnostic tests are also now developed with prompt diagnosis at affordable prices. The diagnostic techniques are classified into two classes: one is molecular assay (RT-PCR) and the second is serologic assay (antigen-antibody reaction) [8]. Based on the above classification, several kits are available in the market for the diagnosis of COVID-19 suspects.

## 5.2 Molecular Assay Techniques

In the molecular assay techniques, the nucleic acid of the virus is detected in the specimen, which is collected from the suspect sputum, throat, or nasal cavity. The nucleic acid is isolated and amplified, and viral load is detected. COVID-19 is a single-strand RNA virus, and genetic information is available at Global initiatives on sharing all influenza data networks. Researchers are making efforts to develop testing kits on available genetic information [8]. The following techniques are employed in the molecular assay techniques.

### *5.2.1 Reverse Transcription-Polymerase Chain Reaction (RT-PCR)*

In 1993, RT-PCR technique was discovered by Nobel laureate Kary Mullis. Usally, a low quantity of desired DNA or RNA is found in any specimen, for detection the amplification of DNA, or RNA is required. PCR is employed for generating several copies of a specific sequence of nucleic acid, and even a single DNA molecule can be amplified with the help of PCR. A considerable quantity of DNA can be generated by using PCR (which can be visualized with the help of gel electrophoresis). PCR generates several replicates of DNA strand exponentially by multiplying a sequence and is catalyzed by a peculiar polymerase enzyme. For amplification, three components are required, like DNA sequence; nucleotide medium, i.e., adenine (A), thymine (T), cytosine (C), and guanine (G); and a primer (DNA fraction). The amplification generates several identical copies of the templates in the presence of polymerase enzyme. The PCR depends on the stability of the polymerase enzyme at a higher temperature [9, 10]. In Mullis's PCR process, in the presence of polymerase enzyme, the in vitro separation of dual helical into single helical DNA sequence occurs by heating it at 96 °C. However, elevated temperature could degrade *E. coli* DNA polymerase; hence Taq DNA polymerase from bacteria *Thermus aquaticus* is used [10, 11].

Real-time RT-PCR (reverse transcription-polymerase chain reaction) is an in vitro method for determining nucleic acid qualitatively from SARS-CoV-2 (severe acute respiratory symptom coronavirus 2) in nasal or throat sample, e.g., oropharyngeal or nasopharyngeal swabs and sputum, collected from suspected individuals of COVID-19, which is used only under the Food and Drug Administration's Emergency Use Authorization.

The RT-PCR test utilized a set of probes and a set of three primers for detecting domains in viral gene and a set of one primer and probe to detect human ribonuclease in the specimen. The nasal or throat sample of suspected individuals is processed; RNA is separated and cleaned (may contain the viral RNA). From RNA mixture, cDNA is produced by reverse transcription and then treated with specially designed primers (marker). The primer is attached to the specific viral RNA segment and amplified by RT-PCR. The annealing of probe to the specific segment takes place betwixt the reverse and forward primer during amplification [11, 12]. In the final step, the Taq polymerase degrades the bound probe, and resulted in the separation of dyes and produce the fluorescence; the fluorescent intensity is recorded, and high fluorescence intensity indicates the presence of SARS-CoV-2 infection (Fig. 5.1) [13]. The outcome detects the infection at an acute level, and other diagnostic information and clinical correlation with patient history are also considered. Negative outcomes should be correlated with the clinical examinations and previous information of the patients [13].

**Advantages**
The RT-PCR has the ability to detect viruses qualitatively and also can quantify the viral load; the RT-PCR amplifies the genetic material many folds; therefore, smaller amount of specimen can be detected easily by using RT-PCR. This technique has high sensitivity without any complexity and also provides results in a short time [14].

**Disadvantages**
The RT-PCR utilized costly sophisticated instruments and thermal cycler, and it uses high thermal heat for processing that can destroy the DNA molecule and enzymes. The carryover contamination is the main disadvantage of this method that can give false readings, and experts are also required to perform and develop new assay methods in the laboratories. It also needs an expensive thermal cycler [14].

### *5.2.2 COBAS 6800/8800*

WHO enlisted COBAS for emergency use for qualitatively detecting novel coronavirus RNA in suspect's specimen – a fully integrated, automated, and improved technique that provides accurate, fast quantitative and qualitative results by using

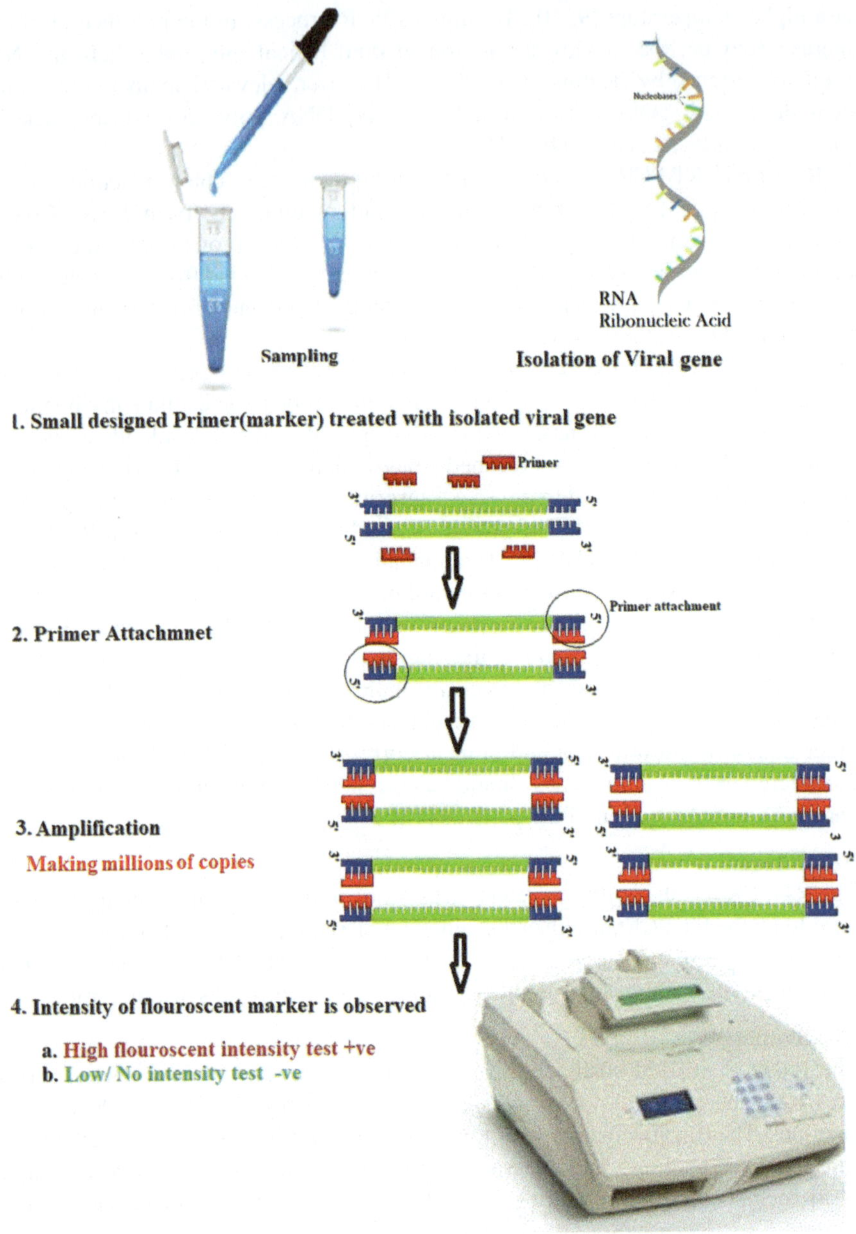


**Fig. 5.1** Viral RNA amplification and detection by RT-PCR

RT-PCR [15]; the previously used RT-PCR is semi-automatic that can cause infection to the person handling the process and can give false result due to carryover contamination. COBAS is the best solution to overcome these problems. It is a software-based program with two versions, COBAS 6800 and 8800, which can test 324 and 960 samples in 8 h, respectively [16]. COBAS is a fast-detecting technique for novel coronavirus devoid of any analytical error; approximately 1200 samples can be detected in a day with a single instrument. The instrument is enabled with the robotics mechanism that removes the chances of getting infected with the personnel handling the specimen. This instrument can also be used in the diagnosis of other diseases, e.g., hepatitis B and C, AIDS, papilloma, MTb, CMV, chlamydia, *Neisseria*, etc. [17].

In COBAS, the viral RNA is extracted and purified automatically from the specimen and then amplified with the help of RT-PCR and detected qualitatively. During the sample processing, the RNA as an internal control is added to each sample for monitoring the preparation of the sample, and that is then amplified in PCR; the external controls (low titer positive control and a negative control) are also added. The automated system is controlled by COBAS 6800/8800 software that is comprised of four integrated modules – (a) supply, (b) transfer, (c) processing, and (d) analysis of the specimen – and provides the outcomes on the computer. The extraction of viral RNA from suspect specimens and added internal control is performed simultaneously. The proteinase and lysate are added to release RNA from specimens and internal control. The released RNA attached to the silica magnetic beads, the unattached material, and the impurities, e.g., denatured protein, cellular junk, and PCR inhibitors, are withdrawn by subsequent washing. The RNA is extracted out from magnetic bead with the help of extraction buffer at high temperature. The same process is also repeated for the external controls for each run. A target region in the virus protein is selected for detecting the coronavirus; a peculiar viral RNA is amplified with the help of target-specific forward and reverse primer. The internal control is amplified by noncompetitive sequence-specific forward and reverse primers that have no homology with the coronavirus genome in the presence of thermostable DNA polymerase. COBAS master mixture contains detecting probes, specific to coronavirus and internal control RNA genome, which are labeled with two dyes (reporter and quencher dye). On not binding to targeted sequence, the quencher suppresses fluorescence of reporter dye. In amplification, the probe hybridized with a peculiar single-strand DNA template, the DNA polymerase breaks down the probe, and the separation of both the dye parts results in the fluorescence. The color intensity increased with per PCR cycle. The coronavirus and RNA internal control representing dye can be distinguished by a UV spectrophotometer. The deoxyuridine triphosphate (dUTP) is also added to the master mixture in newly synthesized cDNA; after each PCR cycle, AmpErase enzyme (uracil-N-glycosylase) is added and heated to remove the carryover impurities formed in the previous cycle [16, 18].

**Advantages**
This technique is more advantageous and better than a semi-automatic system; it saves processing time and provides fast and accurate result. Being a fully automatic system, less labor is required [15]. The integrated system minimizes the chances of contamination [15]. Approximately 1200 samples per day can be tested [15]. AmpErase enzyme is used in the process that removes the carryover impurities [16], and it can perform three assays for the same batch [18].

**Disadvantages**
The disadvantages of this technique are very few, but skilled labor is required for processing the samples, and the daily maintenance of instrument is also required.

### *5.2.3 Loop-Mediated Isothermal Amplification (LAMP)*

Although RT-PCR is a widely employed technique for COVID-19 diagnosis, it requires expensive instruments as well as a well-equipped laboratory [19–21]. To overcome this problem, the molecular diagnostic LAMP method was utilized for the diagnosis of COVID-19. It is a rapid and reliable technique developed for the amplification of a small amount of target sequence that avoids the requirement of ultramodern thermal cycler instruments for detection [22]. This method is widely used as a diagnostic tool in the life sciences and medical field including genetic disorders and contagious disease. The amplification of DNA sequence is performed at a constant temperature, and this technique is based on automated cycling strand displacement DNA synthesis [22], and with the excellent strand displacing and replicating function, the DNA polymerase executed this process with the help of two engineered inner and outer primers; at the start, all primers are employed, but at the final stage, only inner primer is used in the process. The primers have a sense and antisense sequence of DNA. High amplification of DNA sequence is achieved by this method, which is visually detectable with the help of dyes (China green, hydroxy naphthol, and calcein) [23, 24] that react with the by-product of DNA synthesis. pH-dependent dyes could also be utilized; for the addition of dNTP, proton assemblage causes the pH alteration, and that is measured and recorded. Figure 5.2 shows the procedure of the LAMP technique. LAMP techniques are employed in an extensive field survey of *Wolbachia*-infected mosquitos [25] and uroscopy for the Zika virus [26]. LAMP is a visually detectable, portable, easiest, more advantageous, and expeditious novel diagnostic technique [21] but less versatile than RT-PCR.

**Advantages**
LAMP can be effectively used for diagnosis in developing countries; specifically designed primers allow highly specific detection of six distinct sequences in the target DNA. The loop primer accelerates the amplification process that reduces the detection time with excellent sensitivity [27]. The short detection time makes it better than RT-PCR; it provides results in 1 h, whereas RT-PCR takes 4–8 h. It is

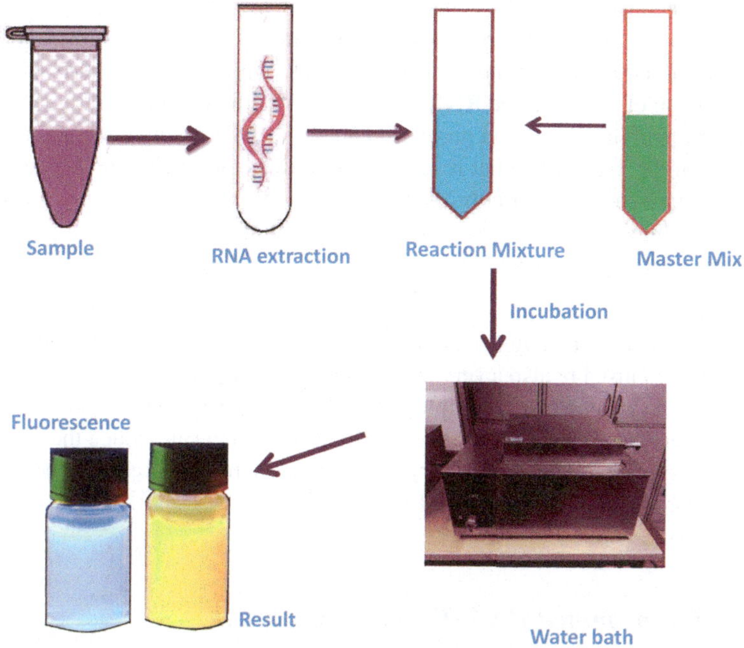


**Fig. 5.2** Loop-mediated isothermal amplification technique

economic and no skilled personnel are required [28]; it has the well-tolerating ability for biological substances than RT-PCR, and removing the DNA isolation step makes it economic. Simple heating apparatus are required (water bath, heating block) for LAMP [29].

**Disadvantages**

The main disadvantage of this technique is the carryover contamination from the previous batch which can give false results, and precaution must be taken while handling the sample vessel; it should not be open. Additional technique is also required to enhance detection values, e.g., fluorescent material, colorimetric material, or lateral flow dipsticks [27].

### *5.2.4 Transcription-Mediated Amplification (TMA)*

A new modified patented technique, more efficient than RT-PCR, is also used for diagnosis purposes [8]. In this method, single probe isothermal amplification of specific sequence of DNA or RNA is done; by using transcription-mediated amplification. The nucleic acid is detected by using the retroviral reverse transcriptase and T7 RNA polymerase enzyme [8]. Hybridization of target RNA with peculiar sequence primer takes place in the presence of RNA polymerase enzyme, and new cDNA is generated. The RNAse destroy the RNA from RNA-cDNA complex, and the primer binds to cDNA, and another duplicate of cDNA is synthesized, and a double-strand DNA is generated containing RNA polymerase that starts RNA transcription from cDNA, and the RNA targets are amplified exponentially [30]. TMA can be used with hybridization protection analysis (HPA) using chemical illuminators (acridinium ester) [31] that react with hybridized amplicon and produce luminescence, whereas the non-hybridized probes were removed by hydrolysis. The intensity of luminescence determines the concentration [30] and the presence of coronavirus infection in suspect.

**Advantages**
The TMA provides benefits over the traditional RT-PCR technique; it provides faster results in just 4 h; also a very small quantity of viral RNA is needed for amplification. Cheap water baths are employed in place of costly thermal cycler to amplify and hybridize. A single tube is utilized in the process that can reduce the chances of contamination. The chances of carryover contamination are reduced because the RNA amplicon is unstable than PCR product [27].

### 5.2.5 *Programmed RNA-Targeted Analysis*

Programmed RNA-targeted analysis is based on a specific nucleic acid strand that is obtained from the bacteria and viruses, that can be identified and trimmed by the enzyme, e.g., Cas9, Cas12, and Cas13 [32]. This is also called CRISPR or specific high-sensitivity enzymatic reporter unlocking (SHERLOCK) platform [6], the latest technique employed for detecting SARS-COVID-19 infection. This technique has high specificity and high sensitivity with visual delectability; in this technique, CRISPR-associated protein 9 (Cas9) is programmed to identify the viral gene strand and trim out the peculiar RNA strands by using simple procedures [33]. For detection of coronavirus, the S gene and Orf1ab gene are targeted [34]; the recombinase polymerase amplification technique (RAT) is used to amplify the synthetic viral RNA, and DNA converted back into RNA. The peculiar strands of RNA were detected with the help of the Cas13 nuclease enzyme, and the extracted RNA is detected visually with the help of antibody-immobilized paper dipstick.

**Advantages**
It is very simple, user-friendly, and cheap and shows high sensitivity and is highly efficient than other gene-modifying technologies; we can analyze the reaction and relation between genetic difference and expression; we can also remove or substitute the undesired gene in genetic therapy [35].

**Disadvantages**
Sometimes the gene editing can be off-targeted that might change the genetic function that can cause genome instability. DNA duplication is a very specific job, but off-targeting can change this process [35].

### 5.2.6 *Rolling Circle Amplification*

Rolling circle amplification is a simplified, economical, expeditious, and highly sensitive nucleic acid (SARS-COVID-19)-detecting technique. It can amplify RNA about $10^{-9}$ time per cycle, and no sophisticated instrument is required [36]. Isolated DNA is denatured by heat shock method, and target DNA is ligated with a circularizable probe and hybridized. DNA ligase is added and amplification done by utilizing a thermal cycler in the presence of dNTP, primers, and DNA polymerase enzyme. The ligation was detected by gel electrophoresis [37]. Enzyme-based biosensor pad can also be prepared for detecting the DNA or RNA [38] in which the immobilized enzyme catalyzes the amplification, and a double effect is produced with RCA to intensify the signal. The DNAzymes can be combined with RCA for detecting the other enzymes, e.g., DNA ligase and polynucleotide kinase phosphate; DNA ligase helps in the generation of cDNA, repairing, and recombination [38].

**Advantages**
Rolling circle amplification is economic than RT-PCR because simple apparatus is used, and it has a high yield.

### 5.2.7 *Microarray*

This technique is more sensitive, efficient, and reproducible with high resolution. Microarray is probed (cDNA) with target DNA to produce gene expression. The microarray is comprised of a solid 3D bed, the bed is segmented in wells, where the radiolabeled cDNA (probe) generated from RNA of the virus through suspended RT [8]. Whereas the target sequence is immobilized with a fluorescent dye, each well contains millions of identical probes. When the target hybridized with probe, the fluorescence is produced and that is measured by the detector. For diagnostic purpose, print or spot technique is also used, where the glass slide printed with a probe is used; it is elegant, cheap, washable and can withstand at high temperature. It also provides good kinetics during the hybridization and has minimum fluorescence in the backdrop [39]. The printing may be non-touching or direct touching; non-touching works similarly to the computer printing; the probe is sprayed onto the glass slide, whereas in direct touching, the printing pins applied the probe solution onto glass slide. It has a high resolution; a nano-liter solution can create a spot in micrometer [39].

**Advantages**
Glass microarray technique is affordable at a low price, and no sophisticated instruments are needed for the hybridization process; data can be processed with a simple laboratory instrument. The instrument has flexible designing that favors the scientific need for experimentation. It also has high sensitivity toward virus detection because of longer target sequences [40].

**Disadvantages**

Although glass microarray is a widely used technique, it also has some disadvantages like skilled persons required for extracting, refining, and collecting the DNA before fabricating microarray. The printing instruments are also costly, and sometimes the false result may appear because of the cross-hybridization of closely related members from the same gene family [40].

### *5.2.8 Metagenomic Next-Generation Sequencing (mNGS)*

In 2014–2016, mNGS proved as a countermeasure for the Ebola virus epidemic in West Africa; now lesser developed areas of Southeast Asia use this for an understanding of COVID-19 sequencing, pathogen, origin, transmission, and evolution [41–43]. For the diagnosis, specimens from the nasal or throat swab of the suspect are collected and separated. RNA is isolated from the specimen via RNA extraction kit, e.g., MoBIO DNA extraction kit and Qiagen DNA microbiome kit. The isolated RNA is then treated with Dnase and amplified in PCR for generating cDNA metagenomic library which is quantified and sequenced by Illumina instrument. A sequenced library is assembled, and annotation is done before bioinformatical analysis [43, 44].

**Advantages**

The metagenomic techniques are very advantageous and powerful techniques employed to evaluate numerous microorganisms simultaneously in one test [45]. This technique has high accuracy and fast testing speed, and this technique can be used in viral load quantification. The metagenomic cloud library could be accessed by everyone from all over the world. Several analytical processes can be performed on the computer with the latest configuration [46].

**Disadvantages**

The main disadvantage of these techniques is its high price; the approximate cost is 500$ to 5000$ for testing [46]. The sequencing data of various microbes is not well known to scientists; therefore, comparison might be complicated because prior information is not available. High technical proficiency is required for testing [46].

## 5.3 Serologic Assay

The serologic assay is based on the antigen-antibody reaction; the serum or plasma is used to detect the presence of infection, the IgM/IgG level is increased in plasma against the infection, is measured in the serological assay. The blood sample, sputum, and other biological fluids are analyzed to detect the infection. The serologic assay determines whether the infection in initial phases or in the advance phase [8]. For any infection, the IgM is detected in the initial phase, and

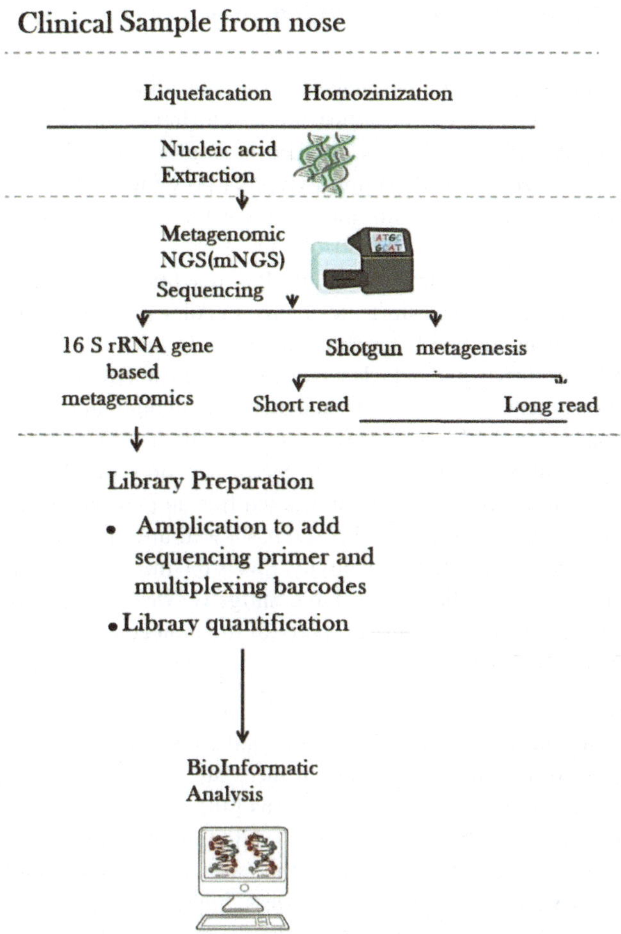


**Fig. 5.3** Metagenomic sequencing technique for COVID-19 detection [47]

IgG can be detected in a later phase. Comparing the result of a serologic and molecular assay, sometimes the results show antilogy; a positive suspect from the RT-PCR technique could be negative in the serologic test, due to delayed antibody production, whereas a positive serologic suspect could be found negative in RT-PCR, due to clearance of milder infection. The sensitivity of the serologic method is limited; ambiguous results are observed some time. The serologic assay is a widespread viral infection diagnostic technique and not exclusive for SARS-CoV-2 infections; for detection of a SARS-COVID-19, spike glycoprotein (S1 and S2) with receptor-binding domain and nucleocapsid protein are used [48]; now various serologic assay-based rapid diagnostic test (RDT) kits are available in the market, and the diagnostic kit exhibits rapid visual result; some serologic assay-based techniques are discussed here.

### 5.3.1 *Enzyme-Linked Immunosorbent Assay (ELISA)*

The ELISA is a robust quantitative analysis technique employed for the detection of antigen or antibody in a composite admixture; this technique allows the detection of protein and peptides. The antigen is fastened in solid surface [48–50]; the micro-plate and tubes are fabricated from polystyrene or polyvinyl. The antigen and antibodies specifically adsorbed onto the micro-plate. ELISA used enzymes and substrate; both react to each other in 30–60 min. To cease this reaction, acid or base are added to the reaction mixture and the result of reaction is recorded with spectrophotometer or visually by recording the change in color [51, 52]. ELISA is categorized into a homogeneous and heterogeneous assay. In the homogeneous assay, the enzyme sticks to antibody and gets deactivated; thus the antigen is isolated from the medium, and this method is utilized to quantify a small amount of drugs. However, it is easiest, but costly and low sensitive method. The heterogeneous technique is based on antigen-antibody interaction with each other and formed a complex, which gets attached to the walls of the tube; unwanted free antigens are also there, which can interfere with the medium, and this setup allowed unwanted molecule to separate during washing. Due to high sensitivity, this is the most widely employed technique for detecting antibodies and soluble antigens. Various types of ELISA are prepared based on construction and property of the molecule to be detected, which are represented in Fig. 5.4.

**Direct Assay**
The macromolecular antigen can be determined using this method in which the antigen is allowed to make an overlay on the plate wall and the enzyme-labeled antibodies are employed for detecting antigens [48, 49]. The unbound antigen can be washed off from the solvent system; on the addition of a suitable substrate to the system, color is produced that quantifies the antigens or antibody [48, 49]. This technique is very valuable because it is errorless, requires few processing steps, and uses minimum reagent; the secondary antibody is also not required. The main

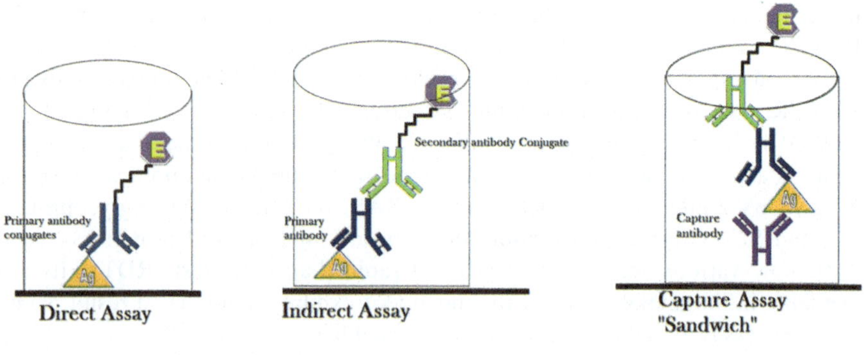


**Fig. 5.4** Various ELISA techniques [48]

demerit of this method is its low specificity due to low immobilization of antigens, minimum flexibility regarding primary antibody, and no signal amplification.

**Indirect**
In this method, the antigen to be detected is measured indirectly; antigen first forms complex with the antibody. Another enzyme-labeled antibody is added to the complex and produces color. In this method [53, 54], the serum of suspect is added to the antigen-overlaid surface of the plate, and then incubation is done; in the course of incubation, the antibodies are developed for the infection or antigen, and an antibody-antigen complex is formed. To reveal the complex formation, another enzyme-labeled antibody having a property of detecting the antibody present in the suspect's serum is introduced with a respective substrate that provides color and quantifies the concentration.

**Sandwich ELISA**
In this technique, the antigen to be detected is sandwiched between two antigen-specific antibodies; this technique is about two- to fivefold more sensitive than other techniques; the plate surface is overlaid with a captured antibody. The serum is added to the antibody-overlaid plates and incubated for a few minutes and then washed, and the unbound antigens are washed off. The specific antigens get bounded to the antibody and remain attached even after washing. The antibodies labeled with antigen-specific enzyme are added, incubated for some time and then washed; the antibody-specific antigen remains bounded with the antibody that can be detected by a color change on the addition of enzyme substrate.

**Advantages**
The serologic assay is a simple, highly sensitive, and specific technique due to antigen-antibody reaction. The procedure is safe, eco-friendly, and economic because cheap reagents are required. It is a handy, rapid, and automated process and also gives results very fast.

**Disadvantages**
Serologic assay needs a sophisticated method for the preparation of antibodies and required skilled personnel and high-priced culture media that increases the price of the test. The results may appear false positive or negative. It also required a species-specific second antibody.

### 5.3.2 *COVID-19 IgM/IgG Antibody Rapid Test*

The Indian Council of Medical Research approved the COVID-19 IgM/IgG antibody rapid test on 16 April 2020, based on lateral flow immunoassay to detect in vitro IgM and IgG antibodies in human plasma, serum, or whole blood qualitatively (Fig. 5.5). RDT is a small movable kit, which shows visual results within 20–30 min. The test kit possesses a colloidal gold-labeled recombinant COVID 19 antigen and a control antibody colloidal gold marker. There are two detection lines

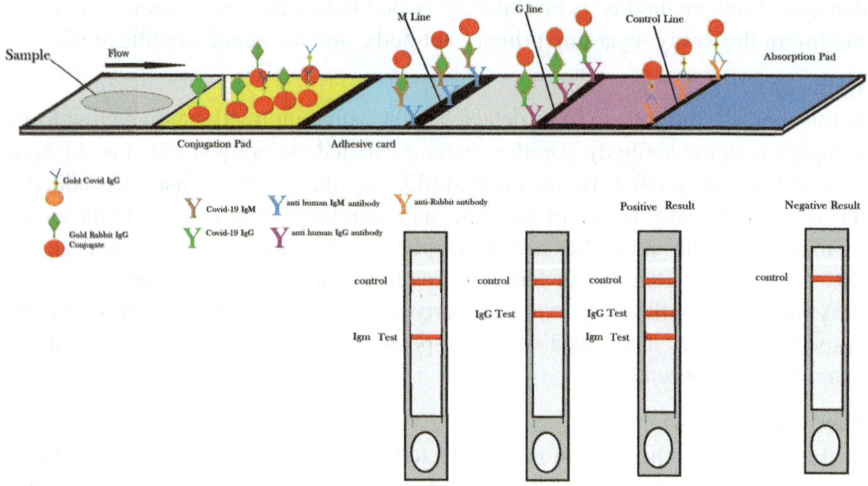


**Fig. 5.5** COVID-19 rapid test kit [55]

(M and G lines, for detecting IgM/IgG) and one control line. The bed is composed of nitrocellulose membrane, in which IgM is immobilized with monoclonal antihuman IgM antibody and IgG immobilized with a monoclonal antihuman IgG antibody for detecting the coronavirus IgM and IgG antibody, respectively. The control anti-rabbit antibody is immobilized on the control line [55], and the results are exhibited by three red lines for a positive and negative response.

**Advantages**

The main advantage of the rapid testing kit is it provides fast results and it is portable and easy to carry and also user-friendly. The blood sample and sweat can easily be used to detect the virus.

**Disadvantages**

Although it is a fast technique for detecting viral infection, it gives the result infection in later stages, and data is needed to be confirmed with RT-PCR.

### 5.3.3 *Chest CT Scan and Chest Radiograph for COVID-19*

X-ray and computed tomography (CT) scanning of the chest is very advantageous as a diagnostic tool for COVID-19 infection and immune-compromised patients [56, 57].

The CT scan and X-ray are the most suitable and sensitive technique for the screening of the symptomatic or asymptomatic suspects [58]. The opaqueness of chest CT scan and X-ray manifest the COVID-19 infection. The CT scan is more preferable than a chest X-ray because of the higher sensitivity of the former, but at the same time, the CT scan has operational convolutions on suspected individuals rather than chest X-rays [57]. The chest CT and X-ray are preferable over RT-PCR; the suspect with moderate symptoms, but negative RT-PCR findings, could be confirmed by these techniques [58]. Various radiology institutes have suggested CT could not be utilized as a diagnostic tool, but few are utilizing this in COVID-19 investigation as an alternative.

**Advantages**
CT scan and radiographic X-rays are widely used for detecting, diagnosing, and assessing the severity of coronavirus; these are also used to follow up on the disease condition. These are rapid, easily available, and economical test than other diagnostic tests [59].

**Disadvantages**
CT and radiographic X-ray scans cannot distinguish between pneumonia and novel coronavirus; therefore, false positives could appear, and RT-PCR is required to confirm the coronavirus. The radiation is also dangerous for patients, and there is a chance of infection from the patient to others. The sensitivity is also lower than other diagnostic techniques [59].

## 5.4 Latest Techniques

Some latest point-of-care diagnostic tests are now introduced with easiest functioning, where no skilled professionals are required to carry out the diagnosis. These can be utilized for the diagnosis of various viruses. These are economic and convenient to handle and also give quick results that help in the prevention of disease. The point-of-care test comprised of different types of biosensor [60].

### *5.4.1 Biosensor*

These biologically sensitive sensors are used for the diagnosis purpose, and the biosensor comprised of a biological receptor [60], a signal convertor, and a detector. The virus reacts with the biological receptor and generates an electronic signal that is converted and amplified by detector and displayed. This system has high sensitivity, specificity, and speedy result in low price. The basic principle of biosensor is similar to the PCR and ELISA. The improved biosensor-based diagnostic techniques have now been employed for fabricating various novel handy tools by using nanotechnology for enhancing the signal amplification and sensitivity, because the nanosize of the virus also favors this technique. The aptamer-based nano-biosensors are a sensitive, speedy, convenient, economic, and influential diagnostic system to diagnose viral disease with respect to traditional techniques. These sensors can be potentially utilized for asymptomatic patients of coronavirus.

### *5.4.2 Aptamer-Based Nano-biosensor*

Aptamers are oligonucleotide of nucleic acid, tiny peptide molecules, immunoglobulin, growth hormone, etc., with high binding affinity to target virus molecule that shows excellent sensitivity and accuracy in diagnosis [60]. The specificity can be enhanced by chemically modifying the surface of aptamers. The aptamers are reproducible, pure, stable, and target specific and can be engineered specifically for coronavirus. The point-of-care test kits are now also in development phase that are claiming fast results in less than 1 min.

### *5.4.3 Paper-Based Detection*

The paper-based diagnostic tools have now also been fabricated; these utilize the integrated system that includes the isolation, elution, refining, amplification, and detection of target substances in a small, economic, disposable paper that is printed with waxy zones [60]; this is a powerless simple system in which the paper is bent into various modes. This is a very advantageous, low-priced, and simplistic and user-friendly technique. This technique precisely diagnosed viruses and can be utilized to detect coronavirus by rapid testing. The paper-based diagnostic test kit can also be used to detect the presence of virus in wastewater.

## 5.5 Summary and Conclusion

The entire world is struggling with the coronavirus pandemic for the survival of humankind. Researchers are continuously working on the development of highly sensitive, efficiently working, affordable, and novel diagnostic techniques and kits for expeditious diagnosis of deadly SARS-COVID-19 as a point of care. In the present chapter, we have discussed several diagnostic approaches that are being employed worldwide for the diagnosis of COVID-19. Here we discussed the molecular and serologic techniques being used in the development of a diagnostic kit. The molecular assay includes RT-PCR, LAMP, and programmed RNA techniques that are more reliable than serologic assay. But a serologic assay-based RDT kit is also popular because of the instant result, without using any sophisticated instruments. Now some latest tools are also fabricated based on the biosensor, aptamers, and paper-based techniques. Different kits approved by the USA, China, India, and other countries are used for SARS-COVID-9 diagnosis and are also under development phases and approval process with the aim of an instant result, high accuracy, and high sensitivity. The chest CT scan and X-ray technology also show promising result, yet a better kit is needed.

**Acknowledgments** We are very thankful to the Department of Pharmaceutical Sciences, Bhimtal Campus, Kumaun University, Nainital, Bhimtal, Uttarakhand, for their kind and valuable support.

## References

1. Padhi, A., Kumar, S., Gupta, E., & Saxena, S. K. (2020). *Laboratory diagnosis of novel coronavirus disease 2019 (COVID-19). Medical virology: from pathogenesis to disease control.* Singapore: Springer. https://doi.org/10.1007/978-981-15-4814-7_0.
2. https://www.who.int/docs/default-source/coronaviruse/situation-reports/20200720-covid-19-sitrep-182.pdf?sfvrsn=60aabc5c.
3. Cascella, M., Rajnik, M., Cuomo, A., et al. (2020). Features, evaluation, and treatment of coronavirus (COVID-19) [Updated 2020 Aug 10]. In: *StatPearls* [Internet]. Treasure Island: StatPearls Publishing. Available from: https://www.ncbi.nlm.nih.gov/books/NBK554776/.
4. Guo, Y. R., Cao, Q. D., Hong, Z. S., Tan, Y. Y., Chen, S. D., Jin, H. J., et al. (2020). The origin, transmission and clinical therapies on corona-virus disease 2019 (COVID-19) outbreak – An update on the status. *Military Medical Research, 7*(11), 2–10. https://doi.org/10.1186/s40779-020-00240-0.
5. Wu, F., Zhao, S., Yu, B., Chen, Y. M., Wang, W., Song, Z. G., et al. (2020). A new corona-virus associated with human respiratory disease in China. *Nature, 579*(7798), 265–269. https://doi.org/10.1038/s41586-020-2008-3.
6. Jia, H. P., Look, D. C., Shi, L., Hickey, M., Pewe, L., Netland, J., et al. (2005). ACE2 receptor expression and severe acute respiratory syndrome corona-virus infection depend on differentiation of human airway epithelia. *Journal of Virology, 79*(23), 14614–14621. https://doi.org/10.1128/JVI.79.23.14614-14621.2005.
7. Wan, Y., Shang, J., Graham, R., Baric, R. S., & Li, F. (2020). Receptor recognition by novel corona-virus from Wuhan: An analysis based on decade-long structural studies of SARS. *Journal of Virology, 94*(7), 1–7. https://doi.org/10.1128/JVI.00127-20.
8. Carter, L. J., Garner, L., Smoot, J. W., Li, Y., Zhou, Q., Catherine, J., et al. (2020). Assay techniques and test development for COVID-19 diagnosis. *ACS Central Science, 6*(5), 591–605. https://doi.org/10.1021/acscentsci.0c00501.
9. Gibbs, R. A. (1990). DNA amplification by the polymerase chain reaction. *Analytical Chemistry, 62*, 1202–1214. https://doi.org/10.1021/ac00212a004.
10. http://www.pcrstation.com/discovery.
11. Joshi, M., & Deshpande, J. D. (2010). Polymerase chain reaction: Methods, principles and application. *International Journal of Biomedical Research, 1–5*, 81–97.
12. Atawodi, S. E., Atawodi, J. C., & Dzikwi, A. A. (2010). Polymerase chain reaction: Theory, practice and application: A review. *Sahel Medical Journal, 2*, 54–63.
13. Tahamtan, A., & Ardebili, A. (2020). Real-time RT-PCR in COVID-19 detection: Issues affecting the results. *Expert Review of Molecular Diagnostics, 20*(5), 453–454. https://doi.org/10.1080/14737159.2020.1757437.
14. https://geneticeducation.co.in/reverse-transcription-pcr-principle-procedure-applications-advantages-and-disadvantages/#Advantages_of_reverse_transcription_PCR.

15. https://www.dialog.roche.com/pk/en_us/products_and_solutions/molecular-lab/cobas-6800-8800-systems.html.
16. Cobb, B., Simon, C. O., Stramer, S. L., Body, B., Mitchell, P. S., Reisch, N., et al. (2017). The cobas® 6800/8800 system: A new era of automation in molecular diagnostics. *Expert Review of Molecular Diagnostics, 17*(2), 167–180. https://doi.org/10.1080/14737159.2017.1275962.
17. Aretzweiler, G., Leuchter, S., Simon, C. O., Marins, E., & Frontzek, A. (2019). Generating timely molecular diagnostic test results: workflow comparison of the cobas® 6800/8800 to Panther. *Expert Review of Molecular Diagnostics, 19*(10), 951–957. https://doi.org/10.1080/14737159.2019.1665999.
18. https://www.who.int/diagnostics_laboratory/eul_0504-04600_cobas_sars_cov2_qualitative_assay_ifu.pdf?ua=1.
19. Huang, C., Wang, Y., Li, X., Ren, L., Zhao, J., Hu, Y., Zhang, L., Fan, G., Xu, J., Gu, X., et al. (2020). Clinical features of patients infected with 2019 novel corona-virus in Wuhan, China. *Lancet, 395*(1023), 497–506. https://doi.org/10.1016/S0140-6736(20)30183-5.
20. To, K. K., Tsang, O. T., Chik-Yan, Y., Chan, K. H., Wu, T. C., Chan, J. M. C., et al. (2020). Consistent detection of 2019 novel corona-virus in saliva. *Clinical Infectious Diseases, 29*(4), 1049–1050. https://doi.org/10.1093/cid/ciaa149.
21. Zhang, Y., Odiwuor, N., Xiong, J., Sun, L., Nyaruaba, R. O., Wei, H., et al. Rapid molecular detection of SARS-CoV-2 (COVID-19) virus RNA using colorimetric LAMP. *Med Rxiv preprint*. https://doi.org/10.1101/2020.02.26.20028373.
22. Notomi, T., Okayama, H., Masubuchi, H., Yonekawa, T., Watanabe, K., Amino, N., & Hase, T. (2000). Loop-mediated isothermal amplification of DNA. *Nucleic Acids Research, 28*(12), E63. https://doi.org/10.1093/nar/28.12.e63.
23. Nzelu, C. O., Gomez, E. A., Caceres, A. G., Sakurai, T., Martini-Robles, L., Uezato, H., et al. (2014). Development of a loop mediated isothermal amplification method for rapid mass-screening of sand flies for Leishmania infection. *Acta Tropica, 132*, 1–6. https://doi.org/10.1016/j.actatropica.2013.12.016.
24. Tomita, N., Mori, Y., Kanda, H., & Notomi, T. (2008). Loop-mediated isothermal amplification (LAMP) of gene sequences and simple visual detection of products. *Nature Protocols, 3*, 877–882. https://doi.org/10.1038/nprot.2008.57.
25. Goncalves, D. D. S., Hooker, D. J., Dong, Y., Baran, N., Kyrylos, P., Iturbe-Ormaetxe, I., et al. (2019). Detecting wMel Wolbachia in field-collected Aedes aegypti mosquitoes using loop-mediated isothermal amplification (LAMP). *Parasites & Vectors, 12*, 404. https://doi.org/10.1186/s13071-019-3666-6.
26. Calvert, A. E., Biggerstaff, B. J., Tanner, N. A., Lauterbach, M., & Lanciotti, R. S. (2017). Rapid colorimetric detection of zika virus from serum and urine specimens by reverse transcription loop-mediated isothermal amplification (RT-LAMP). *PLoS One, 12*, e0185340.
27. Ismail, A., Modh Nor, N., Abdullah, J. M., Acosta, A., & Sarmiento, M. E. (2017). *Sustainable diagnostics for low resources areas*. Gelugor: Penerbit University Sains Malaysia.
28. Kashira, J., & Ahmed Yaqinuddin, A. (2020). Loop mediated isothermal amplification (LAMP) assays as a rapid diagnostic for COVID-19. *Medical Hypotheses, 141*, 109786. https://doi.org/10.1016/j.mehy.2020.109786.
29. Kaneko, H., Kawana, T., Fukushima, E., & Suzutani, T. (2007). Tolerance of loop-mediated isothermal amplification to a culture medium and biological substances. *Journal of Biochemical and Biophysical Methods, 70*(3), 499–501. https://doi.org/10.1016/j.jbbm.2006.08.008.
30. Langabeer, S. E., Gale, R. E., Harvey, R. C., Cook, R. W., Mackinnon, S., & Linch, D. C. (2000). Transcription-mediated amplification and hybridisation protection assay to determine BCR-ABL transcript levels in patients with chronic myeloid leukaemia. *Leukemia, 16*, 393–399.
31. Zannoli, S., Morotti, M., Denicolo, A., Tassinari, M., Chiesa, C., Pierro, A., & Sambri, V. (2018). Chapter 9 – Diagnostics and laboratory techniques: Chikungunya and zika viruses global emerging health threats 2018. *The American Journal of Tropical Medicine and Hygiene, 99*(4), 1105–1106. https://doi.org/10.4269/ajtmh.18-0613.
32. Stower, H. (2018). CRISPR-based diagnostics. *Nature Medicine, 24*, 702.

33. https://www.synthego.com/blog/crispr-Corona-virus-detection.
34. Wang, H., Li, X., Li, T., Zhang, S., Wang, L., Wu, X., et al. (2020). The genetic sequence, origin, and diagnosis of SARS-CoV-2. *European Journal of Clinical Microbiology & Infectious Diseases, 24*, 1–7. https://doi.org/10.1007/s10096-020-03899-4.
35. https://www.taconic.com/taconic-insights/model-generation-solutions/crispr-genome-engineering-advantages-limitations.html.
36. Hamidi, S. V., & Perreault, J. (2019). Simple rolling circle amplification colorimetric assay based on pH for target DNA detection. *Talanta, 201*, 419–425. https://doi.org/10.1016/j.talanta.2019.04.003.
37. Wang, B., Potter, S. J., Lin, Y., Cunningham, A. L., Dwyer, D., Su, Y., et al. (2005). Rapid and sensitive detection of severe acute respiratory syndrome corona-virus by rolling circle amplification. *Journal of Clinical Microbiology, 43*(5), 2339–2344. https://doi.org/10.1128/JCM.43.5.2339-2344.2005.
38. Gu, L., Yan, W., Liu, L., Wang, S., Zhang, X., & Lyu, M. (2018). Research progress on rolling circle amplification (RCA)-based biomedical sensing. *Pharmaceuticals (Basel), 11*(2), 1–19. https://doi.org/10.3390/ph11020035.
39. Melissa, B., & Miller, Y. W. T. (2009). Basic concepts of microarrays and potential applications in clinical microbiology. *Clinical Microbiology Reviews, 22*(4), 611–633. https://doi.org/10.1128/CMR.00019-09.
40. http://grf.lshtm.ac.uk/microarrayoverview.htm.
41. Gire, S. K., Goba, A., Anderson, K. G., Sealfon, R. S. G., Park, D. J., Kanneh, L., et al. (2014). Genomic surveillance elucidates Ebola virus origin and transmission during the 2014 outbreak. *Science, 345*, 1369–1372. https://doi.org/10.1126/science.1259657.
42. Hoenen, T., Groseth, A., Rosenke, K., Fischer, R. J., Hoenen, A., Seth, D., et al. (2016). Nanopore sequencing as a rapidly deployable Ebola outbreak tool. *Emerging Infectious Diseases, 22*, 331–334.
43. Manning, J. E., Bohl, J. A., Lay, S., Chea, S., Sovann, L., Sengdoeurn, Y., et al. (2020). Rapid metagenomic characterization of a case of imported COVID-19 in Cambodia. *bio Rxiv preprint*, 1–7. https://doi.org/10.1101/2020.03.02.968818.
44. Deng, X., Achari, A., Federman, S., Yu, G., Somasekar, S., Bartolo, I., et al. (2020). Metagenomic sequencing with spiked primer enrichment for viral diagnostics and genomic surveillance. *Nature Microbiology, 5*, 1–12. https://doi.org/10.1038/s41564-019-0637-9.
45. https://geneticeducation.co.in/what-is-metagenomics-definition-steps-process-and-applications/#Advantages_of_metagenomics.
46. Jessica, F. D., Natalie, K. C., Jennifer, R., Franco, P., & Aleisha, R. (2017). Metagenomics: The next culture-independent game changer. *Frontiers in Microbiology, 8*, 1069. https://doi.org/10.3389/fmicb.2017.01069.
47. Jacob, J. J., Veeraraghavan, B., Vasudevan, K., (2019). Metagenomic next-generation sequencing in clinical microbiology. *Indian J Med Microbiol. 37*(2), 133–140. doi: 10.4103/ijmm.IJMM_19_401. PMID: 31745012.
48. https://www.thermofisher.com/in/en/home/life-science/protein-biology/protein-biology-learning-center/protein-biology-resource-library/pierce-protein-methods/overview-elisa.html#2
49. https://www.centerforhealthsecurity.org/resources/COVID-19/serology/Serology-based-tests-for-COVID-19.html#sec1.
50. https://microbeonline.com/elisa-test-for-antigenantibody-detection/.
51. https://www.biomedomics.com.
52. Engvall, E., & Perlmann, P. (1971). Enzyme linked immunosorbent assay (ELISA) quantitative assay of immunoglobulin G. *Immunochemistry, 8*, 871–875.
53. Kohler, C., & Milstein, C. (1975). Continuous cultures of fused cells secreting antibody of predefined specificity. *Nature, 256*, 495–497.
54. Avrameas, S., & Uriel, J. (1996). Method of antigen and antibody labeling with enzymes and its immunodiffusion application. *Comptes Rendus Hebdomadaires des Seances de l'Academie des Sciences. D: Sciences Naturelles, 262*, 2543–2545.

55. Aydin, S. (2015). A short history, principles, and types of ELISA, and our laboratory experience with peptide/protein analyses using ELISA. *Peptides, 72*, 4–15.
56. Ye, F., Chen, L., Zhan, Z, et al. (2020). Development and clinical application of a rapid Igm-IgG combined antibody test for SARS-Cov infection diagnosis. *Journal of Medical Virology, 92*, 1518–1524.
57. Jokerst, C., Chung, J. H., Ackman, J. B., Carter, B., Colletti, P. M., Crabtree, T. D., et al. (2018). ACR Appropriateness Criteria® acute respiratory illness in immunocompetent patients. *Journal of the American College of Radiology, 15*(11S), S240–S251. Available at https://acsearch.acr.org/docs/69446/Narrative/.
58. Tenda, E. D., Yulianti, M., Asaf, M. M., Yunus, R. E., Septiyanti, W., Wulani, V., et al. (2020). The importance of chest CT scan in COVID-19: A case series. *Acta Medica Indonesiana-Indonesian Journal of Internal Medicine, 52*(1), 68–73.
59. Zhao, W., Zhong, Z., Xie, Q., Yu, J., & Liu, J. (2020). Relation between chest CT findings and clinical conditions of coronavirus diseases (COVID19) pneumonia: A multicentre study. *AJR. American Journal of Roentgenology, 214*(5), 1072–1077. https://doi.org/10.2214/AJR.20.22976.
60. Li, M. (2020). Chest CT features and their role in COVID-19. *Radiology of Infectious Diseases, 7*(2), 51–54. https://doi.org/10.1016/j.jrid.2020.04.001.
61. Kumar, R., Nagpal, S., Kausik, S., & Mendiratta, S. (2020). COVID-19 diagnostic approaches: Different roads to the same destination. *Virus Disease, 31*, 97–105. https://doi.org/10.1007/s13337-020=00599-7.

# Chapter 6
# COVID-19: AI-Enabled Social Distancing Detector Using CNN

**K. Anitha Kumari, P. Purusothaman, D. Dharani, and R. Padmashani**

## Abbreviations

| | |
|---|---|
| CNN | Convolutional neural networks |
| CUDA | Compute Unified Device Architecture |
| cuDNN | CUDA Deep Neural Network |
| DNNs | Other commonly used algorithms are the deep neural networks |
| GAN | Generative adversarial networks |
| LSTM | Long short-term memory |
| RBM | Restricted Boltzmann machines |
| RNN | Recurrent neural networks |
| SARS | Severe acute respiratory syndrome |
| WHO | World Health Organization |
| YOLO | You Only Look Once |

## 6.1 Introduction

The novel coronavirus (COVID-19) that originated in Wuhan, China, had pushed the universal health into a pandemic situation, and it still seems to be inevitable. The huge number of people from majority of the countries around the world had tested positive within a short span of time, and the mortality rate from this cause also drastically surged. Still many countries are experiencing the outbreaks. Worldwide there have been 12,964,809 confirmed cases and 570,288 deaths reported to the World Health Organization (WHO) due to COVID-19 as of 15 July 2020 [1]. Initially, on 31 December 2019, the WHO gave an alert due to quite a few cases of pneumonia

K. Anitha Kumari (✉) · D. Dharani · R. Padmashani
Department of IT, PSG College of Technology, Coimbatore, TN, India
e-mail: kak.it@psgtech.ac.in

P. Purusothaman
Department of IT, Bannari Amman Institute of Technology, Coimbatore, TN, India



S. Kautish et al. (eds.), *Computational Intelligence Techniques for Combating COVID-19*, EAI/Springer Innovations in Communication and Computing,
https://doi.org/10.1007/978-3-030-68936-0_6

of strange etiology. It was stated that it had been detected much in advance around 8 December 2019. The delay in announcing the incidence of a pandemic and the failure of informing the international authorities in a well-timed manner lead to an abandoned increase of the disease. Hence, at present, this deadly disease is the focus of universal attention. COVID-19 confirmed cases and mortality rate of several countries are depicted in Figs. 6.1 and 6.2, respectively, as per the data collected from WHO COVID-19 Dashboard.

### *6.1.1 Types of Coronavirus*

The coronavirus is a large family (family name, *Coronaviridae*, and subfamily name, *Coronavirinae*) of virus which is known to have an effect on birds and mammals including human beings. This virus could be one of the root causes for an infection ranging from typical cold to severe respiratory track diseases. Out of hundreds of coronaviruses, only seven viruses are identified as human corona virus; thus it can affect human beings as well. Those viruses are listed below:

- 229E
- NL63
- OC43

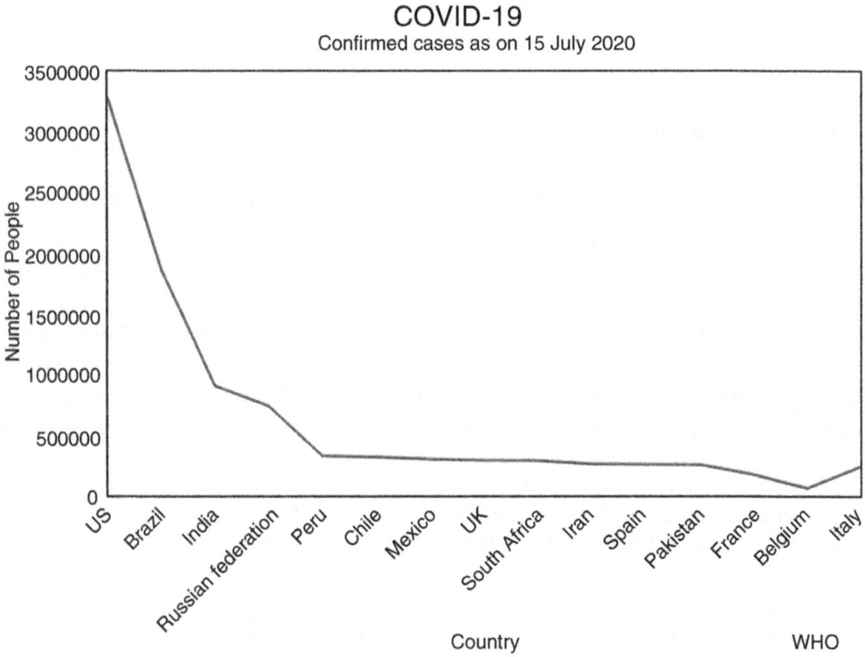


**Fig. 6.1** COVID-19 confirmed cases

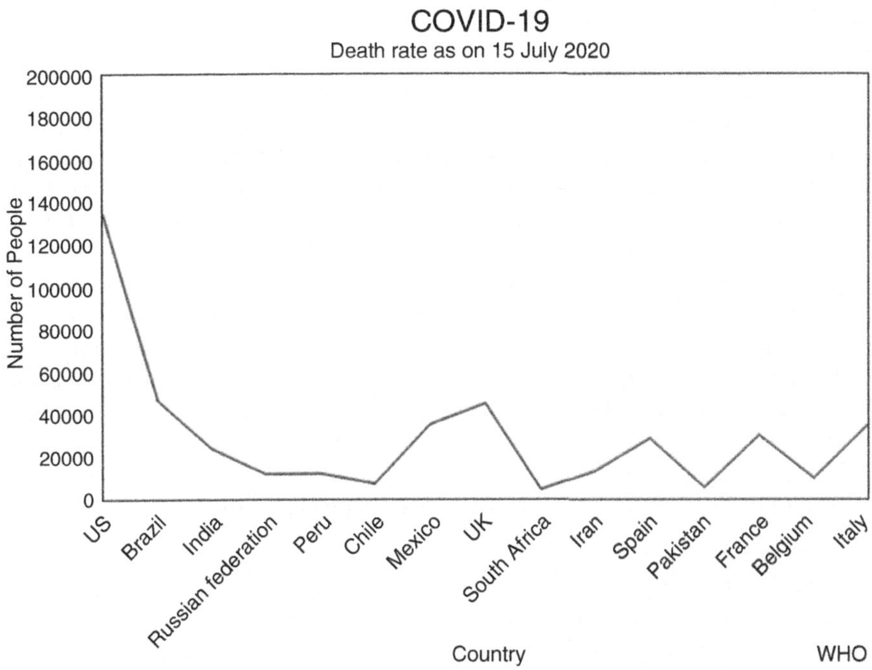


**Fig. 6.2** COVID-19 mortality rate

- HKU1
- SARS-CoV
- MERS-CoV
- SARS-CoV-2

Above all, the 229E, NL63, OC43, and HKU1 viruses can cause moderate symptoms such as nasal congestion, cough, fever, and headaches. The other three viruses are in fact originated from animals and transmitted to humans that can create high risk to the health of the human being. SARS-CoV creates the disease severe acute respiratory syndrome (SARS) in humans and alleged that it was transmitted from bats. The first case was reported in November 2002 in Foshan, Guangdong, China. Consequently, the outbreak ended with around 8096 confirmed cases and 774 deaths reported to WHO. MERS-CoV creates the disease Middle East respiratory syndrome (MERS) in humans suspected that it was transmitted from camels. This contagious disease had become known in September 2012 in Saudi Arabia, and then most of the cases have been identified in and around the countries of Middle East. 2040 laboratory-tested positive cases and 712 mortality rates were reported to WHO since 2012. SARS-CoV-2 is the root cause that creates illness which is called as a COVID-19 as this is a new form of coronavirus that has not affected human being yet [2].

## 6.1.2 Symptoms of COVID-19

The common symptoms of COVID-19-infected patients are depicted in Fig. 6.3.

These symptoms may emerge ranging from 2 to 14 days after the contact of virus. Despite the common indications, people are also experiencing few other rare symptoms such as diarrhea, sore throat, and loss of taste/smell. Many people have experienced these symptoms ranging from very mild to severe in line with their immune level and their medical complications. According to the Centers for Disease Control and Prevention (CDC), people aged above 65 years, frontline workers, and people with serious health issues such as pneumonia, heart problems, and diabetes are at high risk to the exposure of COVID-19 [3]. The disease generally transmits through respiratory droplets from the affected people. Thus it is a mandatory rule being followed worldwide that the affected people must quarantine themselves at least for 14 days to avoid transmission. Breaking the chain has become everyone's responsibility at this time.

The following are the general self-practices to prevent coronavirus exposure:

- Wear masks.
- Wash hands often.
- Avoid direct contact with patients.
- Maintain social distancing.
- Observe good personal hygiene.
- Cover the mouth and nose when coughing/sneezing.
- Disinfect the surrounding.

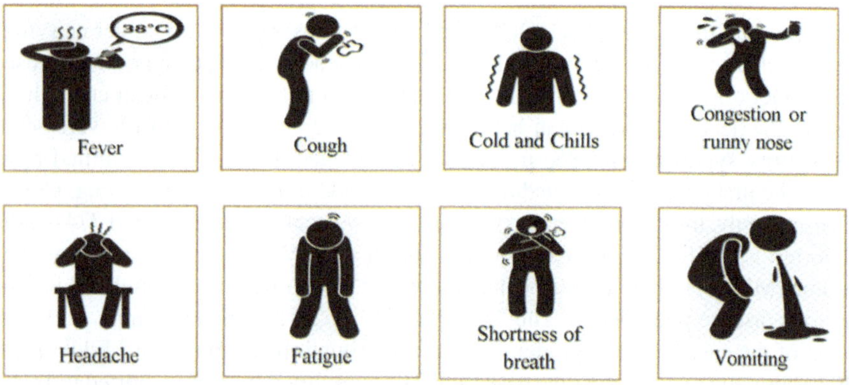


**Fig. 6.3** Symptoms of COVID-19

### 6.1.3 *Impact of Social Distancing*

The death rate and positive cases of COVID-19 rapidly increase across the world. Meanwhile, many authorities of countries are strictly involved in slowing down the outbreak with stringent set of laws including mandatory social distancing. In general, social distancing is keeping up to 6 feet or 2 meter gap among individuals when exposed to public to avoid transmission of the virus. As the vaccines and medicines for COVID-19 are still under research, the only way to protect ourselves from the deadly disease is social distancing along with the self-hygiene [18]. Figure 6.4 depicts several do's and don'ts to maintain social distancing.

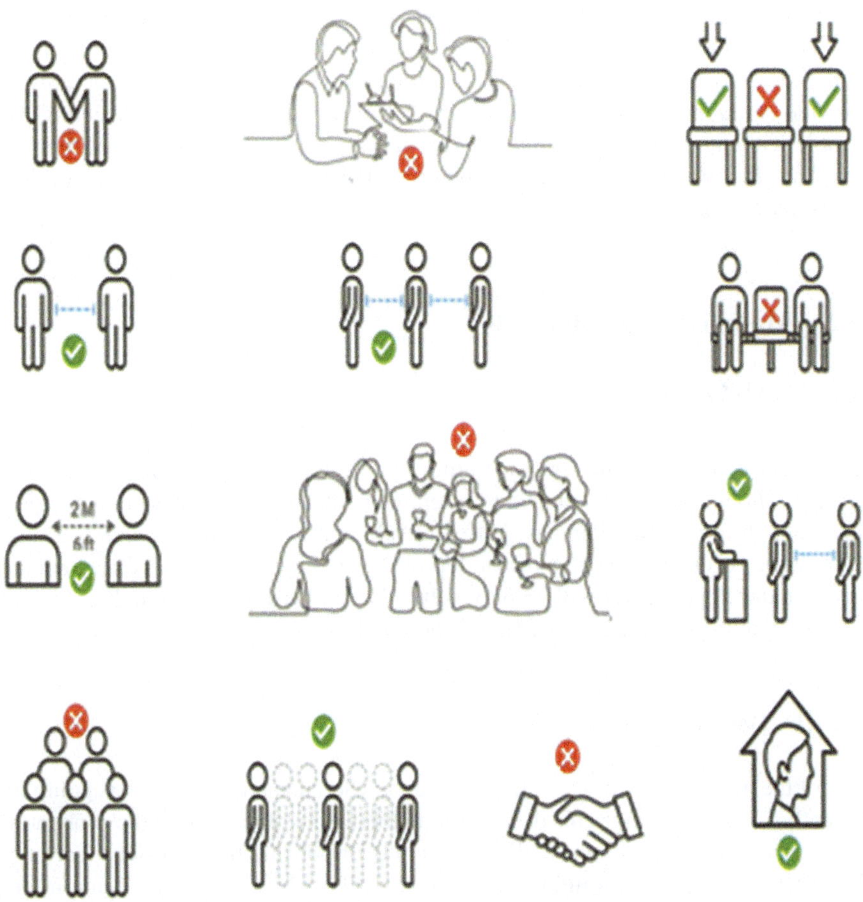


**Fig. 6.4** Icons of social distancing

### 6.1.4 Literature Survey

Although governments have taken a variety of measures and actions to control the disease spread, the human intervention has become an essential one in all the places to monitor the violations of any rules. In order to automate these procedures, few systems have been proposed where artificial intelligence (AI) plays its crucial role. The systems can be designed to focus on various applications including early detection of the disease; prevention of the disease; automatic monitoring of the treatment; tracing contacts of patients; following up and projecting the death rate, positive cases, and cured patient details; drugs and vaccine development; and so on [4]. In addition, reducing the workload of frontline warriors is also one of the fields where AI is leaving its footprints. Every organization is in a compulsion to function with highly sufficient rules to prevent the disease spread. In this regard, every individuals and organizations are acting as frontline warriors. As the task of monitoring mass gatherings has become a difficult task, automatic AI systems help considerably to provide solutions for it. For instance, AI software tools capable of detecting the people without mask are integrated in the surveillance cameras which will help in tracking the rule violations. This system also helps to minimize the transmission and spread of the virus [5].

## 6.2 Materials and Methods

### 6.2.1 Methods

Artificial intelligence is integrated in almost any automated applications in the past decade. Though AI was developed to resemble human being, the system is not perfect enough to replicate humans. Different sub-areas of AI like machine learning, deep learning, etc. have been a research problem in the last few years for which the solution developed today will be only better than yesterday's solution, but it is not complete and is looking for a better solution daily.

#### 6.2.1.1 Deep Learning

Out of the many topics of interest, the one area wherein a lot of research is going on recently is deep learning. This deep learning mainly revolves around the concept of mimicking the human brain [6–8]. Neural networks is the base for deep learning. Human brain consists of millions of individual cells called the neurons. Neurons are the basic unit of any neural network. The information from one neuron to another neuron passes with the help of synapses basically in the form of electrical signals. Information which the brain perceives will be processed and stored in neurons. Learning happens when neurons get trained to similar patterns received. In the future when the same kind of data is seen by the neurons, it will be predicting the data correctly based on what it has learned. This is the base of any deep learning algorithms, and the layers are shown in Fig. 6.5.

Deep learning is a subset of machine learning which in turn is the subset of AI. DNNs are capable to work efficiently without any human intervention. In machine learning, there are different types of data like supervised, unsupervised, and semi-supervised. Supervised data are those wherein the input and the output will be given during the training for the system to learn properly and to predict similar data in the future. When a new type of output is expected, the system will not be able to predict properly.

In case of unsupervised learning mechanism, only the input will be given during the training phase, and then the system is made to predict the output correctly. The accuracy of predicting new data will be less when compared to supervised learning as the system is not capable enough to predict the output correctly because of poor learning ability. In semi-supervised learning, a mix of supervised and unsupervised data will be given as input, and the system should identify the output properly. Again the accuracy is not so good when compared to supervised learning.

Deep learning works perfectly well even with unsupervised data, and the accuracy achieved is highly efficient when compared to other machine learning algorithms. In machine learning, the system is made to think on its own based on its learning capacity, and the system should be updated or trained periodically in order to improve the rate of prediction. It is a lifelong learning process.

Deep learning finds its applications in varied areas like fraud detection, image recognition, pattern recognition, drug discovery, automated vehicles, biometric identification and verification, spatial bodies' exploration, speech recognition, etc. Neural network was an old concept which was there some 50 years back. Deep learning in turn revolves around artificial neural networks only. But the thing which distinguishes itself from ANN is performance. The computing capability of the systems available in those days was not good enough to process lightly complex neural network. But in recent times, the computing capacity has improved drastically in terms of CPU performance, storage space, network connectivity, and other resources. In traditional machine learning technique, when the performance of the system is

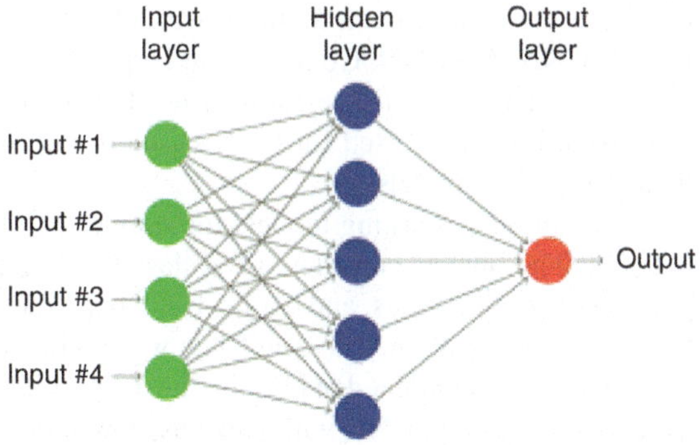


**Fig. 6.5** Basic layers of deep learning algorithms

plotted in the form of a graph, after some threshold value, the performance will not improve irrespective of how many data are being fed for learning. The performance is saturated after some time. In the case of deep learning technique, in conflict to traditional machine learning technique, the more the data fed, the better the performance.

According to LeCun et al. [7], deep learning can be pictured as a model with multiple layers used to represent the data. The methodology basically revolves around the back propagation algorithm which tells the system how to learn the parameters in each layer. The computation and design of the current layer is decided by the previous layer. The paper also proposes two models: the convolutional neural network (CNN) and the recurrent neural network (RNN). CNN finds its applications in a wide range of areas especially in image processing and video and audio processing, whereas RNN finds its role in speech and text processing.

Yoshua Bengio [8] in his paper discusses different deep architectures. He also says about how the representation of the data is going to affect the learning process. The paper focuses on the deep belief networks and has shown that the contrastive divergence update mechanism for restricted Boltzmann machine was giving a better performance in terms of learning.

In a novel approach proposed by Liu et al. [9], three components are used: the CNN, the face localization, and the attribute prediction. This paper mainly focuses on recognizing faces with varying lightings and poses. The CelebA and LFWA datasets are used which in turn are derived from Celeb and LFW datasets, respectively. The proposed feedforward algorithm for locally shared filters results in reduction of computations, thereby increasing the performance of the system. On an average, the overall performance of the approach stands up to 83%.

Zhao et al. [10] in their paper dicussed different object detection algorithms based on deep learning, and they have taken three case studies for doing the comparison being salient object detection, face detection, and pedestrian detection. In salient object detection, the object which is of main importance or coverage is identified. In this paper, CNN is used for implementing the former process. ECSSD, HKUIS, PASCALS, and SOD are the datasets considered. Here in the proposed model, local connections between the CNN models are considered, and the same is extended for the global context for better performance. For face detection too, CNN is used in this paper. Here the FDDB dataset is used, and different variations of CNN are compared, namely, the CascadeCNN, Joint Cascade, DeepIR, HR-ER, Face-R-CNN, MTCNN, Conv3D, and HyperFace, respectively. It is found that the variations of faster CNN perform better. For the pedestrian detection, the Caltech Pedestrian Dataset is used for CNN-based detection, and faster CNN works better than other CNN models.

Different deep learning models for submarine object detection are discussed in [11, 20]. The objects considered for classification and comparison purpose in this paper are fish, planktons, and corals. Here again the CNN and its variations are used for doing classification. The deepCNN was giving an accuracy of 98.57%.

The methods explained in [12] are the deep saliency network, part-based method, adversarial learning, CNN with part-based method, detection by generating images or pixels, fine-grained object detection method, and generation of all possible occlusions and deformations. The datasets considered for detection are Microsoft COCO, ImageNet, CIFAR-10, CIFAR-100, ILSVRC, and Caltech 256.

Even though the backbone of deep learning is ANN, several deep learning algorithms are available. The most popular among that are the CNN and RNN models. Other commonly used algorithms are the deep neural networks (DNNs), generative adversarial networks (GAN), long short-term memory (LSTM), restricted Boltzmann machines (RBM), etc. Each one of this algorithm has advantages and disadvantages on its own. One algorithm which works on an application may or may not go in hand with another application. Selection of the algorithm is directly proportional to the performance of the system.

CNN finds its ability in predicting an output at its best in image processing applications. They are multilayer feedforward neural networks. The most commonly used layers are the convolution layer, pooling layer, normalization layer, and fully connected layer. The placement of the layers varies from one application to another. Another major difference between ANN and CNN is in terms of how it processes the input. Figure 6.6 shows the detailed process of the algorithm.

In case of standard ANN, whatever be the size of the input especially in images, it will be considered as a two-dimensional array input. Thereby some features may be lost during preprocessing step itself thereby affecting the overall working of the system. In case of CNN, the input images are treated as tensors or multidimensional array input, hence preserving all the features of the image. RNN is another most widely used algorithm which is based on time series data and is shown in Fig. 6.7. The network has internal memory which remembers the data for a period of time, thereby making better decisions when predicting the output. RNN finds its application mainly in speech recognition and handwriting recognition.

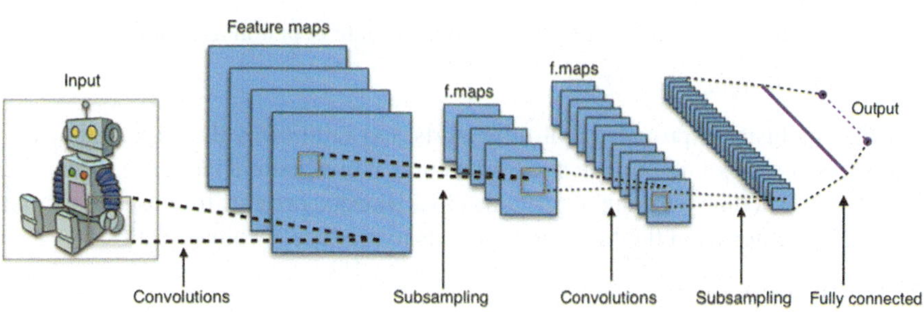


**Fig. 6.6** Process of CNN algorithm

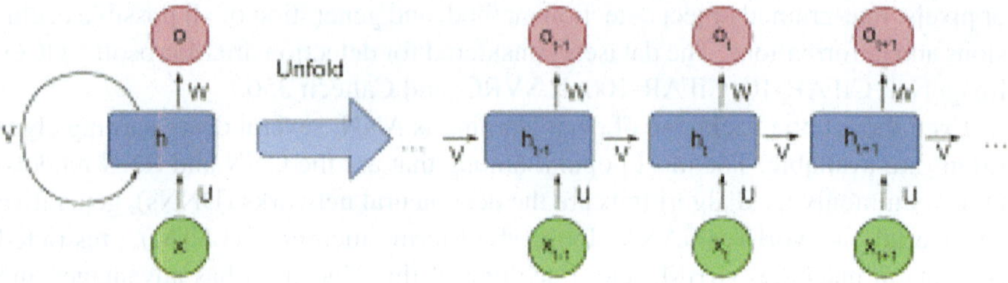


**Fig. 6.7** RNN algorithm

## 6.2.2 *Materials*

Data collection plays a crucial role in any analysis. Many organizations already started to combat this pandemic by using AI-based techniques. However, certain difficulties are involved in gathering data essential for the analysis as follows:

- Lack of data
- Too much noisy data/outlier data
- Data privacy issues
- Public health concerns
- Continuous human-AI interaction

Hence identification of a problem at its grassroots level is highly important as AI can be deployed to diagnosis and prognosis, early warning and alerts, tracking and prediction, treatment and cures, and social control for COVID-19 infections. Prime mandate focus must be given to data collection and a deeper understanding on what it solves. Further data exploration, modeling, validation, and deployment can be carried out.

### 6.2.2.1 Data Collection

Accurate data collection leads to making appropriate decision and analysis.

(a) *Bluedot Insights*

Bluedot Insights provides real-time alerts and minimizes the exposure to diseases to a larger extent. For detection/prediction, it uses natural language processing (NLP) and machine learning algorithms [14]. Bluedot Insights used to collect data every 15 minutes from the following sections to produce accurate result:

- Health organizations
- Digital media
- Airline tickets
- Health report
- Population demographics

(b) *HealthMap*

HealthMap is used to consolidate the report from manifold data sources like expert discussions, reports, and news and validates it [15]. It is an AI-based model developed by Boston Children's Hospital for outbreak predicting and monitoring of emerging diseases.

(c) *Microsoft Bing's AI Tracker*

To track local and global cases of COVID-19, Microsoft Bing created a new tracker with lots of built-in features to stay updated. It gathers data under one roof from different healthcare organizations and presents to the users in a user-friendly manner. The tracker provides trustworthy information collected from Government of India, ICMR, and WHO [22].

(d) *Kaggle*

To attain data science goals, the better platform is kaggle.com. Manifold open dataset and machine learning algorithms were posted related to this global pandemic. For instance, COVID-19 Open Research Dataset Challenge (CORD-19) is posted as an open AI challenge to receive better novel solutions from the young minds. In addition, it provides insight on COVID-19 in India, exclusively a dataset hosted for Indian states and territories. A recent dataset on COVID-19 releases number of confirmed cases, deaths, and recovered cases worldwide. On its part, kaggle.com plays the best role in deriving novel solutions by gathering the data across the globe on daily basis [23].

(e) *Corona Tracker API with ML*

A simple and fast corona tracker API was created by utilizing the virtues of machine learning algorithms. It can be accessed at https://coronavirus-tracker-api.herokuapp.com/v2/locations and used for performing a lot of AI data analysis [16]. Country-wise, corona-confirmed cases, deaths, and recovered cases are identified and used for analysis as shown in Fig. 6.8.

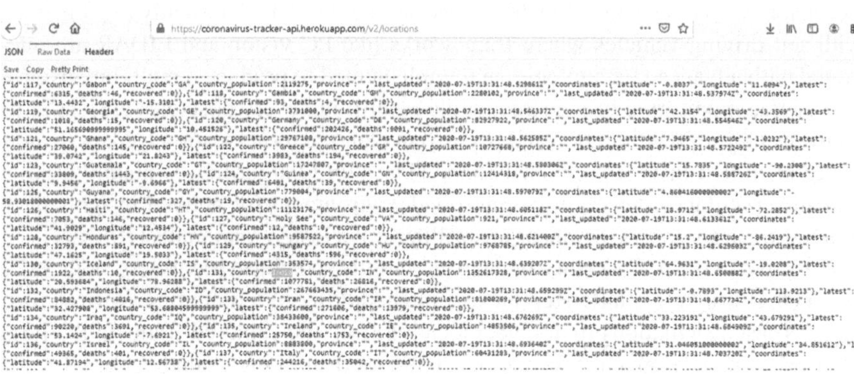


**Fig. 6.8** Corona tracker API

With the help of these forums, data can be collected effectively for COVID-19 for future prediction and analysis. With this chapter, our prime focus is on social control by scanning public/private places to detect potentially infected peoples/ cases, and it can be extended further for analysis. CNN method is employed to ensure the distance between the people.

## 6.3 Social Distancing Detector Algorithm Using Convolution Neural Network

The social distancing detector algorithm involves the following modules as rightly pointed and presented by Punn et al. [19]

- Human detection in live video stream using YOLO objection detection.
- Compute pairwise distance.
- Checking whether the pairwise distance is greater than N pixel.
- Message and alert module.

### *6.3.1 Building YOLO Object Detector*

When it comes to deep learning-based object detection, there are three primary object detection algorithms present in convolution neural network: recurrent convolution neural network (R-CNN) and their variants, single-shot detector (SSD), and YOLO. YOLO is a viable continuous article acknowledgment calculation, first depicted in the fundamental 2015 paper by Joseph Redmon et al. [13]. In this article, we present the idea of item identification, the YOLO calculation itself, and one of the calculation's open-source executions: dark net [21].

Image classification is one of the many energizing uses of convolution neural systems. Besides simple image classification, there are a lot of intriguing issues in PC vision, with object detection being one among them. It is normally implemented with self-driving vehicles where frameworks like PC vision and LIDAR are integrated with advanced technologies and implemented to produce a multidimensional 360-degree monitoring of the street while identifying every obstacles present in its pathway. Object identification and pedestrian identification location is likewise normally identified in video reconnaissance [11]. YOLO algorithm is mainly used in human surveillance detection in controlled environment for general insights or to monitor trespassers' involvement in strolling ways inside strip malls [10, 12].

To improve the performance of deep learning-based object identifiers, both SSDs and YOLO utilize a single-step locator methodology by computing pairwise distance. These calculations treat object location from the captured frame in the form of pixels, taking a given information picture and marking bounding box for the detected object and relating class mark probabilities. Single-stage object detectors are generally less precise than two-phase object detectors; however, they are essentially quicker. YOLO is an exceptionally good algorithm with a single-stage object identifier.

### *6.3.2 Bounding Boxes*

Bounding boxes are imaginary boxes that are utilized to find the existence of objects in a picture or in a video. There are a 2D bounding box framework and a 3D bounding box framework that are both being utilized. In advanced computer vision or image processing algorithms, the bounding box is simply the directions of the rectangular border that completely covers a computerized picture when it is set over a page, a canvas, a screen, or other two-dimensional digital format outputs. Calculations are performed on locating the bounding box and centroid coordinates to measure the distance between two bounding boxes. First it initializes the shade of the bounding box to be green. If YOLO algorithm identifies the presence of multiple objects, then multiple bounding boxes are formed. If two bounding boxes overlap each other, then it updates the shade of the jumping box to red. Draw both the bouncing box of the individual with their item centroid. Each is shading facilitated, so we'll see which individuals are excessively close as shown in Fig. 6.9.

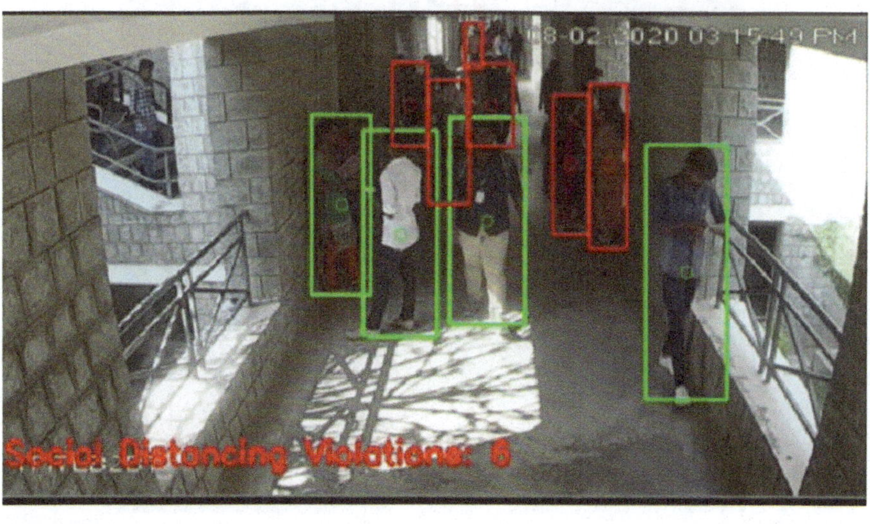


**Fig. 6.9** Accessing video camera and identifying violations

### 6.3.3 Compute Pairwise Distance

It distinguishes the nearness of two individual YOLO object detections within a frame. At that point, it draws all the three medians for a triangle. The center for each of the rectangular frame is called centroid. With the assistance of SciPy.spatial Python library, it discovers the closest neighboring point. Presently once more, it draws all the three medians to discover the centroid of that closest article. At that point, it figures the Euclidean separation between all sets of centroids. Figure 6.10 shows the distance.

### 6.3.4 Checking Whether the Pairwise Distance Is Greater Than N Pixel

In light of the pair separation figured, it verifies whether any two individuals are not as much as N pixels separated. Here the N pixel is the base social separation that one must follow which is gone ahead by WHO public well-being experts. With the assistance of pairwise distance identifier, it verifies whether the two object-identified bounding boxes are separated or not in the middle of the two sets. In the event that two individuals are excessively close, we add them to the abuse set. To distinguish them effectively, the shade of the bounding boxes is changed to red at whatever point the social separating is abused.

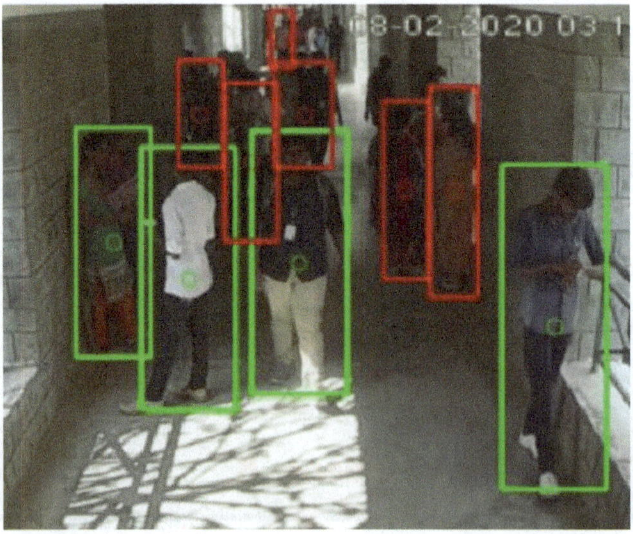

**Fig. 6.10** Change in frame after computing pairwise distance

### *6.3.5 Message and Alert Module*

WhatsApp is the most famous application currently widespread in the world. With the Twilio API for WhatsApp, you can arrive at more than 1.5 billion WhatsApp clients with 1 REST API, which is a piece of Twilio's Programmable Messaging stage. First sign up for (or sign in to) the Twilio Account and initiate the Sandbox. Before you can send a WhatsApp message from web language, you have to pursue a Twilio record or sign in to the current record and enact the Twilio Sandbox for WhatsApp. Here, we need to check the restrictions circling proclamation to check whether the social distance is violated or not. On conditions like social distance is not violated and its value is unchanged and set to zero, it won't send any message. If pairwise centroid metrics is violated, it will send a message to the enlisted WhatsApp mobile number at whatever point the social distancing violator is refreshed and detected. There are a few application interfaces (API) accessible to change over content to discourse in Python. One of such APIs is the Google Text-to-Speech API regularly known as the gTTS API. GTTS (Google Text-to-Speech) is extremely simple to implement which converts over the content entered in the form of text into sound which can be spared as an mp3 document. With the assistance of that API, it sends an alert message "SOCIAL DISTANCE VIOLATED" to the surveillance camera enabled with audio output to alert the peoples present in the surveillance location as shown in Fig. 6.11.

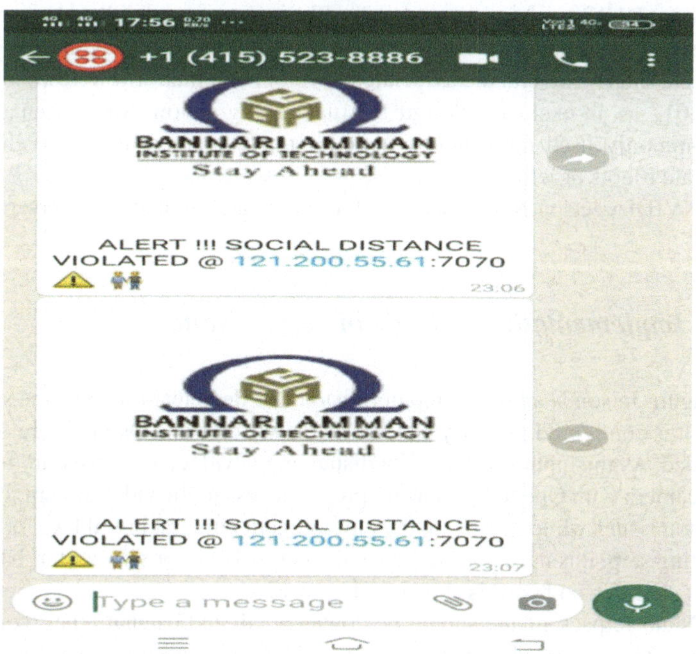


**Fig. 6.11** Alert message with Whatsapp module

## 6.4 Integration of Embedded Hardware Kit with Social Distancing Application

Jetson Nano is a small, powerful computer that lets us to run multiple neural networks in parallel for applications like image classification, object detection, segmentation, and speech processing. More likely, it is an embedded operating system-on-module and developer kit from the NVIDIA Jetson family, including integrated highly potential processing parts [17]. There are various versions and development kits available in NVIDIA store for easy and better choice of embedded hardware based on their computational requirements. It has compatibility to run all AI algorithms and can process high-resolution sensors/images simultaneously. It requires a microSD of a modular memory card for internal storage, which runs the OS in it. It can be connected to camera, display, and USB ports and has Maxwell high-processing GPU in it. It is powered using a 5 V constant power supply that can be powered by the mobile charger.

Using the hardware development kit with abovementioned configuration, it is possible to integrate social distance analyzer imposed upon any camera in the pathways. Install the necessary machine learning libraries used for this social distancing analyzer. Jetson Nano can run various operating systems and software on the Jetson board series. As a default software bundle, it is provided with Jetpack, a software development kit provided by NVIDIA. It is a LINUX for Tegra operating system. Nano has Compute Unified Device Architecture (CUDA) and CUDA Deep Neural Network (cuDNN) package provided by Tegra system provider. As mentioned, QNX operating system is also available for Jetson platform, though it is not widely announced. This board and the associated development platform were announced in March 2017 as an exclusive design for functioning in low-power scenarios. The most commonly used applications include smaller camera drones with various small-scale robots or jetbots.

The NVIDIA Jetson Nano packs 472GFLOPS of computational horsepower.

### *6.4.1 Implementation of Code in Jetson Nano*

To configure Jetson Nano for computer vision and deep learning, test the system to confirm it is configured properly and TensorFlow/Keras and OpenCV are operating as intended. As the input for the social distancing is video, it is necessary to test the Nano's camera with OpenCV to ensure proper access to the video stream. In case of installation issues while setting up the environment either at initial level or with the final testing step, it is necessary to go back and resolve it; or worse, start back at the very first step. Jetson board is shown in Fig. 6.12.

The Nano Jetpack image should be downloaded, and balenaEtcher (software to flash memory) is installed to make it ready to flash the image to a microSD. Loading the microSD card and microSD reader hardware probably with 32GB or 64GB stor-

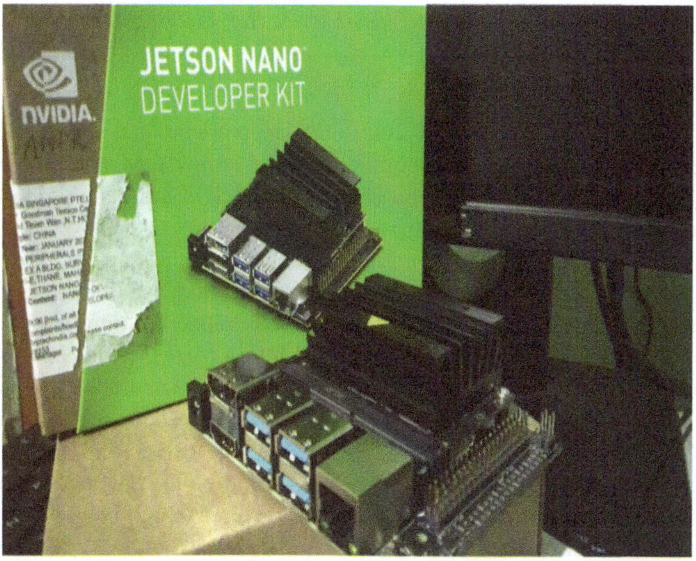


**Fig. 6.12** NVIDIA Jetson Nano Embedded Hardware Kit

age capacity, fire up balenaEtcher and proceed to flash. There are two typical ways to power the Jetson Nano. A 5 V 2.5 A (10 W) microUSB power adapter is a good option. In case of a lot of peripherals utilized being powered by the Nano (keyboards, mice, Wi-Fi, cameras), then consider a 5 V 4 A (20 W) power supply to ensure that the processors can run at their full speeds while powering the peripherals. Technically, there's a third power option too if you want to apply power directly on the header pins. On completing the installation part, check for the system-level dependencies and tools. To configure and resolve troubleshooting issues, Jetson Nano comes with a pre-compiler tool called CMake. CMake is a pre-compiler tool to make successful installation of OpenCV, an image processing library. Create a virtual environment for working with the project, and so you can be aware of the libraries installed and get rid of confusions. Virtual environments allow for isolated installs of different Python packages. Utilizing the virtual environment setup enables us to use one version of a Python library in one environment and another version in a separate environment. On creation of the virtual Python environment, install all the libraries to get the program ready to work. When using the NVIDIA Jetson Nano, there are two options for input camera devices:

1. A CSI camera module, such as the Raspberry Pi camera module (which *is* compatible with the Jetson Nano)
2. A USB web camera

The default camera value is set to −1, implying that an attached CSI camera should be used. To access a USB camera, change the default camera value from −1 to 0 (or whatever the correct V4L2 camera is). Library in Jetson is presented in Fig. 6.13.

## 6.4.2 *Preparing the Jetson Nano with the Hardware Environment*

The NVIDIA Jetson Nano packs 472GFLOPS of computational horsepower. While it is a very capable machine, configuration is little complex. Start the download by ensuring the images as "Jetson Nano Developer Kit SD Card image." Downloaded page and image are shown in Fig. 6.14.

This NVIDIA's Jetpack is a combination of all the necessary requirements for performing deep learning and computer vision techniques. It includes the pre-installed CUDA and cuDNN packed together. Download the .img file and flash it with the memory card before running with the Jetson Nano. While Nano SD image is downloading, go ahead and download and install balenaEtcher, a disk image flashing tool. Once both (1) Nano Jetpack image is downloaded and (2) balenaEtcher is installed, ready to flash the image to a microSD. Insert the microSD into the card reader, and then plug the card reader into a USB port on the computer. From there, fire up balenaEtcher and proceed to flash. In this step, we will power up the Jetson Nano and establish network connectivity.

This step requires the following:

1. The flashed microSD
2. An NVIDIA Jetson Nano dev board
3. HDMI screen

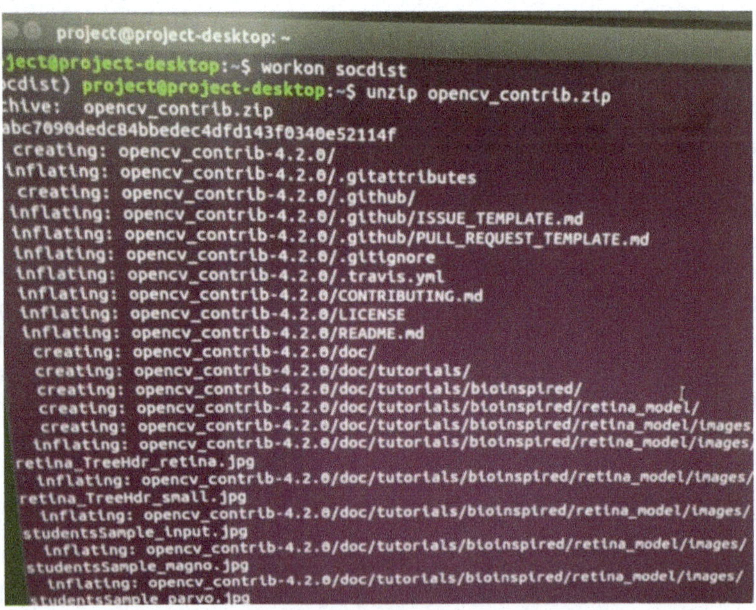


**Fig. 6.13** Trouble library in virtualized environment in Jetson Nano OS

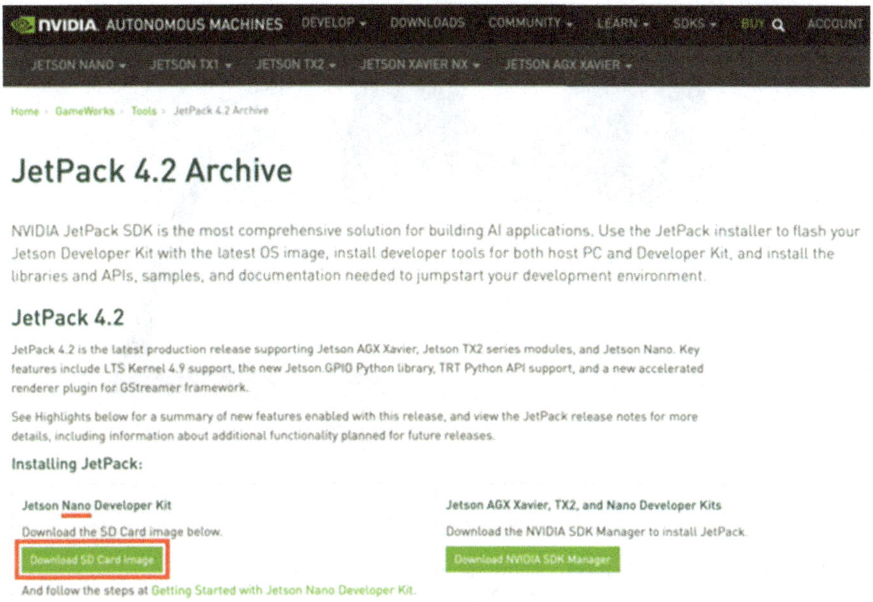


**Fig. 6.14** Jetson Nano Package Downloader from NVIDIA Platform

4. USB keyboard + mouse
5. A power supply—either (1) a 5 V 2.5 A (12.5 W) microSD power supply or (2) a 5 V 4 A (20 W) barrel plug power supply with a jumper at the J48 connector

Network connection may be either as follows: (1) an Ethernet cable connecting the Nano to the network or (2) a wireless module. The wireless module can come in the form of a USB Wi-Fi adapter or a Wi-Fi module installed under the Jetson Nano heat sink.

As a result of performing the Jetson Nano with CUDA and cuDNN libraries, the Nano can able to process 15FPS without parallel processing support, and it accelerates up to 6FPS. For cameras supported with 10FPS, it can be automated and controlled and provides support for decision-making with Jetson Nano. Peripherals used are shown in Fig. 6.15.

## 6.5 Conclusion

Social distancing has become essential in our day-to-day life to fight against the aggressive pandemic COVID-19. Moreover, it is a life-supporting strategy to prevent the spread of COVID-19 in public/private places. For better survival with the pandemic, it is essential to maintain social distancing. To handle the situation effectively, monitoring the people is highly important. And more likely to indulging them

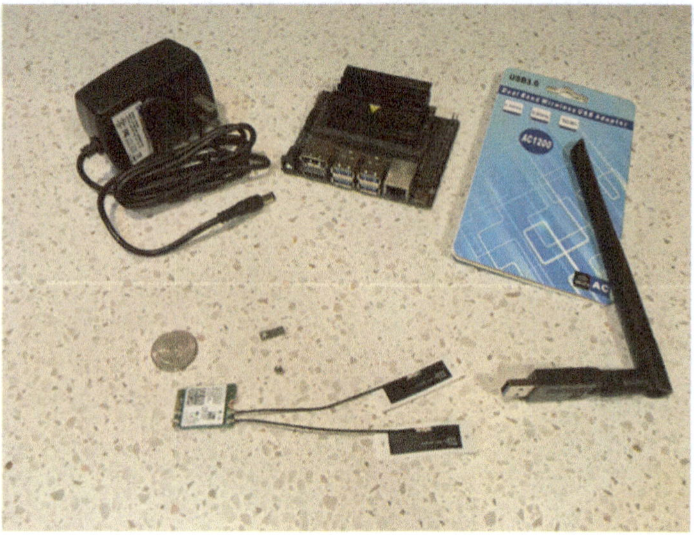


**Fig. 6.15** Electronic peripherals for hardware integration with Jetson Nano

the practice of social distancing. With that notion in this chapter, a detailed literature survey is presented for monitoring the social control via object detection and proposed a methodology for automatic detection of objects via YOLO object detector. When multiple objects are identified by YOLO, it innately results in multiple objects present in a frame and sends alert message to the corresponding authorities via WhatsApp. Thus, violations of rules are avoided, and the integration of social distancing application with Jetson Nano board for the successful execution is elaborated in detail in Sect. 6.4. This proposed kit is going to benefit the society effectively by maintaining social distancing. As future enhancement, the same approach can be tested in various spatial locations to prove its efficacy.

## References


1. WHO Coronavirus Disease (COVID-19) Dashboard. Accessed at https://covid19.who.int/
2. Coronavirus Types. Accessed at https://www.healthline.com/health/coronavirus-types. Online: Accessed 29 Apr 2020.
3. Coronavirus Disease 2019 (COVID-19) – Older Adults. Accessed at https://www.cdc.gov/coronavirus/2019-ncov/need-extra-precautions/older-adults.html
4. Vaishya, R., et al. (2020). Artificial Intelligence (AI) applications for COVID-19 pandemic. *Diabetes & Metabolic Syndrome: Clinical Research & Reviews, 14*, 337–339.
5. Loey, M., et al. (2020). A hybrid deep transfer learning model with machine learning methods for face mask detection in the era of the COVID-19 pandemic. *Measurement, 167*, 108288.
6. Du, X., Cai, Y., Wang, S., & Zhang, L. (2017, January). Overview of deep learning. In *31st youth academic annual conference of Chinese Association of Automation (YAC).*

7. LeCun, Y., Bengio, Y., & Hinton, G. (2015). Deep learning. *Nature, 521*, 436–444. https://doi.org/10.1038/nature14539.
8. Bengio, Y. (2009). Learning deep architectures for AI. *Foundations and Trends® in Machine Learning, 2*(1), 1–127. https://doi.org/10.1561/2200000006.
9. Liu, Z., Luo, P., Wang, X., & Tang, X. (2015). Deep learning face attributes in the wild. In *2015 IEEE international conference on computer vision (ICCV)* (pp. 3730–3738). Santiago. https://doi.org/10.1109/ICCV.2015.425.
10. Zhao, Z., Zheng, P., Xu, S., & Wu, X. (2019, November). Object detection with deep learning: A review. *IEEE Transactions on Neural Networks and Learning Systems, 30*(11), 3212–3232. https://doi.org/10.1109/TNNLS.2018.2876865.
11. Moniruzzaman, M., Islam, S. M. S., Bennamoun, M., & Lavery, P. (2017). *Deep learning on underwater marine object detection: A survey* (pp. 150–160). https://doi.org/10.1007/978-3-319-70353-4_13.
12. Pathak, A. R., Pandey, M., & Rautaray, S. (2018). Application of deep learning for object detection. *Procedia Computer Science, 132*, 1706–1717, ISSN 1877-0509. https://doi.org/10.1016/j.procs.2018.05.144.
13. Redmon, J., Divvala, S., Girshick, R., Farhadi, A., & Once, Y. O. L. (2016, June). Unified, real-time object detection. In *IEEE conference on computer vision and pattern recognition (CVPR).*
14. Bluedot Insights. Accessed at https://bluedot.global/products/insights/
15. HealthMap. Accessed at https://www.healthmap.org/en/
16. Corona Tracker API with ML. Accessed at https://coronavirus-tracker-api.herokuapp.com/v2/locations
17. Jetson Nano Developer Kit. Accessed at https://developer.nvidia.com/embedded/jetson-nano-developer-kit
18. Glass, R. J., Glass, L. M., Beyeler, W. E., & Jason Min, H. (2006). Targeted social distancing designs for pandemic influenza. *Emerging Infectious Diseases, 12*(11), 1671–1681.
19. Punn, N. S., Sonbhadra, S. K., & Agarwal, S. (2020). *Monitoring COVID-19 social distancing with person detection and tracking via fine-tuned YOLO v3 and Deepsort techniques*. arxiv.org
20. Pias. (2020). *Object detection and distance measurement*. https://github.com/paul-pias/Object-Detection-and-Distance-Measurement. Online: Accessed 01 Mar 2020.
21. Sonawane, A. (2020). *Medium: YOLOv3: A huge improvement*. https://medium.com/@anand-sonawane/yolo3. Online: Accessed 6 Dec 2019.
22. Microsoft Bing's AI Tracker. Accessed at: https://www.bing.com/covid/local/india
23. Kaggle Covid-19 Dataset. Accessed at: https://www.kaggle.com/search?q=covid-19

# Chapter 7
# IoT-Enabled Applications and Other Techniques to Combat COVID-19

**N. Renugadevi, S. Saravanan, C. M. Naga Sudha, and Parul Tripathi**

## 7.1 Introduction

According to WHO report, different categories of influenza viruses such as H1N1, H2N2, and H3N3 are responsible for the past pandemic in the decade. Presently, severe acute respiratory syndrome (SARS) named as COVID-19 has emerged as a reason for major outbreak. This virus belongs to a family of the *Coronaviridae* which is a single-stranded, positive-sense RNA virus. It also affects the respiratory system of the humans and causes illnesses like cough, fever, fatigue, and breathlessness. Four stages of COVID-19 are, namely, imported cases only (stage 1), sporadic cases/local transmission (stage 2), clusters of cases (stage 3), and community transmission (stage 4). The first case of COVID-19 was reported in Wuhan city of China at stage 1 in December 2019. Then, it progressed to stage 2, and it started to spread globally which resulted in a pandemic situation [1]. It has made numerous researchers, organizations, scientists, and laboratories around globe to develop vaccines and various treatment methods.

As pandemic outbreaks have emerged, there arises a need of numerous hospitals to take care of the patients. To deal with this great problem, technological developments are spotted into light. Therefore, Internet-connected hospitals, i.e.,

N. Renugadevi
Department of Computer Science and Engineering, Indian Institute of Information Technology, Tiruchirappalli, India

S. Saravanan (✉)
Department of Mechanical Engineering, K. Ramakrishnan College of Technology, Trichy, India

C. M. Naga Sudha
Department of Computer Technology, Anna University MIT Campus, Chennai, India

P. Tripathi
Department of Computer Science, Banasthali Vidyapith, Jaipur, India



S. Kautish et al. (eds.), *Computational Intelligence Techniques for Combating COVID-19*, EAI/Springer Innovations in Communication and Computing,
https://doi.org/10.1007/978-3-030-68936-0_7

hospitals which are integrated with Internet of Things (IoT) devices, are highly assisting clinical staffs during this pandemic time. Also, social distancing plays a key role in reducing the spreading factor. To highlight such precautions, when the social distancing is not obeyed, applications which will automatically inform the medical staffs about the measures to be taken are developed. Telehealth consultations are made available in handling the faraway locality patients. COVID-19 outbreak has highlighted that more researches need to be carried out not only in medical aspects but also in technological aspects. Several research papers have been published on COVID-19 themes. In [2], clinical characteristics such as signs, symptoms, and demographics of COVID-19 patients have been studied in Wuhan, China. The study was performed among 138 patients in which the medical diagnosis was made carefully. A report was also presented in order to explain the effects of SARS-CoV-2 virus in other different vital organs. Out of 99 patients with COVID-19 symptoms, a group of 49 patients were in a direct link to Huanan seafood market in Wuhan which is a COVID-19 epicenter [3]. Report has been published that 17% has developed acute respiratory distress syndrome; among those patients, 11% died due to multiple organ dysfunction syndromes.

In COVID-19 pandemic, various challenges are faced all over the world which can be resolved by an advanced technical platform, the IoT. Real-time information and other required data of the diseased patient can be easily accessed through IoT. IoT execution processes to fight against COVID-19 pandemic are as follows: Initially, health data is monitored in remote location followed by virtual management system through meetings and conferences. Analysis of received data along with controlling activities like immediate sanitation and maintenance of containment zone is processed at the next step, and finally the reports attained are to be followed up [4]. IoT-based smartphone applications are also developed for the benefit of the people who can alert the people to take preventive measures. Proper database of the symptoms and recovered cases are managed by the doctors or the hospital management through which whole quarantine period can be monitored properly. A smart network is formed by interconnecting enormous number of devices with the help of IoT for developing the proper health management system. This system analyzes the data of the patient and the information regarding their symptoms digitally without any human intervention. It helps in appropriate decision-making process also. Key merits of IoT for COVID-19 pandemic are, namely, reduced chances of mistakes, contactless and superior treatment, lesser expenses, effective control, and enhanced diagnosis [5]. Technology and society are shaped with the Internet revolution which began before 30 years as shown in Fig. 7.1 [Source: Deolitte LLP 2018]. Through IoT technologies, healthcare sector and wireless technology are growing rapidly, and therefore, improvements in connected medical devices are taking place. Internet of Medical Things (IoMT) can be initiated by merging a more number of medical devices, large amount of data, IT systems and software, connectivity technologies, and services in the network.

As healthcare domain has attained more focus during the pandemic situation, researchers have made their contributions in treating COVID-19 with several technologies. The organization of the chapter is as follows: IoT in Healthcare and

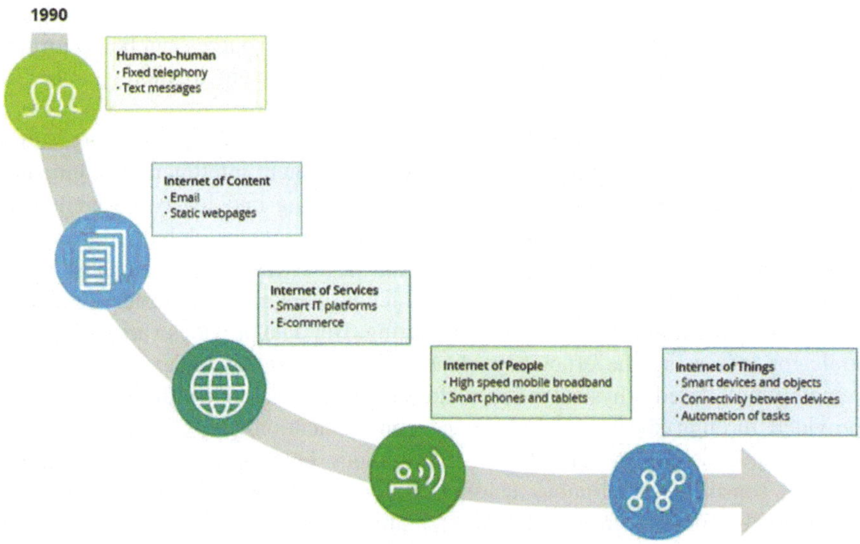


**Fig. 7.1** IoT Revolution

IoMT are highlighted in Sects. 7.2.1 and 7.2.2, respectively. A new category of Internet of Covid Things (IoCT) is proposed in this chapter which is explained in detail under Sect. 7.2.3. Interactive communication between patients and doctors can be provided through telemedicine which is described in Sect. 7.3. Nowadays, industries are coming forward to manufacture Internet of Health Things (IoHT)-related products which are described in Sect. 7.4.

## 7.2 IoT-Based Applications

IoT-based applications are categorized according to their utilization under particular fields. Therefore, in medicinal sectors, IoT is classified as IoT in healthcare and IoT in medical care, and they are explained in the following subsections.

### *7.2.1 IoT in Healthcare*

IoT has attractive applications in medical care and healthcare. Medical care can be provided through various medical devices, imaging devices, and sensors which can be used as smart devices constituting a fundamental part of the IoT. Reduction of cost, increased quality of life, and enrichment of the user experience are attained through the implementation of the IoT in healthcare. It is stated that it can be possible to reduce the downtime of the devices from the remote location through IoT. Hence, through IoT, scheduling of the inadequate resources can be performed for their efficient usage and in providing proper treatment to more number of patients [6].

In Fig. 7.2 [7], various technologies integrated with IoT are, namely, cloud computing, grid computing, big data, networks, ambient intelligence, augmented reality, and wearables. Integration of cloud computing into IoT-based healthcare application gives a facility of accessing the shared resources globally. In order to satisfy the requests and to offer services on the network, applications of cloud computing are essential. Grid computing which is also known as cluster computing is viewed as the foundation of cloud computing. Big data provides various types of tools for increasing the efficiency of applicable health treatment which can be remotely monitored. Physical infrastructure of the IoT-based healthcare network is provided through short- and long-range communications. Also, ultra-wideband, Bluetooth Low Energy, and RFID technologies help in designing low-power medical sensor. As continuous learning is more important for humans to react immediately for any triggered action, ambient intelligence is integrated with IoT-aided healthcare services. IoT-based healthcare application with augmented reality is applied for remote monitoring and surgery.

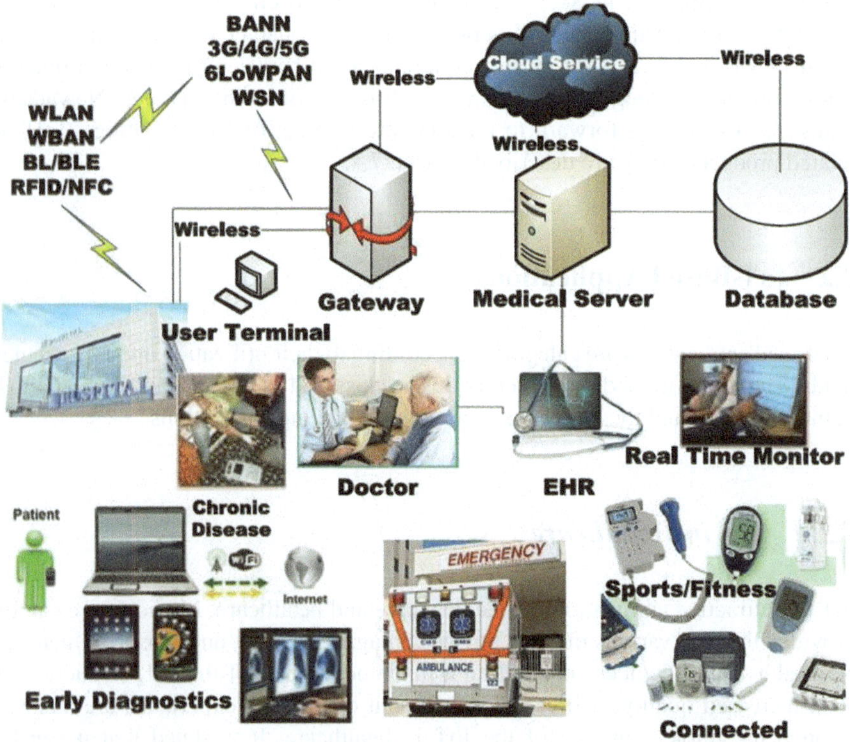


Fig. 7.2 IoT-based healthcare technologies

### 7.2.2 *Internet of Medical Things (IoMT)*

IoHT is also denoted as IoMT if it combines with the medical services and software application which provides additional healthcare services integrated with IT system of healthcare. IoMT is focused on various connected medical devices which are capable to generate, collect, analyze, or transfer health data and images which are connected to healthcare-providing network [8]. IoMT plays an important role in filling the gap between physical world and digital world. The main stakeholders in the IoMT system are shown in Fig. 7.3 [Source: Deolitte LLP 2018]. With the help of IoMT, patient condition can be monitored and modified based on their conditions of asthma, diabetes, and high blood pressure in the real-time environment. Streamlining of many clinical procedures to connect the patients, caretakers, medical staffs, and patients' data with performance and medical devices via mobile applications for enhancement in delivering the healthcare is made possible through IoMT.

In the current pandemic scenario, IoT has provided numerous promising solutions for COVID-19. Hence, with the help of technological advancement, doctors are able to deal with the victims of COVID-19 in a secure way.

### 7.2.3 *Proposed Internet of Covid Things (IoCT)*

IoT technologists have designed a variety of medical equipments as per requirements from the doctors and medical staffs to handle the patients during this critical situation of COVID-19. Depending upon the applications of those devices, a new category on IoCT is proposed in this subsection.

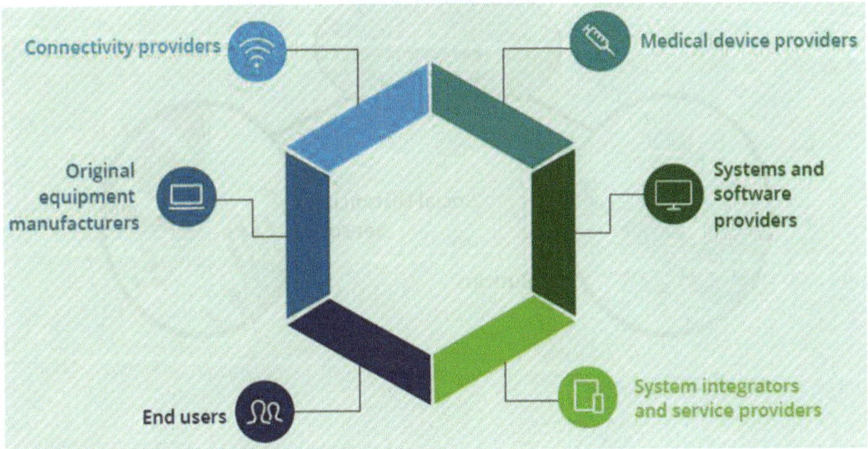


**Fig. 7.3** Main stakeholders in the IoMT system

In COVID-19 scenario, there is an urge in need of numerous reliable diagnoses to break the pandemic chain. Due to the lack of testing kits of COVID-19, preliminary testing cannot be made feasible up to the optimum level. This situation pushes the government in trouble as it is difficult to distinguish the symptoms of COVID-19 from the symptoms of common flu; therefore, with the help of special category of medical devices integrated with IoT, COVID-19 pandemic situation can be handled better. IoT sensors which can sense the symptoms of COVID are categorized as IoCT. Proposed category of IoCT devices is shown in Fig. 7.4, and they are explained in the following subsections.

#### 7.2.3.1 Smart Thermometers

Before 8 years, Kinsa Health a US-based health technology has designed smart thermometers which can screen people with high fevers. Initially, these were used to track only common flu; nevertheless, these are very useful in identifying clusters of COVID-19 around the USA. Now Kinsa Health has launched million to billion smart thermometers which are used in households of the USA. Mobile applications which are integrated with smart thermometers allow the readings to be transmitted

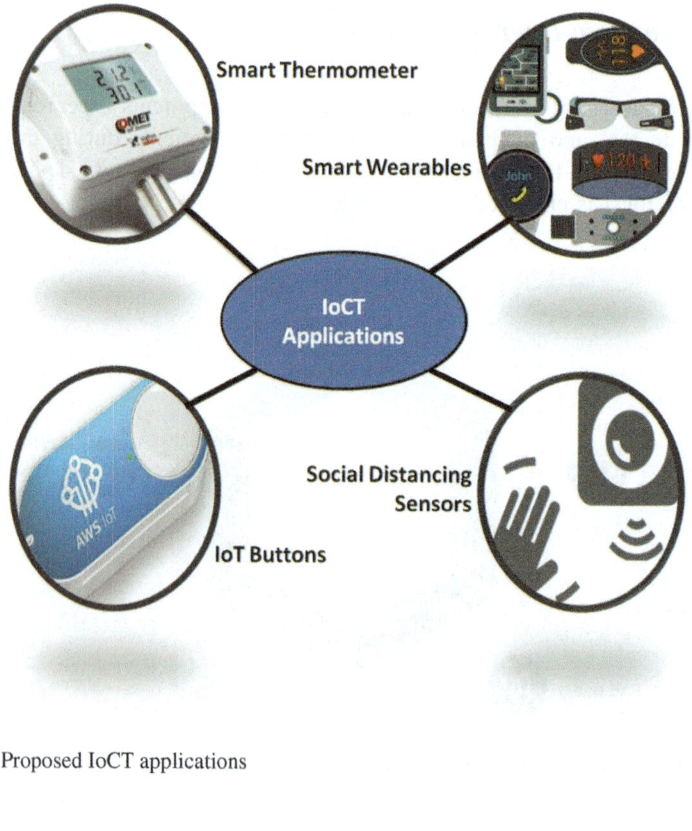


**Fig. 7.4** Proposed IoCT applications

to the company. It can assimilate the data and generate maps showing US regions witnessing high fevers, and it helps the US authorities in identifying hotspots. These interactive maps have proven accuracy in prediction of spreading rates of flu around the USA which outdoes the Centers for Disease Control and Prevention official application in promptness measure of prediction [9].

#### 7.2.3.2 Wearables

Wearables have become ideal technologies which are increasingly adopted in healthcare sector. Wearables are connected to the Internet for communication on tracking the health information. It ranges from fitness trackers like smart headbands Dreem, Apple watch, and many other personal sensors and patches as shown in Fig. 7.5 [10]. Wearables must be able to connect with physiological transducers which can measure patient's body temperature, blood pressure, heartbeat rate, and others. These devices are also used for sensing patient's physical activity and caring of elderly people. Sensors on patient clothes can also be used for monitoring health parameters. A ubiquitous system is designed to take care of elder patients suffering from Alzheimer's disease. Patient can press a button in emergency situation which will send the important data on oxygen saturation, heart rate, and blood pressure to the concerned professionals for analysis [11–13]. In this current scenario, organizations have started to roll out wearable devices for managing the impact of COVID-19.

WHOOP, a Boston-based technology startup, and Central Queensland (CQ) University in Australia have joined to examine the mechanism of COVID-19 identification in its incubation duration. Due to high reproductive factor, COVID-19 has become a severe outbreak in global manner. Therefore, an American academic medical center, Cleveland Clinic, at Ohio and researchers of CQ University's Appleton Institute have carried out a 24/7 study on physiological data gathered through WHOOP in a wrist-mounted mode. Among hundreds of members, people who have identified themselves a victim of COVID-19 volunteered to be a part of study. WHOOP Straps help in monitoring the respiratory rates and to notify the individual about the issues in their health. The data from *WHOOP Journal* is also collected which is an online interface accessed through member's smartphone. It helps in monitoring daily behavior and to make a healthy lifestyle. WHOOP is the only wearables with more accuracy rate to measure cardio respiration validated by third-party study [14, 15].

LifeSignals, a Silicon Valley startup, has designed a life signal biosensor patch which can monitor cardiovascular functionalities. The patches which are shower-proof and lightweight are fixed on chest area to record the person's temperature along with respiration rate, heart rate, and ECG trace. These data are collected and sent to the user's smart device in order to view the results. If data is matched with COVID-19 symptoms, the data are sent to a secure cloud platform to alert the healthcare workers. Single patch can be worn for 5 days, and it can be safely dis-

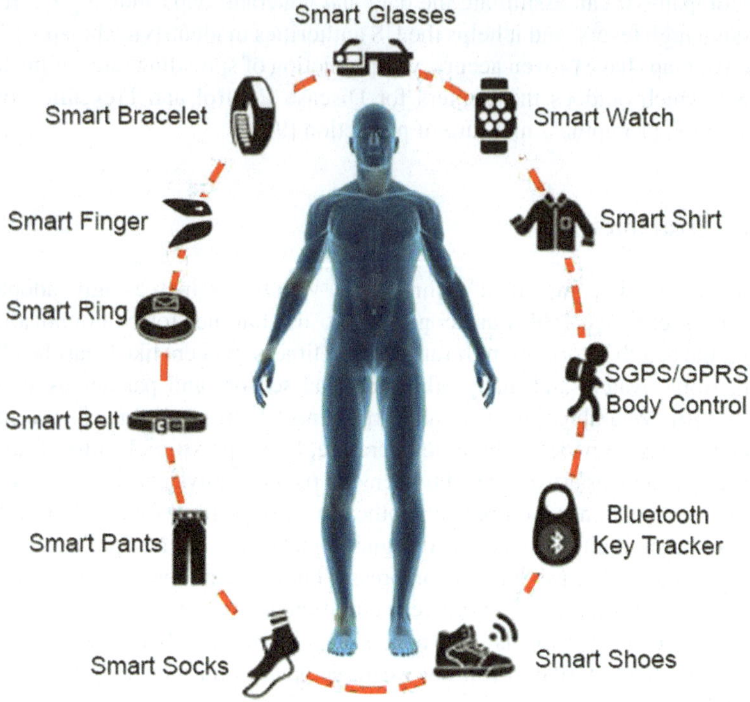


**Fig. 7.5** Various wearable to IoCT

posed. LifeSignals has planned to design a second version of Biosensor Patch 2A which can monitor COVID-19 patients under intensive care units [16, 17].

Some of the challenges of wearables rely on managing the supply chain which is highly critical during lockdown periods, limited power supply in battery mode, and security issues on accumulated data.

IoT buttons are deployed in order to limit the number of hospital-acquired infections and to maintain standards of high cleaning. In Vancouver, which is a city in British Columbia, Canada, hospitals have deployed IoT buttons in battery mode which are named as Wanda QuickTouch. These are designed and deployed rapidly in order to alert the hospital management with prompt signals, which require emergency sanitation and maintenance. The important feature of this IoT button is that it is not necessary to stick to external surface [18, 19].

#### 7.2.3.3 Artificial Intelligence-Based IoCT Applications

Artificial Intelligence is the new electricity.– Dr. Andrew Ng

Humans have made the machines to learn and act to the environment accordingly. Hence, artificial intelligence (AI) has its footprint as a landmark in technological development. In the pandemic situation, the first and foremost application of AI is in busting of fake news and enforcing the lockdown measures. Various other applications of AI are effectively used in COVID-19 such as surveillance of diseases, screening and medical diagnosis of patients, modelling of virus, and host identification. However, there are many challenges in implementing these applications. Some of the limitations mentioned in [20] are as follows: Accurate results can be attained only when AI models have training data in a substantial amount. As there are insufficient historical data in unprecedented pandemic nature, several inefficient AI models are rendered. The major limitation of AI lies in machine learning (ML) models where AI assumes that contingencies will always occur from the trained data. AI also faces challenges not only from the insufficient data but also from the outlier data and noisy data. For instance, the reason behind failure of Google Flu Trends is "big data hubris" which makes algorithm to be vulnerable to overfitting and their functionalities are inhibited. Also, privacy breach is a major concern when AI technique is used for crowd surveillance. Public health is more important during pandemic times than the privacy breach. However, people have the fear that government might monitor their privacy details even after the pandemic. The main drawback of AI application is its dependency on human expertise to provide knowledge on implementing techniques learnt in order to provide a significant change to fight against COVID-19 pandemic situation. However, despite several limitations of AI applications, its contributions during pandemic situations are benefitted to the public. Its advances have made tremendous progress in natural language processing, deep learning, ML, and data analytics which also serve the public during COVID-19.

ML algorithms have been developed for the diagnosis of COVID-19. For instance, screening of SARS-CoV-2 based on ML using CRISPR-based virus detection system has been designed with high sensitivity and speed. Some of the symptoms of COVID-19 were detected through neural networks (respiratory pattern detection) and deep learning models (analyzing thoracic CT images). As there is a worldwide need in developing a vaccine against COVID-19, AI has supported more in repositioning and repurposing the existing drug candidates to fight against SARS-COVID-19. Deep learning-based drug discovery pipeline has been designed for generating novel drug-like compounds to treat against COVID-19.

AlphaFold, which is a deep learning model developed by Google DeepMind, helps in predicting the protein structures for treating COVID-19. In traditional methods, these techniques took longer time to predict the structures. COVID-19 vaccine candidates have been proposed by Vaxign reverse vaccinology which are integrated with ML. AI and ML are in need of real-time data such as timely delivery of patient's data, therapeutic outcomes of patients, physiological data, and data transformation, which are really very challenging for collection. The step-by-step process which is involved in the data collection and processing is depicted in Fig. 7.6 [21]. It includes several steps of AI and ML through which COVID-19 patient data can be managed and processed through databases. But, such tasks are becoming very challenging due to a new infrastructure known as cyber-physical system, which is developed and has invited worldwide collaborations.

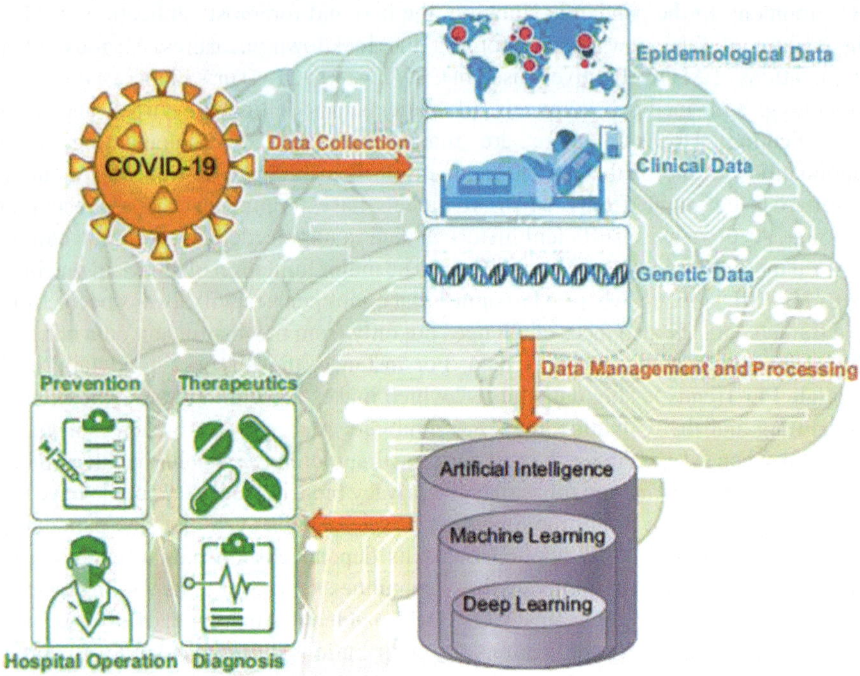


**Fig. 7.6** Application of AI in the fight against COVID-19

#### 7.2.3.4 Blockchain-Based IoCT Applications

In recent times, Blockchain 2.0 and Blockchain 3.0 have made extensive deliberation among researchers and industrialists. Blockchain concept has stepped into almost all the sectors, namely, drone communication technologies, insurance sector, healthcare sector, and transportation industry [22]. Even though it is in prefatory stage, it is gaining more prominence in security aspects. It helps in verifying the party claims in a transaction. Hence, it is continuously an expansion of record transaction among two parties [23]. Utility of blockchain has made various authorities and companies to build their own applications along with blockchain to counter COVID-19. These applications aim to solve an issue which prevails in the integration of verified data sources. Experts are much more interested in the process of validating dynamic data which is a very important criterion in COVID-19 situation [24]. Presently, blockchain has gained a major spotlight in the COVID-19 which is neither centralized nor independent crisis. As blockchain has a property of distributed ledger, it can enable organizations and individuals to connect in an interconnected network which facilitates secure transfer and sharing of data. Blockchain has genuine features like tamper-proof data, consensus algorithms, and smart contracts which can minimize dissemination of fraudulent information and bogus data [25]. Collaboration between connected medical devices and industries is shown in Fig. 7.7 [Source: Deolitte LLP 2018].

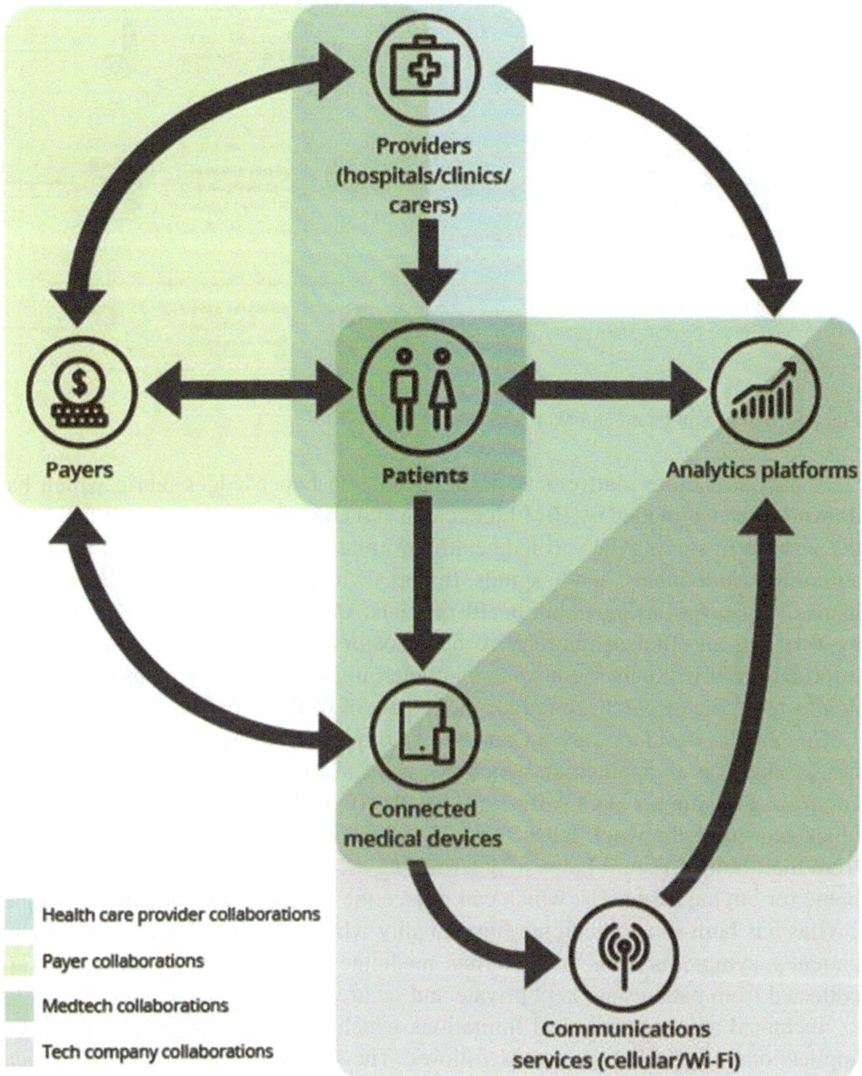


**Fig. 7.7** Industrial collaboration between medical devices

Blockchain applications help in relieving the burdens of hospital staffs and healthcare personnel in significant ways such as facilitating increased testing and reporting, recording the details of the COVID-19 patients, managing the lockdown implementation, preventing the circulation of fake news, enabling an incentive-based volunteer participation platform, enabling a secure donation platform for supporters, and limiting supply chain disruptions. The advantages of using blockchain-based IoCT application are illustrated in Fig. 7.8 [26].

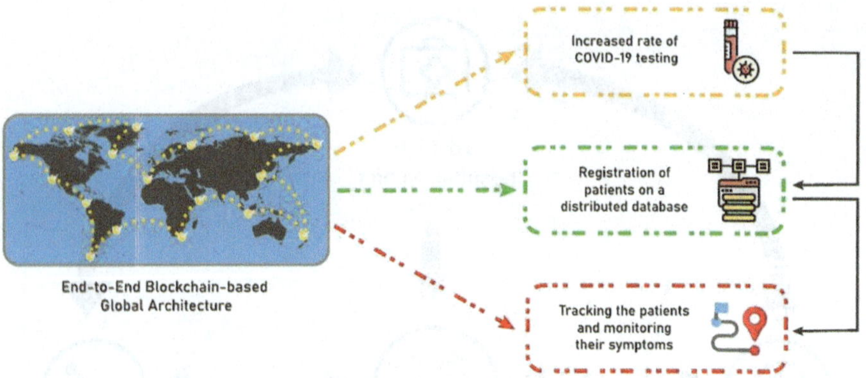


**Fig. 7.8** Blockchain-based global architecture for COVID 19

A data streaming platform, MiPasa is built on hyper-ledger fabric which has drawn services provided by IBM blockchain and IBM cloud platforms. It facilitates the services of sharing the verified health information along with the location to the authorities, individuals, and hospitals. It works with the information collected from medical organizations and public health officials. At the same time, it is acknowledged by WHO as an efficient platform to help doctors in gaining access on verifiable information. It will help the hospitals in determining their future plans and actions in allocating the resources to reduce the impact of COVID-19 [27].

Civitas was developed by a Canadian startup company which is specialized in blockchain. It is an application which assists local authorities of various nations in controlling the impact of COVID-19. It has an official IDs of people associated with blockchain records which helps to verify whether they have permission to leave from their home. Also, it helps in determining the time period for persons to leave home for buying essentials, which can reduce the risks of infection among people. Civitas has built-in telemedicine functionality which allows the doctors in tracing patient's symptoms and to prescribe medicines accordingly. Data which are collected from patients are kept private and secure [28].

Technical and non-technical limitations which prevail in the blockchain-based applications of COVID-19 are as follows: The first and foremost non-technical drawback is lesser awareness on potential impact of blockchain. Several people have reserved their minds on blockchain with fraudulent activities. Another non-technical problem of blockchain lies in scalability issue. As the current pandemic situation is in need of a high-scalable platform to manage data globally, it makes blockchain lesser in use. It can be overcome by the construction of directed acyclic graph. The current pandemic situations need blockchain to get consolidated with various emerging technologies. However, it takes time to be integrated as it is itself a new technology to the world. Absence of central authority can sometimes be a big challenge, which will lead to a necessity of enforcing standards and government regulations in order to ensure their functionalities. Despite these challenges, COVID-19 situation has made an impact on blockchain which has to be explored more in upcoming years.

#### 7.2.3.5 IoCT Security Challenges

In this era of IoCT, medical field is highly expected to have a widespread adoption of IoT. When many eHealth IoT applications are developed which deal with private information, it can become a target for attackers. As these devices are connected to global networks to get access anytime and anywhere, high security measures are to be considered. Challenges in providing healthcare services include mobility, scalability, communications media, and multiplicity of devices, dynamic network topology, multi-protocol network, security updates, and tamper-resistant packages. Also, computational, memory, and energy limitations are still on open issues in security aspect [29].

IoCT-based applications have been very useful among the public. Using these applications, spreading of COVID-19 is reduced to a large scale. Also, with the help of these devices, patients can consult doctors through telemedicine mode which is explained in the following section.

## 7.3 Telemedicine

Telemedicine is the practice of monitoring the patient in remote. It is also known as telehealth, which allows clinicians to diagnose, treat, and evaluate the patients' conditions without their physical interaction. According to JD Health report, due to COVID-19, there is a considerable rise of demand in virtual consultations with doctors. Also, this rise has reflected in share prices by more than 100% in few weeks. Overloads of hospital staffs have lessened, and infection rate is highly reduced through telemedicine [30]. Various telemedicine platforms have been designed all over the world to manage COVID-19 impact as shown in Table 7.1 [31–35]. As telemedicine is in emerging stage, true potential can be realized only when it is integrated with other technologies, namely, smart wearables and robots, as shown in Fig. 7.9 [36].

With this interactive mode of consultation, patients are able to contact their own doctors or medical consultants from home. Treatment provided to the patients along with the patient information is stored in the cloud platform. As the cloud deals with the medical care, it is termed as IoMT cloud [33].

Traditionally, episodic models of care with reactive methods are considered as high cost, and there is a lack of effectiveness to operate. Proactive models which are enabled digitally can care patients effectively. With these changes, companies like MedTech can concentrate on production of IoMT which will connect providers, patients, and payers. These technologies will be more of patient-centric, cost-effective, and productive. The interconnected IoMT health ecosystem is explained in Fig. 7.10 [Source: Deolitte LLP 2018].

Mobile applications have also emerged as a new phase in fighting against COVID-19. As per new requirements from health sector, government and private organizations have stepped into development of application platforms to fight

**Table 7.1** Telemedicine platforms of COVID-19

| Country | Hospital | Measures taken |
|---|---|---|
| USA | George Washington University Hospital | Video consultations, Live Facebook webinars [31] |
| | Rush University Medical Centre | Telemedicine platforms to facilitate on-demand video consultations to provide medical expertise for screening COVID-19 [13] |
| India | Districts of Andhra Pradesh and Assam Government | Telemedicine platforms for remote interaction [14, 15] |
| Israel | Sheba Medical Centre | Telehealth technologies to monitor Israeli passengers who are quarantined in Japan and also to ensure human contact in hospital premises [16, 17] |

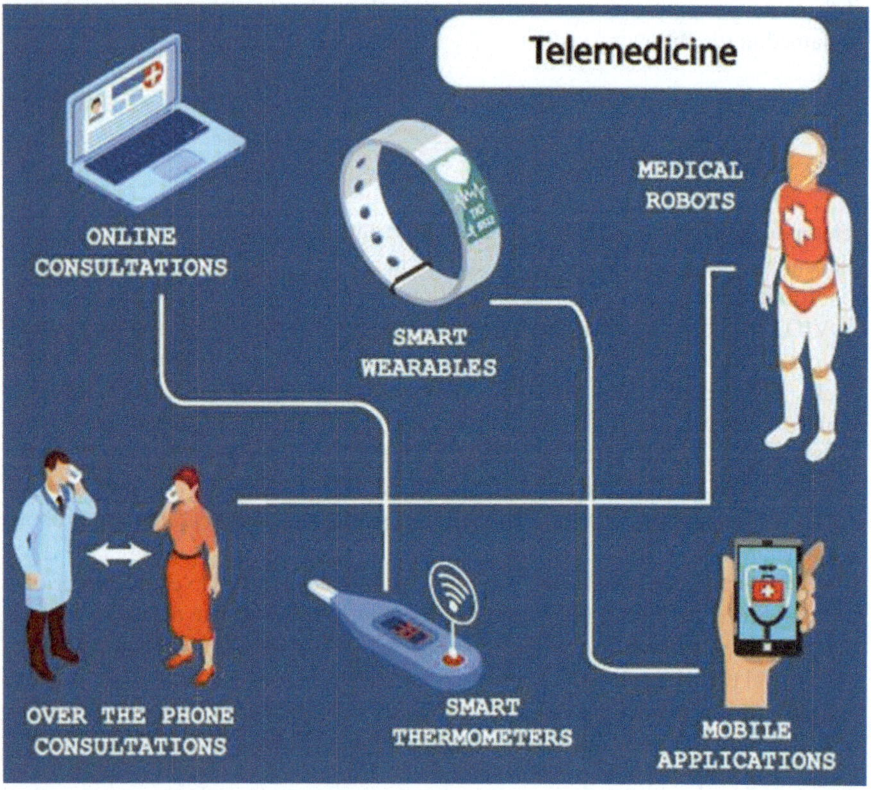


**Fig. 7.9** Various technologies enabling telemedicine

COVID-19 impact globally. Applications such as Aarogya Setu (India), COVIDSafe (Australia), StopTracing (France), and Corona-Warn-App (Germany) are developed to work under various technologies such as GIS, Bluetooth, and GPS, which are basically integrated with smart mobiles. Also, nowadays certain applications are made to adopt blockchain which helps in storing of data as immutable blocks.

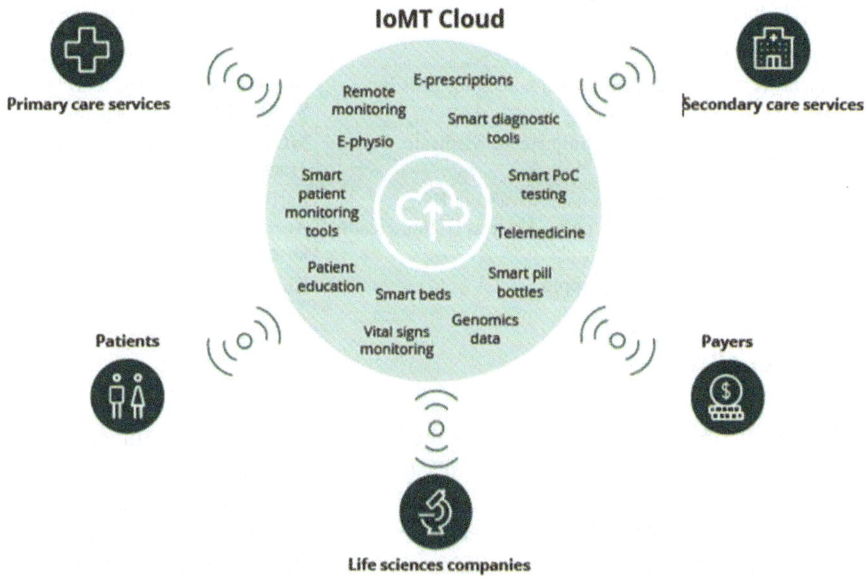


**Fig. 7.10** IoMT cloud health ecosystems

## 7.4 IoHT Industry Status

New startups, multinational corporations, and companies on IoHT named as Industrial IoHT (IIoHT) are stepping into giant market which will yield more profits. Recent IoHT services and solutions which are available are presented in Table 7.2 [36]. A key component of any product is of greater interest if there is more benefit to the public. Industrialists are also more involved in manufacturing the profitable product. Therefore, when IoHT industries are focused, the main considerations are on the necessities, usability constraints, and comfortability.

No matter who you are or where you are, instinct tells you to go home. – Laura Marney

IoHT increases the comfort of patients when they are taken care remotely. Hence, these devices are continuously monitoring the status of the patients, and the data are analyzed by doctors remotely. This comfort zone access not only ensures the patients' accessibility but also decreases cost and reduces the spreading of infection in the hospital. In framework for remote healthcare monitoring, this will reduce admission rates in the hospital [37]. EarlySense is a proactive patient care clinic located in the USA and Israel that works to improve patient's safety in contact-free mode. Heart rate, respiration rate, patient deterioration in an early stage, and preventing pressure ulcer are mainly monitored. Security issues are taken into highlights, where the possibilities of solutions are explored in IoHT. However, EarlySense studies are published in company's website, whereas solutions are available only in two countries, namely, the USA and Israel [38].

**Table 7.2** IoHT services developed by companies [36]

| Health services | Company | Product |
|---|---|---|
| Ambient-assisted living | Assisted Living Technologies Inc., Fade | Be Close Remote Monitoring System, Fade: Fall Detector |
| Smartphone applications | MCare, Safe Heart, Medisafe, On Track | MCare, iOximeter, Medisafe, On Track Diabetes |
| Remote healthcare monitoring | Early Sense, NovaSom, Hi Technologies, Proteus Digital Health Inc. | Early Sense All-in-One, AccuSom, Tele-ECG, Proteus Discover |
| Wearables | MC10, Apple | Bio Stamp RC, Apple Watch |

## 7.5 Conclusion

The year 2020 has made a huge shift in lifestyle of people globally. Importance on cleanliness and healthy diet are being insisted through media in order to safeguard the public. This chapter provides a detailed knowledge exposure on various topics initiating from the COVID-19 followed by emergence of IoT. Section 7.2 discusses about IoT-based applications in specialization to healthcare. IoMT and proposed IoCT are explained in detail under Sects. 7.2.2 and 7.2.3. The main components such as smart thermometers and wearables are illustrated under Sects. 7.2.3.1 and 7.2.3.2, respectively. Recent technologies like AI-based IoCT applications are explained in Sect. 7.2.3.3, and blockchain-based IoCT applications are described under Sect. 7.2.3.4. A security challenge which prevails in IoCT is explained in Sect. 7.2.3.5. Telemedicine which is the most preferable treatment method among public during COVID-19 is described in Sect. 7.3. As industries are stepping into manufacturing of more medical devices, IoHT Industry Status is discussed in Sect. 7.4. Thus, the whole chapter provides an entire map on applications and technologies involved to fight against COVID-19 pandemic times.

## References

1. Sohrabi, C., Alsa, Z., O'Neill, N., Khan, M., Kerwan, A., Al-Jabir, A., Iosidis, C., & Agha, R. (2020, April). World Health Organization declares global emergency: A review of the 2019 novel coronavirus (COVID-19). *International Journal of Surgery, 76*, 71–76.
2. Wang, D., Hu, B., Hu, C., Zhu, F., Liu, X., Zhang, J., Wang, B., Xiang, H., Cheng, Z., Xiong, Y., Zhao, Y., Li, Y., Wang, X., & Peng, Z. (2020, March). Clinical characteristics of 138 hospitalized patients with 2019 novel coronavirus_ infected pneumonia in Wuhan, China. *Journal of the American Medical Association, 323*(11), 1061.
3. Chen, N., Zhou, M., Dong, X., Qu, J., Gong, F., Han, Y., Qiu, Y., Wang, J., Liu, Y., Wei, Y., Xia, J., Yu, T., Zhang, X., & Zhang, L. (2020, February). Epidemiological and clinical characteristics of 99 cases of 2019 novel coronavirus pneumonia in Wuhan, China: A descriptive study. *Lancet, 395*(10223), 507–513.
4. Javaid, M., Vaishya, R., Bahl, S., Suman, R., & Vaish, A. (2020). Industry 4.0 technologies and their applications in fighting COVID-19 pandemic. *Diabetes & Metabolic Syndrome: Clinical Research & Reviews*. https://doi.org/10.1016/j.dsx.2020.04.032.

5. Singh, R. P., Javaid, M., Haleem, A., & Suman, R. (2020). Internet of Things (IoT) applications to fight against COVID-19 pandemic. *Diabetes & Metabolic Syndrome: Clinical Research & Reviews, 14*, 521–524.
6. Pang, Z. (2013, January). *Technologies and architectures of the Internet-of-Things (IoT) for health and well-being* (M.S. thesis). Dept. Electron. Comput. Syst., KTH-Roy. Inst. Technol., Stockholm, Sweden.
7. Vasanth, K., & Sbert, J. Creating solutions for health through technology innovation. *Texas Instruments*. [Online]. Available: http://www.ti.com/lit/wp/sszy006/sszy006.pdf. Accessed 15.7.2020.
8. Zhao, W., Chaowei, W., & Nakahira, Y. (2011, October). Medical application on Internet of Things. In *Proc. IET Int. Conf. Commun. Technol. Appl. (ICCTA)* (pp. 660–665).
9. Mcneil Jr, D. G. (2020, March). Can smart thermometers track the spread of the Coronavirus? *The New York Times*. [Online]. Available: https://www.nytimes.com/2020/03/18/health/coronavirusfever-thermometer%s.html
10. Oliveira, G. A. (2016). *A model for historical management of physiological contexts* (Master thesis). Integrated postgraduate program in applied computing, University of Vale do Rio dos Sinos.
11. Portocarrero, J. M. T., Souza, W. L., Demarzo, M., & Prado, A. F. (2010). Brazilian digital library of computing. In *X Medical Informatics workshop*.
12. Rios, T. S., & Bezerra, R. M. S. (2015). WHMS4: An integrated model for health remote monitoring: A case study in nursing homes for the elderly. In *10th Iberian conference on information systems and technologies*.
13. Raad, M. W., Sheltami, T., & Shakshuki, E. (2015). Ubiquitous tele-health system for elderly patients with alzheimer's. *Procedia Computer Science, 52*, 685–689.
14. Yannone, T. (2020, April). Could fitness wearables help detect early signs of COVID-19? *Boston Magazine*. [Online]. Available: https://www.bostonmagazine.com/health/2020/04/03/_tness-wearablescoro%navirus/
15. Berryhill, S., Morton, C. J., Dean, A., Berryhill, A., Provencio-Dean, N., Patel, S. I., Estep, L., Combs, D., Mashaqi, S., & Gerald, L. B. (2020, February). Effect of wearables on sleep in healthy individuals: A randomized cross-over trial and validation study. *Journal of Clinical Sleep Medicine*, 8356. https://doi.org/10.5664/jcsm.8356.
16. Life Signals. *Covid-19 remote health monitoring in hospitals and at home*. [Online]. Available: https://lifesignals.com/covid19/. Accessed 20 Apr 2020.
17. NS Medical Devices. (2020, April). *LifeSignals to roll out biosensor patch for COVID-19 monitoring*. [Online]. Available: https://www.nsmedicaldevices.com/news/lifesignals-biosensor-patchcovid%-19/
18. Watson, J., & Builta, J. (2020, April). IoT set to play a growing role in the COVID-19 response_Omdia. *OMDIA*. [Online]. Available: https://technology.informa.com/622426/iot-set-to-play-a-growingrole-in%-the-covid-19-response
19. D'mello. (2020, March). First IoT buttons shipped for rapid response to cleaning alerts. *IoT now_how to run an IoT enabled business*. [Online]. Available: https://www.iot-now.com/2020/03/24/101940-_rstiot-buttons-shipped-rap%id-response-cleaning-alerts/
20. Hollister, M. (2020, March). COVID-19: AI can help – But the right human input is key. *World Economic Forum*. [Online]. Available: https://www.weforum.org/agenda/2020/03/covid-19-crisis-arti_cialintel%ligence-creativity/
21. Naude, W. (2020, April). Artificial intelligence against covid-19: An early review. *Medium*. [Online]. Available: https://towardsdatascience.com/arti_cial-intelligence-against-covid-19%-an-early-review-92a8360edaba
22. Alladi, T., Chamola, V., Sahu, N., & Guizani, M. (2020, June). Applications of blockchain in unmanned aerial vehicles: A review. *Vehicular Communications, 23*, 100249.
23. Alladi, T., Chamola, V., Parizi, R. M., & Choo, K.-K.-R. (2019). Blockchain applications for industry 4.0 and industrial IoT: A review. *IEEE Access, 7*, 176935–176951.

24. Miglani, N., Kumar, V. C., & Zeadally, S. (2020, February). Blockchain for Internet of energy management: Review, solutions, and challenges. *Computer Communications, 151*, 395–418.
25. Alladi, T., Chamola, V., Rodrigues, J. J. P. C., & Kozlov, S. A. (2019). Blockchain in smart grids: A review on different use cases. *Sensors, 19*(22), 4862.
26. Hassija, V., Chamola, V., Dara, N. G. K., & Guizani, M. (2020). A distributed framework for energy trading between UAVs and charging stations. *IEEE Transactions on Vehicular Technology*. https://doi.org/10.1109/TVT.2020.2977036.
27. Blockchain Pulse: IBM Blockchain Blog. (2020, March). *MiPasa project and IBM blockchain team on open data platform to support COVID-19 response*. [Online]. Available: https://www.ibm.com/blogs/blockchain/2020/03/mipasa-project-andibm-blo%ckchain-team-on-open-data-platform-to-support-covid-19-response/
28. Wright, T. (2020, April 7). *Blockchain app used to track COVID-19 cases in Latin America*. [Online]. Available: https://cointelegraph.com/news/blockchain-app-used-to-track-covid-19-ca%ses-in-latin-america
29. Alladi, T., Chamola, V., Sikdar, B., & Choo, K.-K.-R. (2020, March). Consumer IoT: Security vulnerability case studies and solutions. *IEEE Consumer Electronics Magazine, 9*(2), 17–25.
30. AMD Telemedicine. *Telemedicine defined*. [Online]. Available: https://www.amdtelemedicine.com/telemedicineresources/telemedicine def%ined.html. Accessed 20 Apr 2020.
31. Shah, M., & Tosto, A. (2020, April). Industry voices-how Rush University Medical Center's virtual investments became central to its COVID-19 response. *FierceHealthcare*. [Online]. Available: https://www.fiercehealthcare.com/hospitals-health systems/industryvoic%es-how-rush-university-system-for-health-s-virtual
32. The Hindu BusinessLine. (2020, April). *Covid-19: AP launches telemedicine facility*. [Online]. Available: https://www.thehindubusinessline.com/news/national/covid-19-ap-launches%-telemedicine-facility/article31332943.ece
33. Chakraborty, A. (2020, April). Assam: Telemedicine, video monitoring for COVID-19 home quarantined people in Dhemaji. *Northeast Now*. [Online]. Available: https://nenow.in/health/assam-telemedicine-videomonitoring-for-covid-1%9-home-quarantined-people-in-dhemaji.html
34. Chauhan, V., Galwankar, S., Arquilla, B., Garg, M., Di Somma, S., El-Menyar, A., Krishnan, V., Gerber, J., Holland, R., & Stawicki, S. P. (2020). Novel coronavirus (COVID-19): Leveraging telemedicine to optimize care while minimizing exposures and viral transmission. *Journal of Emergencies, Trauma, and Shock, 13*(1), 20.
35. Comstock, J. (2020, February). Israel's Sheba Hospital turns to telehealth to treat incoming coronavirus-exposed patients. *MobiHealthNews*. [Online]. Available: https://www.mobihealthnews.com/news/europe/israels-shebahospital-turns%-telehealth-treat-incoming-coronavirus-exposed-patients
36. Chamola, V., Hassija, V., Gupta, V., & Guizani, M. (2020). A comprehensive review of the COVID-19 pandemic and the role of IoT, drones, AI, blockchain, and 5G in managing its impact. *IEEE Access, 8*, 90225–90265.
37. Pourhomayoun, M., Alshurafa, N., Dabiri, F., Ardestani, E., Samiee, A., Ghasemzadeh, H., & Sarrafzadeh, M. (2017). Why do we need a remote health monitoring system? A study on predictive analytics for heart failure patients. In *11th international conference on body area networks*.
38. EarlySense. (2017). *Early Sense One*. Retrieved from http://www.earlysense.com/earlysense-one/

# Chapter 8
# Optimum Distribution of Protective Materials for COVID−19 with a Discrete Binary Gaining-Sharing Knowledge-Based Optimization Algorithm

**Said Ali Hassan, Prachi Agrawal, Talari Ganesh, and Ali Wagdy Mohamed**

## 8.1 Introduction

Currently, the entire world is suffering from a global epidemic of COVID-19 that has infected thousands of people in almost all countries (Sara [21]). In December last year, Wuhan, in China, was the origin of pneumonia of unknown cause. Cases of COVID-19 are not limited to this city, and by January this year, assured cases were detected outside Wuhan [23].

The number of confirmed infected cases in all countries clarifies that this is a vast-evolving case, and new situation changes may not be represented at once [25]. Although the confirmed numbers in some countries are moderate till now, numbers are expected to increase exponentially as new cases are discovered and since the daily increasing rate is about 12% [27].

It is worth noting the importance of protective materials like respirator masks, medical gloves and disinfection fluids to both hospital crews and patients, especially those suspected of having the emerging coronavirus. Countries that have succeeded in slowing the prevalence of the emerging coronavirus have forced their citizens to wear masks in public places.

S. A. Hassan
Department of Operations Research and Decision Support, Faculty of Computers and Artificial Intelligence, Cairo University, Giza, Egypt

P. Agrawal · T. Ganesh
Department of Mathematics and Scientific Computing, National Institute of Technology Hamirpur, Hamirpur, Himachal Pradesh, India

A. W. Mohamed (✉)
Operations Research Department, Faculty of Graduate Studies for Statistical Research, Cairo University, Giza, Egypt

Wireless Intelligent Networks Center (WINC), School of Engineering and Applied Sciences, Nile University, Giza, Egypt



S. Kautish et al. (eds.), *Computational Intelligence Techniques for Combating COVID-19*, EAI/Springer Innovations in Communication and Computing,
https://doi.org/10.1007/978-3-030-68936-0_8

The vast majority of the infected people have contracted the infection in closed environments and in poorly ventilated spaces, such as public places, transportation, restaurants, cinemas, stores, hospitals and homes. Therefore, it is always essential to provide such places with protective materials.

The optimum distribution of protective materials for COVID-19 in network optimization is defined for scheduling the distribution truck with a maximum load capacity to a list of hospitals with known demanded quantities. The objective is to settle the foremost effective route for the distribution truck measured by maximizing the total delivered protective quantities in a certain limited time shift. The route starts from a predetermined store position and next proceeds to each chosen hospital exactly once and returns once more to the store.

The second section includes an overview of the new coronavirus (COVID-19). This information covers the COVID-19 that has infected thousands of people in almost all countries.

Section 8.3 is devoted to demonstrating the importance to provide hospitals with protective materials to protect medical personnel, patients and visitors. This section describes the problem under consideration to distribute protective materials to a group of hospitals in an optimal way so as to meet the needs of each hospital while increasing the total distributed protective materials during a specified time shift.

The mathematical model of the problem is designed in Sect. 8.4 including all needed formulations. The proposed formulation is a nonlinear binary mathematical model with a dimension depending on the number of candidate hospitals to be visited; the steps of the solution procedure are also explained.

A real application case study is presented in Sect. 8.5, and in Sect. 8.6, a novel discrete binary version of a recently developed gaining-sharing knowledge-based optimization technique (GSK) is introduced for solving the problem. GSK cannot solve the problem with discrete binary space; therefore, discrete binary GSK optimization algorithm (DBGSK) is proposed with two new discrete binary junior and senior stages. These stages allow DBGSK to inspect the problem search space efficiently.

Section 8.7 represents the experimental results of the problem obtained by DBGSK, and Sect. 8.8 summarizes the conclusions and the suggested points for future researches.

## 8.2 Coronavirus (COVID-19): An Overview

Nowadays, the new coronavirus (COVID-19) put humans in all countries in front of a huge danger. Its spread all over the world is continuously increasing; the coronavirus disease (COVID-19) is affecting 213 countries and territories around the world and 2 international conveyances. The total number of cases is 22,640,172 in September 1, 2020, the total deaths are 792,204, and the total recovered is 15,356,056. Current number of infected patients is 6,491,912, [31]. Figure 8.1 represents the worldwide daily confirmed cases until August 20, 2020 [28].

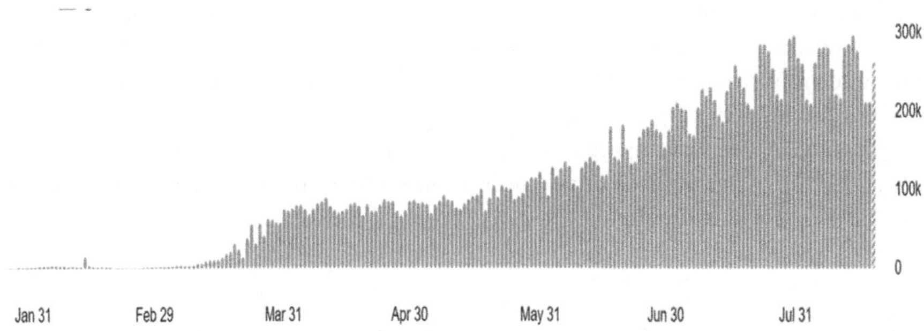


**Fig. 8.1** Worldwide confirmed cases for COVID-19

Current evidence suggests that COVID-19 spreads between people through direct, indirect (through contaminated objects or surfaces) or close contact with infected people via mouth and nose secretions. These include saliva, respiratory secretions or secretion droplets. These are released from the mouth or nose when an infected person coughs, sneezes, speaks or sings. People who are in close contact (within 1 metre) with an infected person can catch COVID-19 when those infectious droplets get into their mouth, nose or eyes.

To avoid contact with these droplets, it is important to stay at least 1 metre away from others, clean hands frequently and cover the mouth with a tissue or bent elbow when sneezing or coughing. When physical distancing (standing 1 metre or more away) is not possible, wearing a fabric mask is an important measure to protect others. Cleaning hands frequently is also critical.

People with the virus in their noses and throats may leave infected droplets on objects and surfaces when they sneeze, cough on or touch surfaces. Other people may become infected by touching these objects or surfaces and then touching their eyes, noses or mouths before cleaning their hands.

To safeguard against disease, various centres of virus disinfection recommend many precautions, among them to stay at home except in cases of necessity and to thoroughly clean hands regularly with soap and water or an alcohol-based hand rub product and to clean surfaces regularly [29].

The Centers for Disease Control and Prevention (CDC) declares the major signs of COVID-19 so that any individual can discover whether or not he/she has such symptoms (Centers for Decease Control and Prevention [3] and Guan et al. [7]).

The risk in these diseases is that there is no vaccine for treatment yet; and antibiotics will not help with them. The matter is further complicated by the fact that the incubation period of the virus is up to 14 days; therefore, officials of the examination at airports and other examination places will not be able to discover all the possible patients carrying the disease.

The greatest risk also lies in travelling from one country to another, (Centers for Disease Control and Prevention [3]). Coronavirus cases, deaths and Recovered cases are declared regularly [32]. The growth factor of daily new cases which is the factor by which a quantity multiplies itself over time shows a growth factor permanently greater than 1 in many countries indicating an exponential growth [33]. Nowadays, it is shown clearly that the current and the near future situations are not quite right if the situation continues as it is now and if strict measures are not taken at the level of governments and peoples.

The rate of the virus spreading is affirmed by its reproductive number, represented by the mean number of people for whom one infected person will transmit the disease. It was estimated in the early stages of the disease to be 2.2 [11].

## 8.3 Distribution of Coronavirus Protective Materials

Protective materials can limit the quantities of viruses that travel through respiratory droplets. They contribute to limiting transmission of infection between people in gatherings, especially on public transport and crowded places.

Frontline workers in medical institutions who wore the "N95" respirator mask did not catch the virus, although they were taking care of the infected patients. That is why it is very important to provide public places and hospital at the top of the list with adequate amounts of these protective materials regularly.

The importance of protective materials and wearing masks in public places is that between 6 and 18 per cent of infected people may not show any symptoms of the disease despite being able to spread the infection. It is worth to mention that the incubation period of the virus may be up to 14 days before symptoms appear. If everyone, especially asymptomatic, wears masks, the number of viruses circulating in the air will decrease, and the risk of transmission will be less. This is because when the newly created coronavirus penetrates and multiplies, viral particles exit from the cells and enter the body fluids in the lungs, mouth and nose. When the person coughs, the tiny droplets that are filled with viruses sprinkle in the air.

About 3000 drops of spray may come out of the mouth of the person during one sneeze, and some fear that the virus will spread through the spray that comes out of the mouth while speaking. Once the spray comes out of the mouth, the larger droplets settle on the surfaces, while the smaller droplets remain suspended in the air for hours, until a healthy person inhales them.

Rothe et al. [20] studied the transmission of 2019-nCoV infection from an asymptomatic contact in Germany, Zou et al. [35] studied the SARS-CoV-2 viral load in upper respiratory specimens of infected patients, Wei et al. [24] studied the Presymptomatic Transmission of SARS-CoV-2 – Singapore, January 23-March 16, 2020 and Li et al. [12] clarify that substantial undocumented infection facilitates the rapid dissemination of novel coronavirus (SARS-CoV-2).

Masks are recommended as a simple barrier to help prevent respiratory droplets from travelling into the air and onto other people; this is called source control. This recommendation is based on what we know about the role respiratory droplets play in the spread of the virus that causes COVID−19, paired with emerging evidence from clinical and laboratory studies that shows masks reduce the spray of droplets when worn over the nose and mouth.

Masks should be used as part of a comprehensive strategy of measures to suppress transmission and save lives; the use of a mask alone is not sufficient to provide an adequate level of protection against COVID−19. People should also maintain a minimum physical distance of at least 1 metre from others, frequently clean hands and avoid touching the face and mask.

Masks can protect people from getting infected, as well as can prevent those who have symptoms from spreading them. WHO recommends the following groups to use medical masks: health workers; anyone with symptoms suggestive of COVID−19, including people with mild symptoms; and people caring for suspect or confirmed cases of COVID−19 outside of health facilities. Medical masks are also recommended for these at-risk people, when they are in areas of widespread transmission and they cannot guarantee a distance of at least 1 metre from others [30]. Davies et al. [4] concluded that masks significantly reduced the number of microorganisms expelled by volunteers, and Konda et al. [9] studied the aerosol filtration efficiency of common fabrics used in respiratory cloth masks. Aydin et al. [1] perform a quantitative mechanistic study of the performance of fabrics for home-made masks against spread of respiratory infection through droplets, Ma et al. [14] demonstrated the potential utilities of mask-wearing and instant hand hygiene for fighting SARS-CoV − 2, and Leung et al. [10] discussed the efficacy of face masks for respiratory virus shedding in exhaled breath.

The conclusion is that if the coronavirus is given favourable opportunities, it may remain suspended in the air for several hours and still be able to transmit to people who inhale the droplets. The virus appears to be able to circulate through the air particularly in closed environments.

Hospitals and health centres are at the top of the list of public places, and attention should be paid to the continuous and timely supply of the required protection materials. The medical teams and employees are the first line of defence in the face of the pandemic, because they are exposed to patients and visitors who may be infected with the virus.

The problem under consideration is how to distribute protective materials to a group of hospitals – as a good example of public places – in an optimal way. A heavy transport vehicle carrying a large amount of these protective materials moves from one of the stores and distributes them to hospitals so as to meet the needs of each hospital. The needed amount is determined according to the number of medical crews, attending patients and the number of visitors. The distribution process takes place within a limited period, the shift of a driver and his companions. The problem begins with considering several hospitals to be supplied and then determining the optimal choice of some or all these hospitals during the limited shift time so that the largest amount of these protective materials are distributed. With the preparation of a new list of hospitals including those that were not provided with protective materials, the process is repeated in the same way till the provision of all hospitals.

## 8.4 Mathematical Model for the Optimum Distribution of Protective Materials

The distribution of protective material problem is designated over a graph $G$ with a set of $n$ nodes $V$ representing the hospitals, and an additional node denotes the store location where the truck starts the job and a set of arcs representing the transportation times between two distinct hospitals. The required quantity of materials for each hospital, the delivery truck capacity, the time of delivery of protective materials to each hospital and the transportation time between two hospitals are specified.

The problem is then defined as:

- Each hospital is visited only once to supply the protective materials.
- The route starts and ends at the store location from where the protective materials are supplied.
- The overall goal of the problem to be achieved is the best utilization of the available time, calculated as the total amount of distributed protective materials.

**Mathematical Model**

*Decision Variables*

Let:

$$x_i^m = \begin{cases} 1, & \textit{if hospital } i \textit{ is approached by the heavy distribution truck on position } m \textit{ of the route, } i \textit{ and } m = 1,2,\ldots,n \\ 0, & \textit{Otherwise} \end{cases}$$

where:

$n$ = number of candidate hospitals.

**Constraints**

(1) *Position Constraints*

Each position $m$ in the optimum chosen route has at most one hospital:

$$\sum_{i=1}^{n} x_i^m \le 1, m = 1,2,\ldots,n. \tag{8.1}$$

(2) *Hospital Constraints*

Each hospital $i$ can be in one position of the truck route or not visited:

$$\sum_{m=1}^{n} x_i^m \le 1, i = 1,2,\ldots,n. \tag{8.2}$$

(3) *Consecutive Position Constraints*

A position ($m$ + 1) cannot exist in the distribution route unless the preceding position $m$ exists; this is achieved by the following set of constraints:

$$\sum_{i=1}^{n} x_i^{m+1} \leq \sum_{i=1}^{n} x_i^{m}, m = 1,2,\ldots,n-1 \tag{8.3}$$

If $\sum_{i=1}^{n} x_i^{m+1} = 1$, then $\sum_{i=1}^{n} x_i^{m} = 1$, $m = 1, 2, \ldots, n - 1$.

If $\sum_{i=1}^{n} x_i^{m+1} = 0$, then there is no restriction on the value of $\sum_{i=1}^{n} x_i^{m}$, $m = 1, 2, \ldots, n - 1$.

(4) *Avoid the Trivial Solution*

(a) In order to avoid the trivial solution that the truck will be saturated with supply for one hospital only, the following condition should hold: The quantity of protective materials to be supplied to any candidate hospital should be smaller than the maximum carrying capacity of the used truck. In case of violation, the truck will travel to that hospital and deliver its total capacity, and there is no need to perform the scheduling process.

(b) In order to avoid the trivial solution that the truck can deliver the needed protective materials to all hospitals, and hence the route is known in advance, and the problem in this case will be to minimize the total transportation distances, the following condition should hold: The total quantities of protective materials to be delivered for all candidate hospitals should be greater than the maximum carrying capacity of the used truck.

These two conditions should be checked before designing the mathematical model.

(5) *Shift Hour Constraint*

The total time $T$ spent in the whole route by the distribution truck is equal to four parts as:

$$T = T_1 + T_2 + T_3 + T_4$$

where:

$T_1$ = time of transportation from the starting store to the first hospital in the route.
$T_2$ = total intermediate transportation times between two adjacent hospitals in the route.
$T_3$ = transportation time spent from the last visited hospital to the starting store.
$T_4$ = total time for delivery, counting and inspection in visited hospitals

$$T_1 = \sum_{i=1}^{n} t_{0,i} x_i^1 \tag{8.4}$$

where:

$t_{0i}$ = transportation time between the starting store and hospital $i$, $\forall\, i \in V$.

$$T_2 = \sum_{i=1}^{n} \sum_{\substack{j=1 \\ j \neq i}}^{n} t_{i,j} \cdot \left( \sum_{m=1}^{n-1} x_i^m . x_j^{m+1} \right) \tag{8.5}$$

where:

$t_{i,j}$ = transportation time between the two adjacent hospitals $i$ and $j$, $\forall i, j \in V$.

Before adding $T_3$, it is necessary at first to determine exactly which hospital is the last visited one in the route of the truck taking into consideration (after avoiding the first trivial solution) that the first visited position hospital in the solution route will not be the last visited hospital.

The last visited hospital position in the determined route is characterized by a unique particularity not available in other hospitals. The last visited hospital doesn't have any adjacent subsequent positions except the case where the $n$ hospitals are visited. This property will be used to determine the hospital $i$ which is located at the last position of the truck route.

The hospital following directly to any position ($m > 1$) in the route is one of the following sets of decision variables:

$$F^{m+1} = \sum_{i=1}^{n} x_i^{m+1} \tag{8.6}$$

The expression ($x_i^m$).($1 - F^{m+1}$) = 1 is only for the last position in the truck route and equals 0 for all other positions; then:

$$T_3 = \sum_{m=2}^{n-1} \sum_{i=1}^{n} \left( t_{0,i} . x_i^m \right) . \left( 1 - \sum_{i=1}^{n} x_i^{m+1} \right) + \sum_{i=1}^{n} t_{i,0} . x_i^n \tag{8.7}$$

where:

$t_{0,i}$= transportation time between the starting store and hospital $i$ and $\forall\, i \in V$.

The second term in (8.7) is added such that in case the route will visit all the candidate $n$ hospitals. In that case the corresponding distance between the hospital in position $n$ of the route and the starting store will be added; otherwise it will not be added since in such a case $x_i^n = 0\ \forall i \in V$.

$$T_4 = \sum_{m=1}^{n} \sum_{i=1}^{n} \left( t_i x_i^m \right) \tag{8.8}$$

From (8.4), (8.5), (8.6), (8.7) and (8.8), the total time of the whole route will have the form:

$$\begin{aligned}&\left\{\sum_{i=1}^{n} t_{0i} x_i^1\right\}+\left\{\sum_{i=1}^{n}\sum_{\substack{j=1\\ j\neq i}}^{n} t_{i,j}\cdot\left(\sum_{m=1}^{n-1} x_i^m . x_j^{m+1}\right)\right\}\\&+\left\{\sum_{m=2}^{n-1}\left[\sum_{i=1}^{n}\left(t_{i,0}.x_i^m\right).\left(1-\sum_{i=1}^{n} x_i^{m+1}\right)\right]\right\}\\&+\left\{\sum_{i=1}^{n} t_{i,0}.x_i^n\right\}+\left\{\sum_{m=1}^{n}\sum_{i=1}^{n}(t_i x_i^m)\right\}\leq T\end{aligned} \tag{8.9}$$

This is a quadratic inequality in two variables; the first part is for the transportation distance from the starting airport to the first position airport in the route, the second part is the total travelled distance between intermediate airports in the route, the third part is the distance between the positions in the route and the starting airport (except the case where all the n airports are visited), and the fourth part is the distance between the starting airport and the airport number $n$ if it is in the last positions in the route.

(6) *Maximum Load Constraints*

The maximum quantity distributed to all visited hospital in any time shift should not exceed the maximum load of the transportation truck measured in weight.

$$\sum_{i=1}^{n} q_i\cdot\left(\sum_{m=1}^{n} x_i^m\right)\leq Q \tag{8.10}$$

where:

$q_i$ = quantity of protective materials required for hospital $i$, $i = 1, 2, \ldots, n$.
$Q$ = maximum load of the transportation truck.

(7) *Binary Constraints*

All the decision variables are 0–1.

$$x_i^m == 0 \text{ or } 1; i, m = 1, 2, \ldots, n. \tag{8.11}$$

(8) *The Objective Function*

The objective function is formulated to maximize the total amount of delivered protection materials as follows:

$$Maximize\ Z=\sum_{i=1}^{n} q_i\cdot\left(\sum_{m=1}^{n} x_i^m\right) \tag{8.12}$$

where:

$q_i$ = quantity of protective materials required by hospital number $i$, $i = 1, 2, \ldots, n$.

Finally, we have a suggested a model that contains ($n^2$) binary variables and ($4n + 1$) constraints.

An optimal solution to the problem will produce two distinct situations:

1. If $\sum_{m=1}^{n} x_i^m = 1$, $i = 1, 2, \ldots, n$, then all the $n$ hospitals are supplied by the needed protective materials in one shift, and the problem is completed.
2. If $\sum_{m=1}^{n} x_i^m = 0$ for any $i$, then the corresponding hospital $i$ is not supplied by the needed materials in the first considered shift. In this case, it is needed to eliminate the visited hospitals, add other candidate hospitals to be supplied, consider one more shift and then repeat the procedure once more.

The solution procedure is presented in Fig. 8.2.

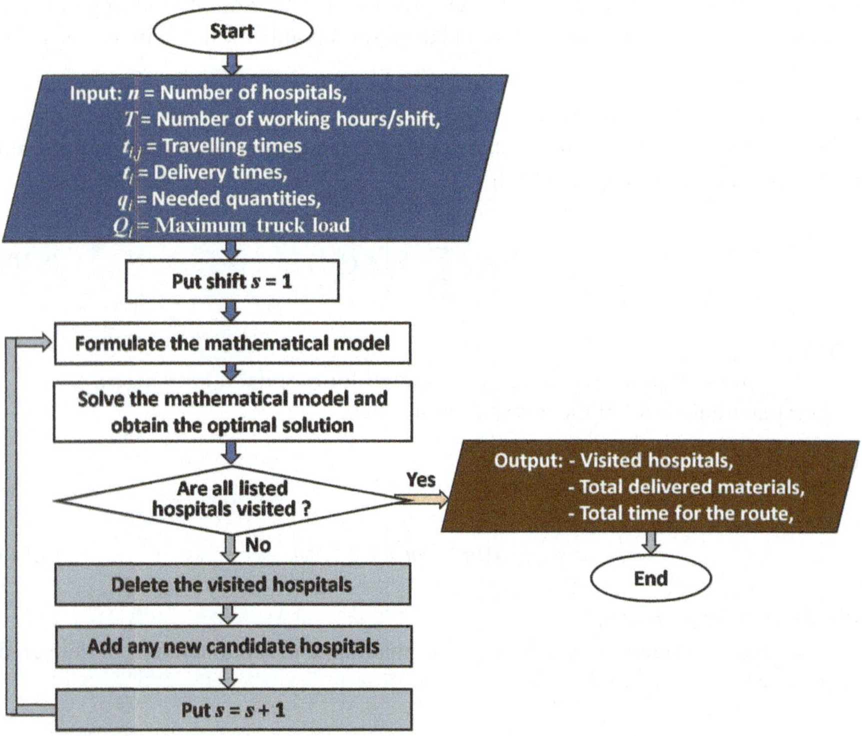


**Fig. 8.2** Steps of the solution procedure of the problem

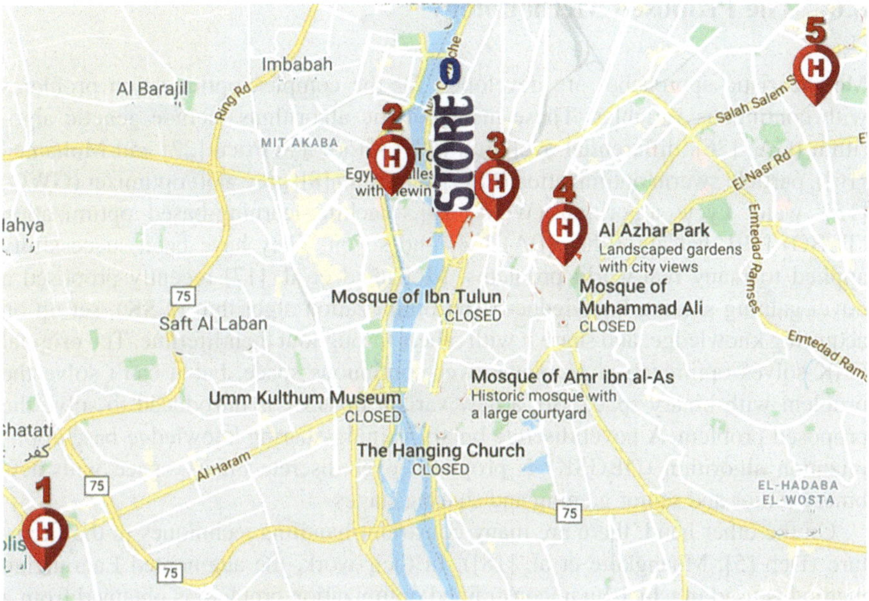


**Fig. 8.3** Locations of the store and hospitals for the example tour

**Table 8.1** Data for the Case Study Example

| $q_i$ | $i$ $j$ | 1 | 2 | 3 | 4 | 5 |
|---|---|---|---|---|---|---|
| **(×100 kg)** | **0** | 1.30 | 0.25 | 0.15 | 0.75 | 1.0 |
| 5 | **1** | | 1.5 | 1.5 | 1.65 | 1.7 |
| 1 | **2** | | | 0.167 | 0.7 | 0.6 |
| 5 | **3** | | | | 0.65 | 0.5 |
| 3.5 | **4** | | | | | 0.7 |
| 2 | **5** | | | | | |

## 8.5 Real Application Case Study

In this case, a real example is presented for the mathematical model application that a heavy truck starts its route from the store of protective materials in location (STORE) in Fig. 8.3. In one shift that lasts 9 hours, five hospitals are identified to choose between them; these hospitals are denoted by serial numbers (1, 2, …, 5), where the store is denoted by (0), and all are located at different places in Great Cairo Governorate with the data given in Table 8.1, where numbers inside the cells $(i, j)$ represent the transportation times $t_{ij}$. For simplicity, the time of delivery, counting and inspection for all hospitals is considered to be equal, $t_i = 1$ hour, $i = 1, 2, \ldots, 5$.

The mathematical formulation for the given case is worked out by substituting in the previously described model, formulas 8.1, 8.2, 8.3, 8.9, 8.10, 8.11, and 8.12.

## 8.6 The Proposed Methodology

Metaheuristic approaches are developed for the complex optimization problems with continuous variables. These metaheuristic algorithms include genetic algorithm (GA) [26], differential evolution (DE) (Storn and Price [22] and Mohamed [16]), particle swarm optimization (PSO) algorithm [8], grey wolf optimizer (GWO) [15], water cycle algorithm (WCA) [6], teaching-learning-based optimization (TLBO) [19], bat algorithm (BA) [34] and so on. They have been successfully applied to many real-world problems. Mohamed et al. [17] recently proposed a novel gaining-sharing knowledge-based optimization algorithm (GSK), set up on acquiring knowledge, and share it with others throughout their lifetime. The original GSK solves optimization problems over continuous space, but it can't solve the problem with binary space. So, a new variant of GSK is introduced to solve the proposed problem. A novel discrete binary gaining-sharing knowledge-based optimization algorithm (DBGSK) is proposed over discrete binary space with new binary junior and senior gaining and sharing stages.

On the other hand, there are many constraint-handling techniques in the literature (Deb [5], Muangkote et al. [18]). In their work, the augmented Lagrangian method is used in which an unconstrained optimization problem is obtained from a constrained optimization one (Long et al. [13], Bahreininejad [2]). The proposed methodology is described below:

### *8.6.1 Gaining-Sharing Knowledge-Based Optimization Algorithm (GSK)*

An optimization problem with constraints can be formulated as:

$$\begin{aligned} \min \quad & f(X);\ X = [x_1, x_2, \ldots, x_{\dim}] \\ s.to. \quad & g_i(X) \le 0;\ i = 1, 2, \ldots, m \\ & X \in [\alpha_p, \beta_p];\ p = 1, 2, \ldots, \dim \end{aligned}$$

where $f$ denotes the objective function; $X = [x_1, x_2, \ldots, x_{\mathrm{Dim}}]$ are the decision variables; $g_i(X)$ are the inequality constraints; and $\alpha_p$, $\beta_p$ are the lower and upper bounds of decision variables, respectively, and Dim represents the dimension of individuals. If the problem is in maximization form, then consider minimization = − maximization.

The human-based algorithm GSK is of two stages: junior and senior gaining and sharing stage. All persons acquire knowledge and share their views with others. The people from early stage gain knowledge from their small networks such as family members, relatives, neighbours, etc. and want to share their opinions with the others who might not be from their networks, due to curiosity of exploring others. These may not have the experience to categorize the people. In the same way, the people from the middle or later age enhance their knowledge by interacting with friends, colleagues, social media friends, etc. and share their views with the most suitable person, so that they can improve their knowledge. These people have the experience to judge other people and can categorize them (good or bad). The process mentioned above can be formulated mathematically in the following steps:

*Step 1*: To get a starting point of the optimization problem, the initial population must be obtained. The initial population is created randomly within the boundary constraints as:

$$x_{tp}^{0} = \alpha_p + rand_p\left(\beta_p - \alpha_p\right) \tag{8.13}$$

where $t$ is for the number of populations and $rand_p$ denotes random number uniformly distributed between 0 and 1.

*Step 2*: At this step, the dimensions of junior and senior stages should be computed through the following formula:

$$\mathrm{Dim}_J = \mathrm{dim} \times \left( \frac{\mathrm{Gen}^{\max} - G}{\mathrm{Gen}^{\max}} \right)^k \tag{8.14}$$

$$\mathrm{Dim}_S = \mathrm{dim} - \mathrm{Dim}_J \tag{8.15}$$

where $k$ (>0) denotes the learning rate that monitors the experience rate. $\mathrm{Dim}_J$ and $\mathrm{Dim}_S$ represent the dimension for the junior and senior stage, respectively. $\mathrm{Gen}^{\max}$ is the maximum count of generations, and G is the count of generation.

```
for t=1:NP
    for p=1:Dim
        if rand≤ k_r (knowledge ratio)
            if f(x_t) > f(x_r)
                x_tp^new = (x_t + k_f * ((x_{t-1} - x_{t+1}) + (x_r - x_t)))
            else
                x_tp^new = (x_t + k_f * ((x_{t-1} - x_{t+1}) + (x_t - x_r)))
            end
        else  x_tp^new = x_tp^old
    end
end
end
```

**Fig. 8.4** Pseudocode for junior gaining-sharing knowledge stage

*Step 3*: Junior gaining-sharing knowledge stage. In this stage, the early aged people gain knowledge from their small networks and share their views with the other people who may or may not belong to their group. Thus, individuals are updated as follows:

(i) According to the objective function values, the individuals are arranged in ascending order. For every $x_t$ $(t = 1,2,\ldots,NP)$, select the nearest best $(x_{t-1})$ and worst $(x_{t+1})$ to gain knowledge; also choose randomly $(x_r)$ to share knowledge. Therefore, to update the individuals, the pseudocode is presented in Fig. 8.4, where $k_f(>0)$ is the knowledge factor.

*Step 4*: Senior gaining-sharing knowledge stage. This stage comprises the impact and effect of other people (good or bad) on the individual. The updated individual can be determined as follows:

(i) The individuals are classified into three categories (best, middle and worst) after sorting individuals into ascending order (based on the objective function values).
(ii) Best individual=100 $p\%$ $(x_{\text{best}})$, middle individual=Dim $- 2 * 100p\%$ $(x_{\text{middle}})$, and worst individual=100 $p\%(x_{\text{worst}})$.
(iii) For every individual $x_t$, choose the top and bottom 100 $p\%$ individuals for gaining part, and the third one (middle individual) is chosen for the sharing part. Therefore, the new individual is updated through the following pseudocode dictated in Fig. 8.5.

where $p \in [0, 1]$ is the percentage of best and worst classes.

```
for t=1:NP
  for p=1:Dim
    if rand≤ k_r (knowledge ratio)
        if f(x_t) > f(x_r)
            x_tp^new = (x_t + k_f * ((x_{t-1} - x_{t+1}) + (x_r - x_t)))
            else
            x_tp^new = (x_t + k_f * ((x_{t-1} - x_{t+1}) + (x_t - x_r)))
        end
      else  x_tp^new = x_tp^old
    end
  end
end
```

**Fig. 8.5** Pseudocode of senior gaining-sharing knowledge stage

### 8.6.2 *Discrete Binary Gaining-Sharing Knowledge-Based Optimization Algorithm (DBGSK)*

For solving problems in discrete binary space, a novel discrete binary gaining-sharing knowledge-based optimization algorithm (DBGSK) is suggested. In DBGSK, the new initialization and the working mechanism of both stages (junior and senior gaining-sharing stages) are introduced over discrete binary space, and the remaining algorithms remain the same as the previous one. The working mechanism of DBGSK is presented in the following subsections:

**Discrete Binary Initialization**

The initial population is obtained in GSK using Eq. (8.13), and it must be updated using the following equation for binary population:

$$x_{tp}^{0} = \text{round}\left(rand\left(0,1\right)\right) \tag{8.16}$$

where the round operator is used to convert the decimal number into the nearest binary number.

**Discrete Binary Junior Gaining and Sharing Stage**

The discrete binary junior gaining and sharing stage is based on the original GSK with $k_f = 1$. The individuals are updated in original GSK using the pseudocode (Fig. 8.6) which contains two cases. These two cases are defined for discrete binary stage as follows:

**Case 1. When** $f(x_r) < f(x_t)$: There are three different vectors $(x_{t-1}, x_{t+1}, x_r)$, which can take only two values (0 and 1). Therefore, a total of $2^3$ combinations are possible, which are listed in Table 8.2. Furthermore, these eight combinations can be categorized into two different subcases [(a) and (b)], and each subcase has four combinations. The results of each possible combination are presented in Table 8.2.

```
Start
|    Initialize the value of parameters (Gen^max, NP, k_r, k , p)
|    Initialize the generation (G = 0)
|    Create discrete binary population using equation (11)
|    Evaluate f(x_t).
|    For G = 1 to Gen^max
|    |    Compute the dimensions of both stages (Discrete Binary junior
|    |    and senior gaining sharing stage)
|    |    Apply Discrete Binary Junior gaining sharing stage
|    |    Apply Discrete Binary Senior gaining sharing stage
|    |    Update the population
|    |    Select the global best solution
|    End
End
```

**Fig. 8.6** Pseudocode for DBGSK

**Table 8.2** Results of the discrete binary junior gaining and sharing stage of Case 1 with $k_f = 1$

| | $x_{t-1}$ | $x_{t+1}$ | $x_r$ | Results | Modified results |
|---|---|---|---|---|---|
| Subcase (a) | 0 | 0 | 0 | 0 | 0 |
| | 0 | 0 | 1 | 1 | 1 |
| | 1 | 1 | 0 | 0 | 0 |
| | 1 | 1 | 1 | 1 | 1 |
| Subcase(b) | 1 | 0 | 0 | 1 | 1 |
| | 1 | 0 | 1 | 2 | 1 |
| | 0 | 1 | 0 | −1 | 0 |
| | 0 | 1 | 1 | 0 | 0 |

**Table 8.3** Results of the discrete binary junior gaining and sharing stage of Case 2, $k_f = 1$

| | $x_{t-1}$ | $x_t$ | $x_{t+1}$ | $x_r$ | Results | Modified results |
|---|---|---|---|---|---|---|
| Subcase (c) | 1 | 1 | 0 | 0 | 3 | 1 |
| | 1 | 0 | 0 | 0 | 1 | 1 |
| | 0 | 1 | 1 | 1 | 0 | 0 |
| | 0 | 0 | 1 | I | −2 | 0 |
| Subcase (d) | 0 | 0 | 0 | 0 | 0 | 0 |
| | 0 | 1 | 0 | 0 | 2 | 1 |
| | 0 | 0 | 1 | 0 | −1 | 0 |
| | 0 | 0 | 0 | 1 | −1 | 0 |
| | 1 | 0 | 1 | 0 | 0 | 0 |
| | 1 | 0 | 0 | 1 | 0 | 0 |
| | 0 | 1 | 1 | 0 | 1 | 1 |
| | 0 | 1 | 0 | 1 | 1 | 1 |
| | 1 | 1 | 1 | 0 | 2 | 1 |
| | 1 | 0 | 1 | 1 | −1 | 0 |
| | 1 | 1 | 0 | 1 | 2 | 1 |
| | 1 | 1 | 1 | 1 | 1 | 1 |

*Subcase (a)*: If $x_{t-1}$ is equal to $x_{t+1}$, the result is equal to $x_r$.

*Subcase (b)*: When $x_{t-1}$ is not equal to $x_{t+1}$, then the result is the same as $x_{t-1}$ by taking −1 as 0 and 2 as 1.

The mathematical formulation of Case 1 is as follows:

$$x_{tp}^{\text{new}} = \begin{cases} x_r; & if\ x_{t-1} = x_{t+1} \\ x_{t-1}; & if\ x_{t-1} \neq x_{t+1} \end{cases}$$

**Case 2. When $f(x_r) \geq f(x_t)$:** There are four different vectors $(x_{t-1}, x_t, x_{t+1}, x_r)$ that consider only two values (0 and 1). Thus, there are $2^4$ possible combinations that are presented in Table 8.3. Moreover, the 16 combinations can be divided into 2 subcases [(c) and (d)] in which (c) and (d) have 4 and 12 combinations, respectively.

*Subcase (c)*: If $x_{t-1}$ is not equal to $x_{t+1}$, but $x_{t+1}$ is equal to $x_r$, the result is equal to $x_{t-1}$.

*Subcase (d)*: If any of the condition arise $x_{t-1} = x_{t+1} \neq x_r$ or $x_{t-1} \neq x_{t+1} \neq x_r$ or $x_{t-1} = x_{t+1} = x_r$ , the result is equal to $x_t$ by considering −1 and −2 as 0 and 2 and 3 as 1.

The mathematical formulation of Case 2 is as follows:

$$x_{tp}^{\text{new}} = \begin{cases} x_{t-1}; & \text{if } x_{t-1} \neq x_{t+1} = x_r \\ x_t; & \text{Otherwise} \end{cases}$$

**Discrete Binary Senior Gaining and Sharing Stage**

The working mechanism of discrete binary senior gaining and sharing stage is the same as the binary junior gaining and sharing stage with value of $k_f = 1$. The individuals are updated in the original senior gaining-sharing stage using pseudocode (Fig. 8.7) that contains two cases. The two cases are further modified for binary senior gaining-sharing stage in the following manner:

**Case 1.** $f(\mathbf{x}_{\text{middle}}) < f(x_t)$: It contains three different vectors ($x_{\text{best}}$, $x_{\text{middle}}$, $x_{\text{worst}}$), and they can assume only binary values (0 and 1); thus a total of eight combinations are possible to update the individuals. These eight combinations can be classified into two subcases [(a) and (b)], and each subcase contains only four different combinations. The obtained results of this case are presented in Table 8.4.

*Subcase (a)*: If $x_{\text{best}}$ is equal to $x_{\text{worst}}$, then the obtained results are equal to $x_{\text{middle}}$.

*Subcase (b)*: On the other hand, if $x_{\text{best}}$ is not equal to $x_{\text{worst}}$, then the results are equal to $x_{\text{best}}$ by assuming −1 or 2 is equivalent to their nearest binary value (0 and 1, respectively).

Case 1 can be mathematically formulated in the following way:

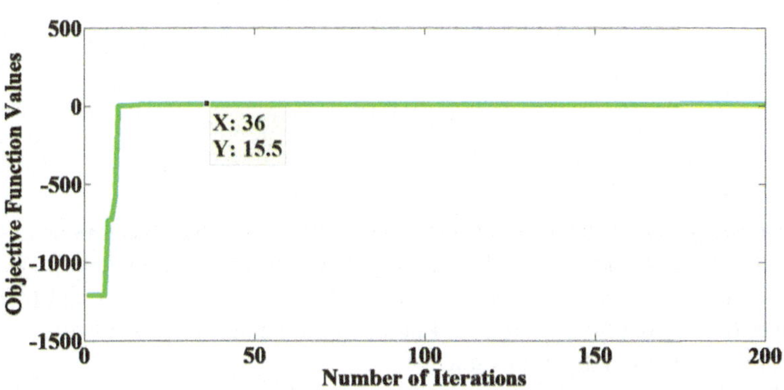


**Fig. 8.7** Convergence graph of DBGSK

**Table 8.4** Results of discrete binary senior gaining and sharing stage of Case 1 with $k_f = 1$

| | $x_{best}$ | $x_{worst}$ | $x_{middle}$ | Results | Modified results |
|---|---|---|---|---|---|
| Subcase (a) | 0 | 0 | 0 | 0 | 0 |
| | 0 | 0 | 1 | 1 | 1 |
| | 1 | 1 | 0 | 0 | 0 |
| | 1 | 1 | 1 | 1 | 1 |
| Subcase (b) | 1 | 0 | 0 | 1 | 1 |
| | 1 | 0 | 1 | 2 | 1 |
| | 0 | 1 | 0 | −1 | 0 |
| | 0 | 1 | 1 | 0 | 0 |

**Table 8.5** Results of discrete binary senior gaining and sharing stage of Case 2 with $k_f = 1$

| | $x_{best}$ | $x_t$ | $x_{worst}$ | $x_{middle}$ | Results | Modified results |
|---|---|---|---|---|---|---|
| Subcase (c) | 1 | 1 | 0 | 0 | 3 | 1 |
| | 1 | 0 | 0 | 0 | 1 | 1 |
| | 0 | 1 | 1 | 1 | 0 | 0 |
| | 0 | 0 | 1 | 1 | −2 | 0 |
| Subcase (d) | 0 | 0 | 0 | 0 | 0 | 0 |
| | 0 | 1 | 0 | 0 | 2 | 1 |
| | 0 | 0 | 1 | 0 | −1 | 0 |
| | 0 | 0 | 0 | 1 | −1 | 0 |
| | 1 | 0 | 1 | 0 | 0 | 0 |
| | 1 | 0 | 0 | 1 | 0 | 0 |
| | 0 | 1 | 1 | 0 | 1 | 1 |
| | 0 | 1 | 0 | 1 | 1 | 1 |
| | 1 | 1 | 1 | 0 | 2 | 1 |
| | 1 | 0 | 1 | 1 | −1 | 0 |
| | 1 | 1 | 0 | 1 | 2 | 1 |
| | 1 | 1 | 1 | 1 | 1 | 1 |

$$x_{tp}^{new} = \begin{cases} x_{middle}; & \text{if } x_{best} = x_{worst} \\ x_{best}; & \text{if } x_{best} \neq x_{worst} \end{cases}$$

**Case 2.** $f(x_{middle}) > f(x_t)$**:** It consists of four different binary vectors ($x_{best}$, $x_{middle}$, $x_{worst}$, $x_t$), and with the values of each vector, a total of 16 combinations are presented. The 16 combinations are also divided into 2 subcases [(c) and (d)]. The subcases (c) and (d) further contain 4 and 12 combinations, respectively. The subcases are explained in detail in Table 8.5.

*Subcase (c)*: When $x_{best}$ is not equal to $x_{worst}$ and $x_{worst}$ is equal to $x_{middle}$, then the obtained results are equal to $x_{best}$.

*Subcase (d)*: If any case arises other than (c), then the obtained results are equal to $x_t$ by taking −2 and −1 as 0 and 2 and 3 as 1.

The mathematical formulation of Case 2 is given as:

$$x_{tp}^{new} = \begin{cases} x_{best}; & \text{if } x_{best} \neq x_{worst} = x_{middle} \\ x_t; & \text{Otherwise} \end{cases}$$

The pseudocode of DBGSK is presented in Fig. 8.6.

## 8.7 Experimental Results

The problem is handled by using the proposed novel DBGSK algorithm, and the used parameters are presented in Table 8.6.

DBGSK runs over personal computer Intel® CoreTM i5-7200U CPU at 2.50 GHz and 4 GB RAM and coded on MATLAB R2015a. To get the optimal solutions, 30 independent runs are complete, and the obtained statistics are provided in Table 8.7, including the best, median, average and worst solutions and the DBGSK standard deviations. Moreover, Fig. 8.7 shows the convergence graph of the solutions using DBGSK. From the figure, it can be observed that after the 36th iteration, it converges to the global optimal solution (15.50), which shows the robustness of the DBGSK.

The route provided by the optimum solution can be seen in Fig. 8.8. The route begins in the store location (S) and then is composed of four hospital numbers 5, 4, 1 and 3 and finally returns to the store once more. The total protective materials supplied to the four hospitals is 1550 kg, and the total time for the route is 8 hours, which means that all the available working time shift is completely utilized.

The remaining unsupplied hospital (number 2) will be added to the new list of candidate hospitals, and the procedure is repeated once more for the next shift.

**Table 8.6** Numerical values of parameters

| Parameters of DBGSK | Considered values |
|---|---|
| NP | 800 |
| k | 10 |
| *Kr* | 0.9 |
| p | 0.1 |
| $k_f$ | 1 |
| Max number of iterations | 200 |

**Table 8.7** Statistical results using DBGSK

| Algorithm | Best (maximum) | Median | Average | Worst (minimum) | Standard deviation |
|---|---|---|---|---|---|
| DBGSK | 15.50 | 15.50 | 15.50 | 15.50 | 0.00 |

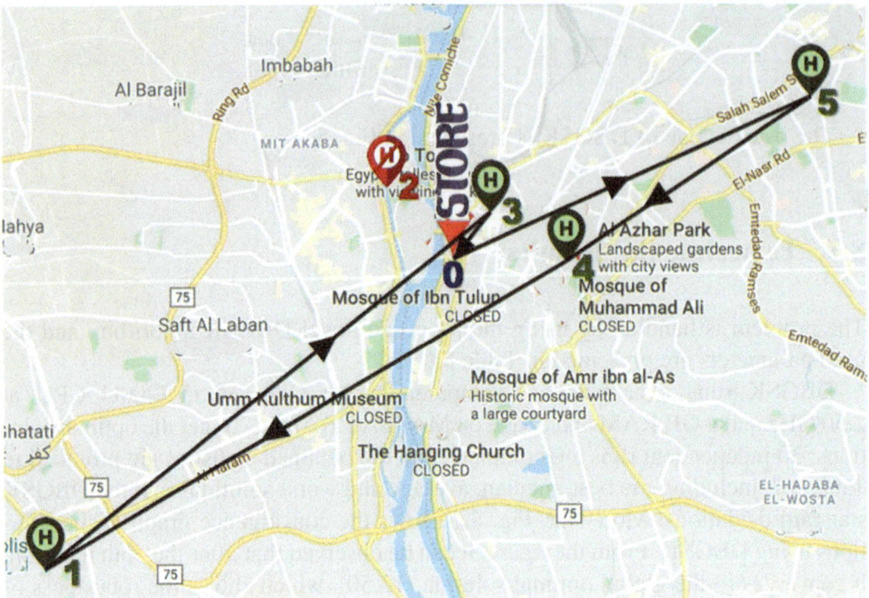


**Fig. 8.8** Optimum solution for the case study example

## 8.8 Conclusions and Points for Future Researches

The main conclusions for this paper can be summarized as follows:

1. An optimum distribution of COVID-19 protective materials which recently placed humans in front of a huge danger is presented. The distribution aims at achieving the maximum utilization of the available shift time, which is evaluated by maximizing the total distributed protective materials to hospitals in a specific time shift.
2. A nonlinear integer constrained mathematical programming model is formulated for the given problem. The integer decision variables represent the delivered quantities of protective materials to hospitals in the chosen route.
3. The mathematical model and the solution method are used to solve a real application case study for five hospitals in Cairo. Many application problems like this one are formulated as nonlinear integer mathematical programming models which are hard to be solved using exact algorithms especially in large dimensions.
4. The proposed problem is solved by a novel discrete integer gaining-sharing knowledge-based optimization algorithm (DBGSK), which involves two main stages: discrete binary junior and senior gaining and sharing stages with a knowledge factor $k_f = 1$. DBGSK is a discrete binary variant of GSK that solves the problem with binary decision variables.

5. DBGSK shows that it has the ability of finding the solutions of the introduced problem, and the obtained results demonstrate the robustness and convergence of DBGSK towards the optimal solutions.

The points for future researches can be stated in the following points:

1. To propose other mathematical models' formulation for the same problem comprising the designing of the objective function, the decision variables and the constraints and then comparing the effectiveness of computations for each model.
2. To apply the same problem formulation to other similar fields that can show up in many other material delivery domains like industry, agriculture, business, education, telecommunications, investing, quality assurance, social and community services, pollution, medical, tourism, marketing, sales, advertising, sports, arts, cooking and others. The only difference is the actual working time of the group in the considered field of study.
3. To check the performance of the DBGSK approach in solving different complex optimization problems, and further works can be investigated by the extension of DBGSK with different kinds of constraint-handling methods.

## References


1. Aydin, O., Emon, B., & Saif, M. T. A. (2020). Performance of fabrics for home-made masks against spread of respiratory infection through droplets: a quantitative mechanistic study. medRxiv preprint. https://doi.org/10.1101/2020.04.19.20071779, posted April 24, 2020.
2. Bahreininejad, A. (2019). Improving the performance of water cycle algorithm using augmented Lagrangian method. *Advances in Engineering Software, 132*, 55–64.
3. Centers of Disease Control and Prevention (CDC) website. (2020). Coronavirus disease 2019, retrieved on April 11, 2020 at: https://www.cdc.gov/
4. Davies, A., Thompson, K. A., Giri, K., Kafatos, G., Walker, J., & Bennett, A. (2013). Testing the efficacy of homemade masks: Would they protect in an influenza pandemic? *Disaster Medicine and Public Health Preparedness, 7*(4), 413–418.
5. Deb, K. (2000). An efficient constraint handling method for genetic algorithms. *Computer Methods in Applied Mechanics and Engineering, 186*(2–4), 311–338.
6. Eskandar, H., Sadollah, A., Bahreininejad, A., & Hamdi, M. (2012). Water cycle algorithm–A novel metaheuristic optimization method for solving constrained engineering optimization problems. *Computers & Structures, 110*, 151–166.
7. Guan, W., Ni, Z., Hu, Y., Liang, W., Ou, C., He, J., Liu, L., Shan, H., Lei, C., Hui, D. S. C., Du, B., & Li, L. (2019, February 28). Clinical characteristics of coronavirus disease 2019 in China. *The New England Journal of Medicine*. https://doi.org/10.1056/NEJMoa2002032. https://www.nejm.org/doi/full/10.1056/NEJMoa2002032.
8. Kennedy, J., & Eberhart, R. (1995). Particle swarm optimization. In *Proceedings of ICNN'95-International Conference on Neural Networks* (Vol. 4, pp. 1942–1948), November 1995, IEEE.
9. Konda A, Prakash A, Moss GA, Schmoldt M, Grant GD, & Guha S. (2020). Aerosol Filtration Efficiency of Common Fabrics Used in Respiratory Cloth Masks. ACS Nano. 2020 Apr 24.
10. Leung, N. H. L., Chu, D. K. W., Shiu, E. Y. C., et al. (2020). Respiratory virus shedding in exhaled breath and efficacy of face masks. *Nature Medicine, 26*(5), 676–680.
11. Li, J., Li, W. and Wang, H. (2015). The multiple knapsack problem with compatible bipartite graphs. *The 12th International Symposium on Operations Research and its Applications*

*in Engineering, Technology and Management (ISORA 2015)*, Luoyang, China, August 21–24, 2015.
12. Li, R., Pei, S., Chen, B., et al. (2020). Substantial undocumented infection facilitates the rapid dissemination of novel coronavirus (SARS-CoV2). *Science (New York, N.Y.), 368*(6490), 489–493.
13. Long, W., Liang, X., Huang, Y., & Chen, Y. (2013). A hybrid differential evolution augmented Lagrangian method for constrained numerical and engineering optimization. *Computer-Aided Design, 45*(12), 1562–1574.
14. Ma, Q. X., Shan, H., Zhang, H. L., Li, G. M., Yang, R. M., & Chen, J. M. (2020). Potential utilities of mask-wearing and instant hand hygiene for fighting SARS-CoV-2. *Journal of Medical Virology, 92*(9), 1567–1571.
15. Mirjalili, S., Mirjalili, S. M., & Lewis, A. (2014). Grey wolf optimizer. *Advances in Engineering Software, 69*, 46–61.
16. Mohamed, A. W. (2016). A new modified binary differential evolution algorithm and its applications. *Applied Mathematics & Information Sciences, 10*(5), 1965–1969.
17. Mohamed, A. W., Hadi, A. A., & Mohamed, A. K. (2020). Gaining-sharing knowledge-based algorithm for solving optimization problems: A novel nature-inspired algorithm. *International Journal of Machine Learning and Cybernetics, 11*, 1501–1529.
18. Muangkote, N., Photong, L., & Sukprasert, A. (2018). Effectiveness of Constrained Handling Techniques of Improved Constrained Differential Evolution Algorithm Applied to Constrained Optimization Problems in Mechanical Engineering, 3rd Technology Innovation Management and Engineering Science International Conference (TIMES-iCON), December 2018, https://doi.org/10.1109/TIMES-iCON.2018.8621654
19. Rao, R. V., Savsani, V. J., & Vakharia, D. P. (2011). Teaching–learning-based optimization: A novel method for constrained mechanical design optimization problems. *Computer-Aided Design, 43*(3), 303–315.
20. Rothe, C., Schunk, M., Sothmann, P., et al. (2020). Transmission of 2019-nCoV infection from an asymptomatic contact in Germany. *The New England Journal of Medicine, 382*(10), 970–971.
21. Cleemput, S., Dumon, W., Fonseca, V., Karim, W. A., Giovanetti, M., Alcantara, L. C., Deforche, K., & de Oliveira, T., (2020). Genome Detective Coronavirus Typing Tool for rapid identification and characterization of novel coronavirus genomes, Bioinformatics, btaa145, 28 February 2020. Retrieved at https://doi.org/10.1093/bioinformatics/btaa145
22. Storn, R., & Price, K. (1997). Differential evolution–a simple and efficient heuristic for global optimization over continuous spaces. *Journal of Global Optimization, 11*(4), 341–359.
23. THE LANCET website. (2020). A novel coronavirus outbreak of global health concern, retrieved on March 30, 2020 at: https://www.thelancet.com/journals/lancet/article/PIIS0140-6736(20)30185-9/fulltext
24. Wei, W. E., Li, Z., Chiew, C. J., Yong, S. E., Toh, M. P., & Lee, V. J. (2020) Presymptomatic transmission of SARS-CoV-2 — Singapore, January 23–March 16, 2020. *MMWR Morbidity and Mortality Weekly Report*. 2020; ePub: 1 April 2020.
25. Wikimedia Commons website. (2020). retrieved on April 15, 2020 at: https://commons.wikimedia.org/wiki/File:COVID-19_Outbreak_World_Map.svg
26. Wright, A. H. (1991). Genetic algorithms for real parameter optimization. In *Foundations of genetic algorithms* (Vol. 1, pp. 205–218). Amsterdam, Netherlands: Elsevier.
27. World Health Organization website. (2020a). Coronavirus disease 2019 (COVID-19) Situation Report – 85, Retrieved on 25 April 2020 at: https://www.who.int/docs/default-source/coronaviruse/situation-reports/20200414-sitrep-85-covid-19.pdf?sfvrsn=7b8629bb_4
28. World Health Organization website (2020b). WHO Coronavirus Disease (COVID-19) Dashboard, Retrieved on 28 August 2020 at: https://covid19.who.int/
29. World Health Organization website (2020c). WHO Coronavirus Disease (COVID-19) Dashboard, Retrieved on 27 August 2020 at: https://www.who.int/emergencies/diseases/

novel-coronavirus-2019/question-and-answers-hub/q-a-detail/q-a-how-is-covid-19-transmitted?gclid=EAIaIQobChMI1pubiOKq6wIVwu7tCh03dwbZEAAYASAAEgJVsvD_BwE
30. World Health Organization website (2020d). Masks and COVID-19, Retrieved on 28 August 2020 at: https://www.who.int/emergencies/diseases/novel-coronavirus-2019/question-and-answers-hub/q-a-detail/q-a-on-covid-19-and-masks
31. Worldometer Website. (2020). COVID-19 Coronavirus Pandemic website, Last updated: August 20, 2020, 14:22 GMT, retrieved on August 27, 2020 at: https://www.worldometers.info/coronavirus/
32. Worldometer website. (2020b). COVID-19 Coronavirus pandemic, retrieved on April 30, 2020 at: https://www.worldometers.info/coronavirus/#ref-13
33. Worldometer website. (2020c). Coronavirus Cases, retrieved on April 30, 2020 at: https://www.worldometers.info/coronavirus/coronavirus-cases/#total-cases
34. Yang, X. S., & Gandomi, A. H. (2012). Bat algorithm: a novel approach for global engineering optimization. *Engineering Computations, 29*, 464–483.
35. Zou, L., Ruan, F., Huang, M., et al. (2020). SARS-CoV-2 viral load in upper respiratory specimens of infected patients. *The New England Journal of Medicine, 382*(12), 1177–1179.

# Chapter 9
# Developing COVID-19 Vaccines by Innovative Bioinformatics Approaches

**Renu Jakhar, Neelam Sehrawat, and S. K. Gakhar**

## 9.1 Introduction

In December 2019, a disease named as COVID-19 spreads from Wuhan city of China to the entire world [1]. The disease is having a very high rate of transmission, and millions of people get affected from this. Due to its serious effects on mankind, the WHO (World Health Organization) declared it a public health emergency on 30 January 2020. As of 14 July 2020, the total numbers of reported cases and deaths for COVID-19 infection are 12,964,809 and 570, 288 globally, while the actual rate of infection is very high because of the emergence of asymptomatic coronavirus infection. The high mortality and transmission of COVID-19 infection cause a huge burden on health organizations and the economy of the countries, and the condition remains hypercritical throughout the world [2, 3]. The efforts are underway to find the finest medical products to prevent infection and diagnose and treat patients during the coronavirus disease 2019 pandemic. WHO confirmed COVID-19 infection is an airborne disease, which makes it more complicated to control its transmission in the human population. Many drugs such as remdesivir, chloroquine, lopinavir, ritonavir, etc. are being used for the treatment of COVID-19 [4–6]. However till date it is not clear which drug or medicine works better against the virus. It's a challenge to develop an effective vaccine and drug to combat this disease [7].

There are seven known human coronaviruses; four of them are HCoV-NL63, HCoV-HKU1, HCoV-229E, and HCoV-OC43 [8–10], and other two types that

R. Jakhar (✉)
Centre for Medical Biotechnology, Maharshi Dayanand University, Rohtak, Haryana, India

N. Sehrawat
Department of Genetics, Maharshi Dayanand University, Rohtak, Haryana, India

S. K. Gakhar
Indira Gandhi University, Rewari, Haryana, India



S. Kautish et al. (eds.), *Computational Intelligence Techniques for Combating COVID-19*, EAI/Springer Innovations in Communication and Computing,
https://doi.org/10.1007/978-3-030-68936-0_9

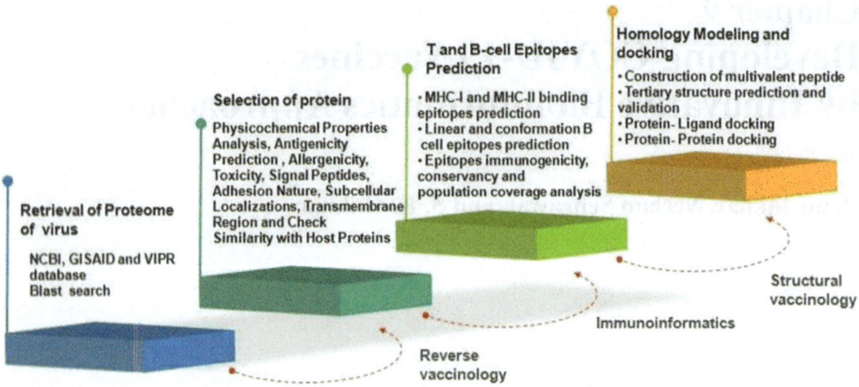


**Fig. 9.1** The methodology discussed in the study; arrows indicate flow of information and transition from one step to another

caused outbreak in 2003 and 2012 are severe acute respiratory syndrome coronavirus (SARS-CoV) and Middle East respiratory syndrome coronavirus (MERS-CoV), respectively. By comparison, 2500 MERS cases are reported worldwide in 2012 with 858 deaths, and 8100 SARS cases are reported worldwide in 2002–2003 with 774 deaths. Coronavirus is a positively stranded, enveloped RNA virus of approximately 29.9 kb and belongs to the family *Coronaviridae*. SARS-CoV-2 is a beta-coronavirus, and the genome of the SARS-CoV-2 encoded for total (6–11) peptides (open reading frame 1ab (ORF1ab), S protein, ORF3a, envelope protein, membrane glycoprotein, ORF6, ORF7a, ORF8 protein, nucleocapsid phosphoprotein, ORF10) [11, 12]. The availability of the COVID-19 genome had opened the new pathway to develop a vaccine against this devastating disease [13]. The conventional approaches do not work effectively for rapid vaccine development, so the different bioinformatics approaches, i.e., reverse vaccinology, immunoinformatics, and structural vaccinology, are used to search the target for vaccine development (Fig. 9.1).

## 9.2 Concepts of Reverse Vaccinology and Immunoinformatics

An approach known as reverse vaccinology with immunoinformatics has been used to develop new vaccines [14, 15]. The immunological efficacy of peptide-based vaccines has already been reported [16, 17]. Identification of specific epitopes from pathogenic protein has significantly advanced the development of peptide-based vaccines. The prediction of immunogenic cytotoxic T lymphocyte (CTL), helper T lymphocyte (HTL), and B-cell epitopes have been performed from tissue-specific proteins of organisms to construct a vaccine to elicit both innate and acquired immunities [17–19]. A memory-based T-cell-based cell-mediated immunity is essential against SARS-CoV-2 infection [20]. Moreover, in silico approach has become handy in vaccine designing as it provides clues to select the target protein sequences [21]. Today, vaccinologists can move beyond traditional conventional methods to reverse vaccinology for vaccine design because of advancements in genomics and computational studies [22–25]. Bioinformatics-based approaches for designing peptide-based vaccines are less time-consuming, easy to produce, cost-effective, safe, and more specific as compared to the conventional vaccines [23, 26]. The multi-epitope peptide vaccines using immunoinformatics have high degree of accuracy [27].

### *9.2.1 Previous Studies on Reverse Vaccinology with Immunoinformatics*

Firstly reverse vaccinology is employed for the vaccine development against group B *Meningococcus* [28], because the scientists are unable to develop a vaccine with conventional approaches, so the scientists focus on the bioinformatics approaches to overcome this problem. After the success to develop a vaccine against group B *Meningococcus*, this approach was also used for other organisms such as group A *Streptococcus* and group B *Streptococcus* and later employed for *Staphylococcus aureus* and *Streptococcus pneumoniae* [28, 29]. Reverse vaccinology has been successfully applied to vaccine discovery for pathogens such as group B *Meningococcus* and led to the license Bexsero vaccine [30, 31]. A vaccine against the serogroup B *Neisseria meningitidis*, which was designed via an immunoinformatics, was successfully produced [32, 33]. Afterward based on immunoinformatics approaches, numerous vaccines were developed, comprising efficient vaccines against *Streptococcus pneumoniae*, *Chlamydia pneumoniae*, *Rickettsia prowazekii* [34], *enterotoxigenic Escherichia coli* [35], *H. pylori* [24, 36], *Klebsiella pneumoniae* [37–39], *Vibrio cholerae* [25], *Staphylococcus aureus* [40], *Campylobacter jejuni* [41], *Pseudomonas aeruginosa* [42], and *Shigella* [43]. Studies also include *Brucella melitensis* [44] and *Mycobacterium tuberculosis* [45] which are some pathogens that mark some epitopes having a potential of being a vaccine. Recent studies on viruses using reverse vaccinology and immunoinformatics include hepatitis C virus (HCV) [46], herpes virus [47], influenza virus [48], chikungunya virus [49], Zika virus [50–52], Nipah virus [53–55], HIV [56], norovirus [57], Lassa virus [58], Ebola virus [22, 59], dengue virus [60], and MERS [17, 43, 61–63]. Moreover, the design of therapeutic antibodies that is guided by computational simulation of antibody-antigen complexes has been reported. Also, epitopes against leishmaniasis [64], malaria [65–67], meningitis [68], tuberculosis [69], filariasis [70], and Kaposi sarcoma [71] diseases help the researchers to target the most potential target for vaccine development.

## 9.3 Bioinformatics Strategies for Emergent Peptide-Based Vaccines Against SARS-CoV-2

There are a number of immunoinformatics-based vaccines which are under the clinical trial/produced [32, 33], so the reverse vaccinology, immunoinformatics, and structural vaccinology can help the researchers to target the new coronavirus. The usage of these in silico approaches for the prediction of antigenic determinants in the various proteins of SARS-CoV-2 is a very important and primary approach. These strategies reduce the time for the identification of potentially immunogenic peptides and are useful to provide a subunit vaccine against SARS-CoV-2. Some published studies on computational multi-epitope vaccine designs against SARS-CoV-2 are mentioned in Table 9.1. However, continuous efforts are being made to predict epitopes against SARS-CoV-2 spike protein [11, 81, 82, 86], nucleocapsid [80], 3Clpro [77], envelope [85] and membrane proteins [84], and ORF1ab [80].

### *9.3.1 Reverse Vaccinology*

The reverse vaccinology approach uses different immunogenic proteins to design/construct a potential subunit vaccine. In the case of COVID-19, reverse vaccinology is an easy and simple way to screen the whole genome of the pathogen and targets the functional protein that is antigenic in nature from 11 open reading frames [88]. With the availability of the whole proteome and genome, the reverse vaccinology approach can help the researcher to examine different characteristics of proteins. With the help of different bioinformatics approaches, the protein sequences are targeted in a precise manner. Each protein must be analyzed in the proteome to select the best proteins. Reverse vaccinology targets the protein/antigen based on its physicochemical properties, extracellular localization, adhesion properties, signal peptide, no transmembrane regions, antigenicity, non-allergenicity, nontoxicity, and lack of any sequence similarity with host proteins (otherwise it generates an immune response against its own cells). The list of various tools considered during reverse vaccinology is mentioned in Table 9.2.

#### 9.3.1.1 Retrieval of Proteome of SARS-CoV-2

The genome and protein sequences of novel severe acute respiratory syndrome coronavirus 2 from different geographic regions are available on NCBI, GISAID, and VIPR database [89]. Perform sequence similarity searches using Blastp to reveal the orthologs in different strains [89]. The ClustalW/MAFFT program can be used for multiple sequence alignment of protein sequences. MEGA6.02 or Unipro UGENE 1.16.1 tools are used to construct the phylogenetic tree [90, 91]. These tools are used to predict the identity, relationship, and conservation of the proteins.

**Table 9.1** Potential candidate peptide-based vaccines against SARS-CoV-2 designed with the aid of bioinformatics tools

| S no. | COVID-19 protein analyzed | Database/resource | Outcome | Refs. |
|---|---|---|---|---|
| 1. | Surface spike glycoprotein, nucleocapsid protein | IEDB, PatchDock, HawkDock, HADDOCK | Multivalent vaccine construct | [72] |
| 2. | 3C-like proteinase, 2'-O-ribose methyltransferase, helicase, 3′ to 5′ exonuclease, endoRNAse, and RNA-dependent RNA polymerase | IEDB, NetCTL, ABCpred, RaptorX, HADDOCK, GROMACS, C-ImmSim server | Multivalent vaccine construct | [73] |
| 3. | Surface spike glycoprotein, nucleocapsid, envelope, ORF1ab, membrane, ORF3a, ORF6, ORF7a, ORF7b, ORF8, and Orf10 | IEDB, I-TASSER, SWISS-MODEL, PatchDock, YASARA | Multivalent vaccine construct | [74] |
| 4. | Envelope, nucleocapsid, spike protein, and RNA-dependent | IEDB and ProPred-I, SWISS-MODEL, HEX | Multivalent vaccine construct | [75] |
| 5. | Nucleocapsid, ORF3a, and membrane protein | Rankpep, BepiPred, IEDB, GalaxyWEB server, PatchDock, GROMACS | Multivalent vaccine construct | [76] |
| 6. | 3C-like proteinase | NetCTL 1.2, IEDB, SWISS-MODEL, HEX | Multi-epitope vaccine construct | [77] |
| 7. | Spike glycoprotein | NetCTL 1.2, IEDB, ABCpred 2.0, I-TASSER, GRAMM-X simulation, GROMACS | Multi-epitope vaccine construct | [78] |
| 8. | Spike glycoprotein | NetCTL 1.2 server, IEDB, NetMHCIIpan 3.2, HADDOCK 2.4, C-ImmSim server | Multi-epitope vaccine construct | [79] |
| 9. | Spike glycoprotein, nucleocapsid, Orf1ab | IEDB, BepiPred, NetCTL | Analysis of T- and B-cell epitopes | [80] |
| 10. | Spike glycoprotein | SWISS-MODEL server, BepiPred 2.0, ABCpred, IEDB, CTLPred | Multi-epitope vaccine construct | [81] |
| 11. | Surface glycoprotein | TepiTool, BepiPred 2.0 IEDB, 3Dpro, HADDOCK | Multi-epitope vaccine construct | [82] |
| 12. | ORF1ab polyprotein | IEDB, SWISS-MODEL, HEX | Multi-epitope vaccine construct | [83] |
| 13. | Surface glycoprotein | NetCTL 1.2 server, CTLPred, NetMHCpan 4.0, BepiPred 2.0, ABCpred, Zdock 3.0.2, RaptorX | Analysis of T- and B-cell epitopes | [11] |
| 14. | Surface spike glycoprotein, nucleocapsid, and membrane glycoprotein | BepiPred, ABCpred, LBtope, NetMHCpan 4.0, nHLAPred, CTLPred, SCWRL, AutoDock Vina | Analysis of T- and B-cell epitopes | [84] |
| 15. | Envelope protein | IEDB, RaptorX, AutoDock 4.0 | Analysis of T- and B-cell epitopes | [85] |
| 16. | Spike glycoprotein | IEDB and ABCpred, ProPred-I, ProPred, HPEPDOCK | Analysis of T- and B-cell epitopes | [86] |
| 17. | Spike glycoprotein | BepiPred 2.0, IEDB | Analysis of T- and B-cell epitopes | [87] |

**Table 9.2** Main characteristics and list of various tools considered during reverse vaccinology

| S no. | Characteristic | Software/database | URL |
|---|---|---|---|
| 1. | Retrieval of proteome | NCBI | https://www.ncbi.nlm.nih.gov/labs/virus/vssi/#/ |
| | | GISAID | https://www.epicov.org/epi3/frontend#6a3f4 |
| | | VIPR | https://www.viprbrc.org/brc/home.spg?decorator=vipr |
| 2. | Antigenicity | VaxiJen | http://www.ddgpharmfac.net/vaxijen/VaxiJen/VaxiJen.html |
| | | ANTIGENpro | http://scratch.proteomics.ics.uci.edu/ |
| 3. | Allergenicity | AllerTOP | http://www.pharmfac.net/allertop |
| | | AlgPred | http://www.imtech.res.in/raghava/algpred/submission.html |
| | | AllergenFP | http://ddg-pharmfac.net/AllergenFP/ |
| 4. | Toxicity | ToxinPred | http://crdd.osdd.net/raghava/toxinpred/ |
| 5. | Secondary structure | SOPMA | https://npsa-prabi.ibcp.fr/cgi-bin/npsa_automat.pl?page=/NPSA/npsa_sopma.html |
| | | PSIPRED | http://bioinf.cs.ucl.ac.uk/psipred/ |
| 6. | Physicochemical properties | ProtParam | http://web.expasy.org/protparam |
| 7. | Disulfide bonds | DIANNA v1.1 | http://bioinformatics.bc.edu/clotelab/DiANNA/ |
| 8. | Protein solubility | SOLpro | http://scratch.proteomics.ics.uci.edu/ |
| 9. | Adhesion nature | SPANN | – |
| 10. | Subcellular localizations | Virus-mPLoc | http://www.csbio.sjtu.edu.cn/bioinf/virus-multi/ |
| 11. | Transmembrane region | TMHMM | http://www.cbs.dtu.dk/services/TMHMM/ |
| 12. | Signal peptides | SIGNAL-BLAST | http://sigpep.services.came.sbg.ac.at/signalblast.html |
| 13. | Similarity with host proteins | Blastp | https://blast.ncbi.nlm.nih.gov/Blast.cgi |
| 14. | Conserved domain | Conserved domain database | https://www.ncbi.nlm.nih.gov/cdd/ |
| | | Pfam | https://pfam.xfam.org/ |
| | | InteProScan | https://www.ebi.ac.uk/interpro/search/sequence/ |
| 15. | Multiple sequence alignment | ClustalW/Clustal omega | https://www.ebi.ac.uk/Tools/msa/clustalo/ |
| 16. | Phylogenetic tree | Unipro UGENE 1.16.1 | http://ugene.unipro.ru/ |

#### 9.3.1.2 Antigenicity Prediction

The antigenicity of the proteins against different bacterial and viral pathogens can be analyzed with the various online tools, i.e., VaxiJen [92] and ANTIGENpro. The proteins of the highest antigenicity are selected for further analysis. ANTIGENpro, a protein antigenicity prediction server, is a part of Scratch Protein Predictor.

#### 9.3.1.3 Allergenicity and Toxicity

AllerTOP [93], AlgPred [94], Allermatch, AllerHunter, and AllergenFP tools predict the non-allergic nature of the sequences. The proteins which are allergic and non-immunogenic in nature should be discarded. Toxicity assessment of epitopes has been predicted by ToxinPred [95]. Features including digestion have been accessed by Protein Digest. The protein selected based on its immunogenicity and allergenicity is further analyzed for the prediction of physicochemical properties.

#### 9.3.1.4 Physicochemical Property Analysis

The next step is to predict the secondary structure of protein using SOPMA [96]/PSIPRED/GOR. The secondary structure prediction includes the percentage of the helix, extended strand, coiled structure, and the beta-turn. ExPASy's online tool ProtParam can be used to determine the various physicochemical properties of the proteins [97]. Secondary structural characteristics of the proteins are analyzed that included solvent accessibility, the total number of amino acids, molecular weight, theoretical pI, molecular formula, estimated half-life, number of charged residues, extinction coefficient, etc. Residues that are predominately present in the beta-sheet indicate the protein's antigenicity. If the grand average of the hydrophobicity rule (GRAVY) value of the linear protein sequence is negative, it indicates its hydrophilic nature and shows the presence of residues mostly on the surface. Instability index less than 40 shows stable nature of protein, and the aliphatic index could have a higher value. The high aliphatic index seems to be a positive factor for increasing the thermostability of globular proteins, and the higher proportions of the coiled regions provide more stability. The proteins are analyzed to identify hydrophilic regions and amino acids exposed to the exterior region for interactions. The prevalence of disulfide bonds has been examined through the use of DIANNA v1.1. Protein solubility on overexpression in *E. coli* was predicted using SOLpro [98].

#### 9.3.1.5 Adhesion Nature

Peptides having adhesion-like properties are selected for vaccine candidates. The physicochemical properties of molecules and length of peptide decide the adhesion nature of molecules. Adhesion molecules located on the surface which helps them to contact antibodies. SPANN has been used for adhesion property prediction, and the proteins having threshold higher or equal to 0.4 are selected for further studies [99].

#### 9.3.1.6 Subcellular Localizations

Proteins localized extracellularly/on the cell have good antigens because they are exposed to the host cells to generate an immune response. Virus-mPLoc software could be used to evaluate the localization [100].

#### 9.3.1.7 Transmembrane Region

Low and very less transmembrane helix is the property of good antigen. The transmembrane helix is the region that spans through the cell membrane, and it is difficult to purify. The software TMHMM and TMpred provide the information about transmembrane helices [101].

#### 9.3.1.8 Signal Peptides

Signal peptides in protein sequences are known to impact protein sequences and possess high epitope densities. Signal-BLAST and SignalP online web servers are used to predict the signal peptides [102].

#### 9.3.1.9 Similarity with Host Proteins

Blastp is available through NCBI to check the similarities of the selected proteins to the host proteins as the antigen could cause autoimmune reactions and could induce cross-protection. All sequences should be submitted individually to the Blastp server to check the homology of viral proteins with the human proteome [89].

#### 9.3.1.10 Conserved Domain Identification

The conservation of the domains can be predicted using various available databases, e.g., the Conserved Domain Database (CDD), Pfam, and InteProScan [103–105]. The conserved domain regions are further used to identify conserved epitope candidates.

### *9.3.2 Immunoinformatics*

Epitope is the segment of the protein which is an antigenic determinant to activate the immune response. To develop a potential vaccine, it is important to remove the non-antigenic segments for the target proteins. The immunological system mainly classified as cellular and humoral and it is triggered by B- and T-cell epitopes against the pathogen. These epitopes activate both innate and acquired immunities. The selection procedures for the B-cell and T-cell epitopes are not identical. Linear B-cell epitope is selected based on its surface accessibility, flexibility, position in beta-turn region, and antigenicity. Conformational B-cell epitope prediction is based on the structure of the protein. The selection of the T-cell epitope is based on its binding affinity with MHC-I and MHC-II molecules. The list of various tools available to search for B- and T -cell epitope is mentioned in Table 9.3.

**Table 9.3** Main characteristics and list of various tools considered during immunoinformatics studies

| S no. | Characteristic | Software/database | URL |
|---|---|---|---|
| 1. | B-cell epitope prediction | BCPREDS (linear) | http://www.imtech.res.in/raghava/bcepred/ |
| | | BepiPred (linear) | http://www.cbs.dtu.dk/services/BepiPred/ |
| | | ABCpred (linear) | http://www.imtech.res.in/raghava/abcpred/ |
| | | IEDB (linear) | http://tools.immuneepitope.org/ |
| | | BEST (linear) | http://biomine.ece.ualberta.ca/BEST/ |
| | | MIMOX (linear) | http://immunet.cn/mimox/ |
| | | Pepsuf (both linear and conformational) | http://pepitope.tau.ac.il |
| | | EPITOpia (both linear and conformational) | http://epitopia.tau.ac.il/ |
| | | ElliPro (both linear and conformational) | http://tools.immuneepitope.org/tools/ElliPro/iedb_input |
| | | DiscoTope (conformational) | http://www.cbs.dtu.dk/services/DiscoTope/ |
| | | EpiSearch (conformational) | http://curie.utmb.edu/episearch.html |
| | | SEPPA (conformational) | http://lifecenter.sgst.cn/seppa/index.php |
| | | EPCES (conformational) | http://sysbio.unl.edu/services/EPCES/ |
| | | BePro (conformational) | http://pepito.proteomics.ics.uci.edu/ |
| | | Pep-3D-search (conformational) | http://kyc.nenu.edu.cn/Pep3DSearch |

(continued)

**Table 9.3** (continued)

| S no. | Characteristic | Software/database | URL |
|---|---|---|---|
| 2. | T-cell epitope prediction | IEDB (both MHC-I and MHC-II) | http://tools.immuneepitope.org/analyze/html/mhc_processing.html |
| | | Rankpep (both MHC-I and MHC-II) | http://bio.dfci.harvard.edu/RANKPEP/ |
| | | MHCPred (both MHC-I and MHC-II) | http://www.ddg-pharmfac.net/mhcpred/MHCPred/ |
| | | EpiVax (both MHC-I and MHC-II) | http://www.epivax.com/ |
| | | SYFPEITHI (both MHC-I and MHC-II) | http://www.syfpeithi.de/bin/MHCServer.dll/EpitopePrediction.htm |
| | | SVMHC (both MHC-I and MHC-II) | http://abi.inf.uni-tuebingen.de/Services/SVMHC |
| | | SVRMHC (both MHC-I and MHC-II) | http://svrmhc.biolead.org/ |
| | | ProPred-I (MHC-I) | http://www.imtech.res.in/raghava/propred1/ |
| | | BIMAS (MHC-I) | http://www-bimas.cit.nih.gov/molbio/hla_bind/ |
| | | NetMHC (MHC-I) | http://www.cbs.dtu.dk/services/NetMHC/ |
| | | NetCTL (MHC-I) | http://www.cbs.dtu.dk/services/NetCTL |
| | | KISS (MHC-I) | http://cbio.ensmp.fr/kiss/ |
| | | MMBPred (MHC-I) | http://www.imtech.res.in/raghava/mmbpred/ |
| | | ANNPRED (MHC-I) | http://www.imtech.res.in/raghava/nhlapred/neural.html |
| | | EpiJen (MHC-I) | http://www.ddg-pharmfac.net/epijen/EpiJen/EpiJen.htm |
| | | PREDEP (MHC-I) | http://margalit.huji.ac.il/Teppred/mhc-bind/index.html |
| | | nHLAPred (MHC-I) | http://www.imtech.res.in/raghava/nhlapred/ |
| | | CTLPred (MHC-I) | http://www.imtech.res.in/raghava/ctlpred/ |
| | | ProPred (MHC-I) | http://www.ddg-pharmfac.net/mhcpred/MHCPred/ |
| | | IMTECH (MHC-II) | http://www.imtech.res.in/raghava/mhc |
| | | MHC2Pred (MHC-II) | http://www.imtech.res.in/raghava/mhc2pred/ |
| | | ProPred (MHC-II) | http://www.imtech.res.in/raghava/propred/ |
| | | IFNepitope prediction (II) | http://crdd.osdd.net/raghava/ifnepitope/ |

| | | | |
|---|---|---|---|
| 3. | Cluster analysis of the MHC alleles | MHCcluster 2.0 | http://www.cbs.dtu.dk/services/MHCcluster/ |
| 4. | Epitope conservation analyses | IEDB | http://tools.iedb.org/conservancy/ |
| 5. | Population coverage calculation | IEDB | http://tools.iedb.org/population/ |

#### 9.3.2.1 B-Cell Epitope Prediction

B-cell epitope interacts with B lymphocytes/antibodies and differentiates them into the memory cell and an antibody-secreting plasma cell. The tools like IEDB, ABCpred, BepiPred, BcePred, BEST, EPCES, BCPREDS, EPITOpia, IgPred, Pepsuf, MIMOX, etc. [8] are available to predict linear/continuous B-cell epitope from the protein. The protein sequence is subjected to search for linear B-cell epitope from the protein, and the IEDB tool predicts epitopes based on six methods (including physiochemical properties): BepiPred linear epitope (predicts the regions that bind to B-cell receptor), Chou and Fasman beta-turn (predicts the residues present in a beta-turn region), Parker hydrophilicity (predicts the residues in hydrophilic region), Karplus and Schulz flexibility (flexible regions), Kolaskar and Tongaonkar antigenicity (predicts the regions being immunogenic), and Emini surface accessibility prediction (predicts the region being in the surface of protein) [106]. Similarly, the BcePred tool shortlists the epitopes based on hydrophilicity, surface accessibility, flexibility, and polarity. The ABCpred tool is based on neural networks. The BepiPred tool uses hidden Markov and propensity scale methods. ElliPro, DiscoTope, BePro (PEPITO), EPCES, SEPPA, and Pep-3D-Search are the tools used to predict potential conformational/discontinuous B-cell epitope [107]. These epitopes are predicted by submitting the tertiary structure of the protein. Discontinuous B-cell epitopes are situated on the surface making them accessible to interact with immune receptors to induce a humoral immune response [67].

#### 9.3.2.2 T-Cell Epitope Prediction

T-cell epitopes interact with MHC molecules to elicit cell-mediated immunity that is memory-based. CTLs and HTLs bound to MHC-I and MHC-II alleles, respectively. The primary sequence of amino acid is required to identify putative T-cell epitopes. There are a number of tools available for the search of MHC-I and MHC-II epitope from the protein including IEDB, Rankpep, BIMAS, NetCTL, TEpredict, NetMHCStab, TepiTool, CTLPred, MHC2MIL, nHLAPred, KISS, ProPred-I, PickPocket, MAPPP, SVMHC, FRED2, iVAX, GPS-MBA, Epitopemap, POPI, PREDIVAC, SVMHC, NetMHC, MHC2Pred, etc. (Table 9.3). These tools are used to predict the stability of epitope binding with MHC. These tools are based on computational training with the previously identified epitopes and nonepitopes [108]. In order to provide values for new protein and to predict whether or not it is an epitope, there are various computational techniques and predictive methods: hidden Markov models (HMMs), Epimatrix algorithm, position-specific scoring matrices (PSSMs), machine learning, multi-step algorithm, published coefficient tables, published motifs, artificial neural networks (ANNs), ANN regression, quantitative matrix, and support vector machines (SVMs). Each computational method possesses different advantages and accuracy levels [109].

MHC Class I Binding Epitope Prediction

The NetCTL, IEDB, Rankpep, CTLPred, ProPred-I, and nHLAPred are the very commonly used tools to predict MHC class I binding epitopes. By using neural networks and weight matrix-based systems, a combined algorithm of MHC-I binding, transporter of antigenic peptide (TAP) transport efficiency, and proteasomal cleavage efficiency are used to predict the overall scores. Epitopes are selected on the basis of the combined score. IEDB MHC-I binding prediction tool based on the consensus SVM/ANN method was used to screen out different types of MHC-I alleles that interacted with CTL epitope. The CTL epitopes that interact with the maximum number of MHC-I alleles with higher affinity IC50 < 200 with lower percentile rank are selected as potential epitopes [110, 111]. An epitope having higher immunogenicity scores is selected as potential candidate antigen [112].

Rankpep uses position-specific scoring matrix (PSSM) method to predict MHC class I and II peptide binder. The nHLAPred uses a quantitative matrix and artificial neural networks (ANNs) as a hybrid approach. NetMHC and NetCTLpan server predict CTLs based on ANN method. CTLPred uses a combined prediction method of ANNs and support vector machine (SVM) methods. ProPred-I uses a quantitative matrix method. MHCPred and EpiJen server predict CTLs based on the additive method and multi-step algorithm approach, respectively.

MHC Class II Binding Epitope Prediction

NetMHCIIpan 3.0 prediction tool at IEDB uses SMM-based method to predict peptide binding to MHC-II molecules [113]. The HTL epitopes that interact with the maximum number of MHC-II alleles with higher affinity IC50 < 200 are selected as potential epitopes. Further, these MHC-II binding epitopes have been checked to induce the IFN-$\gamma$ using IFN epitope server [114].

ProPred-I and IMTECH tools use quantitative matrix method to predict MHC class II peptide binder [115]. The tool MHC2Pred predicts HTLs based on SVM-based method.

There can be several overlapping amino acid sequences that are present between MHC-I and MHC-II epitopes, which shows antigen presentation to immune cells via both MHC class I and II pathways [77]. The potential CTL and HTL epitopes may have overlapping B-cell epitope (linear and discontinuous) region, suggesting the possibility of generation of cellular and humoral immunity for further in vivo and in vitro assays.

#### 9.3.2.3 Epitope Conservation Analyses

The selected epitopes should be conserved among all its variants. The conservancy analysis of selected epitopes has been performed by the IEDB conservancy analysis resource at IEDB [116]. The conservancy analysis of epitopes has been carried out among all the SARS-CoV-2 protein sequences submitted at NCBI from various countries.

#### 9.3.2.4 Population Coverage Calculation

HLA distribution of alleles varies among different geographic regions around the world. Thus, to obtain an effective vaccine, population coverage must be taken into a different set of alleles to cover 16 identified geographic regions of the world. Population coverage of the whole world for epitope has been assessed by the IEDB population coverage calculation tool [117]. Calculations are achieved using the selected MHC-I and MHC-II interacted alleles by the IEDB population coverage calculation tool. The selected epitopes must have a binding affinity with the maximum number of MHC alleles to achieve higher population coverage.

### *9.3.3 Structural Vaccinology*

Structural vaccinology involves homology modeling and molecular docking to analyze the interactions between epitopes and antibodies/MHC receptors. More interaction of epitopes with receptors makes them good candidate antigens. The conformational features of proteins have been studied by this approach. Structural vaccinology focused on the binding grooves or pockets/active sites of receptor where the designed peptide vaccine/epitopes bind. This approach has been used mainly to select or design peptide-based vaccines or cross-reactive antigens with the capability of generating immunity against different antigenically divergent pathogens [118]. List of various tools considered during structural vaccinology is mentioned in Table 9.4.

#### 9.3.3.1 Homology Modeling

3D structure of proteins can be obtained from the PDB server [119]. The 3D structures of some proteins are not available on the PDB server. So by using protein sequence, the 3D structure has been generated by Modeller, SWISS-MODEL [120], RaptorX [121], I-TASSER [122], Robetta [123], and 3Dpro servers. These servers use homology detection methods to build 3D models. The 3D structure visualization and minimization could be performed with UCSF Chimera [124], Swiss-PdbViewer [125], PyMOL, and YASARA. The minimized structure can be further validated by RAMPAGE [126], PROCHECK, WhatIF, ERRAT, Verify3D, and ProSA web servers [127]. Further the QMEAN server can be used to asses and verify the quality of the model [128]. The 3D structures of the protein are necessary to predict conformational B-cell epitopes, to visualize all predicted T-cell epitopes in the structural level, as well as to further verify predicted B-cell epitopes for surface accessibility and hydrophilicity. Also, the 3D structures predicted are used for docking studies.

**Table 9.4** Main characteristics and list of various tools considered during structural vaccinology

| S no. | Characteristic | Software/database | URL |
|---|---|---|---|
| 1. | Protein structure retrieval | PDB server | https://www.rcsb.org/ |
| 2. | Tertiary structure prediction | SWISS-MODEL | https://swissmodel.expasy.org/ |
| | | RaptorX | http://raptorx.uchicago.edu/StructurePropertyPred/predict/ |
| | | I-TASSER | https://zhanglab.ccmb.med.umich.edu/I-TASSER/ |
| 3. | Tertiary structure validation | RAMPAGE | http://mordred.bioc.cam.ac.uk/_rapper/rampage.php |
| | | PROCHECK | https://servicesn.mbi.ucla.edu/PROCHECK/ |
| | | ERRAT | http://services.mbi.ucla.edu/ERRAT/ |
| | | Verify3D | https://servicesn.mbi.ucla.edu/Verify3D/ |
| | | ProSA web server | https://prosa.services.came.sbg.ac.at/prosa.php |
| 4. | Quality check of protein structure | QMEAN | https://swissmodel.expasy.org/qmean/ |
| | | GalaxyRefine server | http://galaxy.seoklab.org/cgi-bin/submit.cgi?type%C2%BCREFINE |
| 5. | Epitope structure prediction | PEP-FOLD | https://mobyle.rpbs.univ-paris-diderot.fr/cgi-bin/portal.py#forms::PEP-FOLD3 |
| 6. | *Docking* | *ClusPro* | *http://cluspro.bu.edu/login.php* |
| | | PatchDock | https://bioinfo3d.cs.tau.ac.il/PatchDock/ |
| | | HawkDock | http://cadd.zju.edu.cn/hawkdock/ |
| | | HDOCK | http://hdock.phys.hust.edu.cn/ |
| | | HPEPDOCK | http://huanglab.phys.hust.edu.cn/hpepdock/ |
| | | HADDOCK | http://milou.science.uu.nl/services/HADDOCK2.2/haddockserver-easy.html |
| 7. | Immune dynamics simulation | C-ImmSim | https://www.iac.rm.cnr.it/~filippo/c-immsim/index.html |
| 8. | In silico codon adaptation | GenScript rare codon analysis | https://www.genscript.com/tools/rarecodonanalysis |

#### 9.3.3.2 Protein-Ligand Docking Studies

Molecular docking is carried out to screen out whether or not these epitopes will bind with HLA molecules when applied in vivo. To carry out the docking simulations, the three-dimensional structures of HLA classes I and II have been obtained from PDB. Before docking simulation, already bound epitope, complexed in the binding groove of these alleles, has to be removed by using AutoDockTools and PyMOL. For some alleles, three-dimensional structures are not available on PDB, so they have to be modeled. T-cell epitopes that bind with good binding affinity with MHC-I and MHC-II alleles have been selected as the ligands. These epitopes are modeled using peptide modeling tool PEP-FOLD, RPBS MOBYL portal [129]. AutoDock Vina [130], ClusPro [131], PatchDock [132], HawkDock [133], HDOCK [134], HPEPDOCK, HEX [135], HADDOCK [136], and GOLD servers are used for dockings and show the suitable epitope binding with the minimal binding energy. The residues from the R group side chains of epitopes show interaction within the binding grooves/pockets of MHC-I and MHC-II alleles. Chimera, Pymol, Swiss-PdbViewer, and Discovery Studio are used to visualize the docked complex and analyze the binding sites/residues. The interacting residues between the vaccine and the TLRs were mapped using Ligplus 1.2 software (Ligplot) [137].

#### 9.3.3.3 Protein-Protein Docking

**The multivalent vaccine with fused peptides** The predicted B- and T-cell epitope from single protein or multiple proteins are fused with the linkers GPGPG and AAY [138]. To enhance immune response, some adjuvant sequences are also added at the C-terminal of the vaccine construct. The first CTL of Vaccine construct is connected with adjuvant at the N-terminal by EAAAK linkers. The various physicochemical properties, secondary structure, antigenicity, toxicity, allergenicity, and similarity with the human genome of the multi-epitope peptide have been evaluated. The 3D structure of the vaccine construct is generated and validated by the tools discussed above. The refinement of the obtained model can be performed by the GalaxyRefine tool [139]. At structural level, conformational B-cell epitopes are also being predicted from the peptide vaccine.

The host produces an efficient immune response if an antigen or a vaccine interacts accurately with the target immune cells. So, molecular docking studies are performed to predict the binding of a multivalent vaccine to the human immune receptors. For docking studies, the multivalent vaccine is used as a ligand, and TLR is used as a receptor. To analyze the binding interactions between TLR-2, TLR-3,

TLR-4, and TLR-8 and vaccine construct, a protein-protein docking can be assessed by docking tools, e.g., ClusPro, PatchDock, GOLD, HADDOCK, etc.

#### 9.3.3.4 Molecular Dynamics (MD) Simulations

MD simulation has been employed to assess the stability of the complexes. GROMACS, AMBER, CHARM, and Schrodinger simulation software can be used for MD simulation [140].

## 9.4 Immune Dynamics Simulation

C-ImmSim server is available to use to generates an in silico immunological response for the peptide vaccine. The software uses different algorithms to analyze the complete response against specific antigens [141]. For immune dynamics simulation, the time and number of doses have to be set according to study, where each time is expressed in a unit of 8 h and initially injection time is 0 [142, 143]. The output file is the graphical representation of each immune cell type against the given antigen. These given cell types include the immunoglobulin and the immunocomplex response against antigen, B-cell population, cytotoxic T-cell population, helper T-cell population, concentration of cytokines and interleukins, macrophage population, and dendritic cell population, arising during vaccination. Also, inset in the plot shows a danger signal together with leukocyte growth factor IL-2.

## 9.5 In Silico Codon Adaptation and Cloning

Reverse translation of the multivalent peptide vaccine into the nucleotide sequence is being carried out by Java Codon Adaptation Tool (JCAT) and GenScript Rare Codon Analysis Tool [144]. Further, the obtained cDNA can be used for codon optimization for in silico cloning. The GC contents together with the codon adaptation index (CAI) are evaluated. The codons are adapted as per the codon usage of the human expression system. cDNA of multivalent vaccine is generated according to mammalian host cell line [145]. The ideal range of CAI is from >0.8 to 1, GC content is 30–70%, and CFD <30% is required to achieve a high expression level in the host. After the development of the vaccine construct, it is very important to express the sequence in the expression vector (*E. coli*) and then analyze its immunogenic response against the pathogen COVID-19. The adapted and optimized nucleotide sequence of the vaccine construct has to be cloned into the vector like pET28a (+) of *E. coli* by using the restriction cloning module of the SnapGene software.

Thus, the predicted multivalent peptide vaccine produced by computational approach could be cloned, expressed, and tested for in vitro and in vivo analysis and considered as a safe, protective, and prophylactic vaccine against COVID-19. To support the predicted universal peptide-based vaccines for this type of SARS-CoV-2 required to be validated by in vitro and in vivo studies.

## References


1. Lu, H., Stratton, C. W., & Tang, Y. W. (2020). Outbreak of pneumonia of unknown etiology in Wuhan, China: The mystery and the miracle. *Journal of Medical Virology, 92*(4), 401–402.
2. World Health Organization. (2020). Novel Coronavirus (2019-nCoV), Situation Report:12.
3. Kock, R. A., Karesh, W. B., Veas, F., Velavan, T. P., Simons, D., Mboera, L. E., Dar, O., Arruda, L. B., & Zumla, A. (2020). 2019-nCoV in context: Lessons learned? *The Lancet Planetary Health, 4*(3), e87–e88.
4. Agostini, M. L., Andres, E. L., Sims, A. C., Graham, R. L., Sheahan, T. P., Lu, X., Smith, E. C., Case, J. B., Feng, J. Y., Jordan, R., & Ray, A. S. (2018). Coronavirus susceptibility to the antiviral remdesivir (GS-5734) is mediated by the viral polymerase and the proofreading exoribonuclease. *MBio, 9*(2).
5. Aguiar, A. C., Murce, E., Cortopassi, W. A., Pimentel, A. S., Almeida, M. M., Barros, D. C., Guedes, J. S., Meneghetti, M. R., & Krettli, A. U. (2018). Chloroquine analogs as antimalarial candidates with potent in vitro and in vivo activity. *International Journal for Parasitology: Drugs and Drug Resistance, 8*(3), 459–464.
6. Cvetkovic, R. S., & Goa, K. L. (2003). Lopinavir/ritonavir. *Drugs, 63*(8), 769–802.
7. World Health Organization. (2014). *Infection prevention and control of epidemic-and pandemic prone acute respiratory infections in health care*. WHO Guidelines.
8. Ong, E., Wong, M. U., Huffman, A., & He, Y. (2020). COVID-19 coronavirus vaccine design using reverse vaccinology and machine learning. *Frontiers in Immunology, 11*, 1581.
9. Cabeça, T. K., Granato, C., & Bellei, N. (2013). Epidemiological and clinical features of human coronavirus infections among different subsets of patients. *Influenza and Other Respiratory Viruses, 7*(6), 1040–1047.
10. Cui, J., Li, F., & Shi, Z. L. (2019). Origin and evolution of pathogenic coronaviruses. *Nature Reviews Microbiology, 17*(3), 181–192.
11. Baruah, V., & Bose, S. (2020). Immunoinformatics-aided identification of T cell and B cell epitopes in the surface glycoprotein of 2019-nCoV. *Journal of Medical Virology, 92*(5), 495–500.
12. Wu, F., Zhao, S., Yu, B., Chen, Y. M., Wang, W., Song, Z. G., Hu, Y., Tao, Z. W., Tian, J. H., Pei, Y. Y., & Yuan, M. L. (2020). A new coronavirus associated with human respiratory disease in China. *Nature, 579*(7798), 265–269.
13. Hui, D. S., Azhar, E. I., Madani, T. A., Ntoumi, F., Kock, R., Dar, O., Ippolito, G., Mchugh, T. D., Memish, Z. A., Drosten, C., & Zumla, A. (2020). The continuing 2019-nCoV epidemic threat of novel coronaviruses to global health—The latest 2019 novel coronavirus outbreak in Wuhan, China. *International Journal of Infectious Diseases, 91*, 264–266.
14. Funston, G., & Young, A. (2000). Rino Rappuoli. *Current Opinion in Microbiology, 3*, 445–450.
15. Purcell, A. W., McCluskey, J., & Rossjohn, J. (2007). More than one reason to rethink the use of peptides in vaccine design. *Nature Reviews Drug Discovery, 6*(5), 404–414.
16. Graham, R. L., Donaldson, E. F., & Baric, R. S. (2013). A decade after SARS: Strategies for controlling emerging coronaviruses. *Nature Reviews Microbiology, 11*(12), 836–848.

17. Shi, J., Zhang, J., Li, S., Sun, J., Teng, Y., Wu, M., Li, J., Li, Y., Hu, N., Wang, H., & Hu, Y. (2015). Epitope-based vaccine target screening against highly pathogenic MERS-CoV: An in silico approach applied to emerging infectious diseases. *PLoS One, 10*(12), e0144475.
18. Davidson, E., & Doranz, B. J. (2014). A high-throughput shotgun mutagenesis approach to mapping B-cell antibody epitopes. *Immunology, 143*(1), 13–20.
19. Steers, N. J., Currier, J. R., Jobe, O., Tovanabutra, S., Ratto-Kim, S., Marovich, M. A., Kim, J. H., Michael, N. L., Alving, C. R., & Rao, M. (2014). Designing the epitope flanking regions for optimal generation of CTL epitopes. *Vaccine, 32*(28), 3509–3516.
20. Ahmed, S. F., Quadeer, A. A., & McKay, M. R. (2020). Preliminary identification of potential vaccine targets for the COVID-19 coronavirus (SARS-CoV-2) based on SARS-CoV immunological studies. *Viruses, 12*(3), 254.
21. Wang, L., Shi, W., Joyce, M. G., Modjarrad, K., Zhang, Y., Leung, K., Lees, C. R., Zhou, T., Yassine, H. M., Kanekiyo, M., & Yang, Z. Y. (2015). Evaluation of candidate vaccine approaches for MERS-CoV. *Nature Communications, 6*(1), 1–11.
22. Ullah, A., Sarkar, B., & Islam, S. S. (2020). Exploiting the reverse vaccinology approach to design novel subunit vaccine against ebola virus. *Immunobiology*, 151949.
23. Farhani, I., Nezafat, N., & Mahmoodi, S. (2019). Designing a novel multi-epitope peptide vaccine against pathogenic Shigella spp. based immunoinformatics approaches. *International Journal of Peptide Research and Therapeutics, 25*(2), 541–553.
24. Nezafat, N., Eslami, M., Negahdaripour, M., Rahbar, M. R., & Ghasemi, Y. (2017). Designing an efficient multi-epitope oral vaccine against Helicobacter pylori using immunoinformatics and structural vaccinology approaches. *Molecular BioSystems, 13*(4), 699–713.
25. Nezafat, N., Karimi, Z., Eslami, M., Mohkam, M., Zandian, S., & Ghasemi, Y. (2016). Designing an efficient multi-epitope peptide vaccine against Vibrio cholerae via combined immunoinformatics and protein interaction based approaches. *Computational Biology and Chemistry, 62*, 82–95.
26. Mahendran, R., Jeyabaskar, S., Sitharaman, G., Michael, R. D., & Paul, A. V. (2016). Computer-aided vaccine designing approach against fish pathogens Edwardsiella tarda and Flavobacterium columnare using bioinformatics softwares. *Drug Design, Development and Therapy, 10*, 1703.
27. Davies, M. N., & Flower, D. R. (2007). Harnessing bioinformatics to discover new vaccines. *Drug Discovery Today, 12*(9–10), 389–395.
28. Seib, K. L., Zhao, X., & Rappuoli, R. (2012). Developing vaccines in the era of genomics: A decade of reverse vaccinology. *Clinical Microbiology and Infection, 18*, 109–116.
29. Kazi, A., Chuah, C., Majeed, A. B. A., Leow, C. H., Lim, B. H., & Leow, C. Y. (2018). Current progress of immunoinformatics approach harnessed for cellular-and antibody-dependent vaccine design. *Pathogens and Global Health, 112*(3), 123–131.
30. Folaranmi, T., Rubin, L., Martin, S. W., Patel, M., & MacNeil, J. R. (2015). Use of serogroup B meningococcal vaccines in persons aged ≥ 10 years at increased risk for serogroup B meningococcal disease: Recommendations of the Advisory Committee on Immunization Practices, 2015. *MMWR. Morbidity and Mortality Weekly Report, 64*(22), 608.
31. Doytchinova, I. A., & Flower, D. R. (2007). Identifying candidate subunit vaccines using an alignment-independent method based on principal amino acid properties. *Vaccine, 25*(5), 856–866.
32. Adu-Bobie, J., Capecchi, B., Serruto, D., Rappuoli, R., & Pizza, M. (2003). Two years into reverse vaccinology. *Vaccine, 21*(7–8), 605–610.
33. Narula, A., Pandey, R. K., Khatoon, N., Mishra, A., & Prajapati, V. K. (2018). Excavating chikungunya genome to design B and T cell multi-epitope subunit vaccine using comprehensive immunoinformatics approach to control chikungunya infection. *Infection, Genetics and Evolution, 61*, 4–15.
34. Caro-Gomez, E., Gazi, M., Goez, Y., & Valbuena, G. (2014). Discovery of novel cross-protective Rickettsia prowazekii T-cell antigens using a combined reverse vaccinology and in vivo screening approach. *Vaccine, 32*(39), 4968–4976.

35. Mehla, K., & Ramana, J. (2016). Identification of epitope-based peptide vaccine candidates against enterotoxigenic Escherichia coli: A comparative genomics and immunoinformatics approach. *Molecular BioSystems., 12*(3), 890–901.
36. Naz, A., Awan, F. M., Obaid, A., Muhammad, S. A., Paracha, R. Z., Ahmad, J., & Ali, A. (2015). Identification of putative vaccine candidates against Helicobacter pylori exploiting exoproteome and secretome: A reverse vaccinology based approach. *Infection, Genetics and Evolution, 32*, 280–291.
37. Farhadi, T., Nezafat, N., Ghasemi, Y., Karimi, Z., Hemmati, S., & Erfani, N. (2015). Designing of complex multi-epitope peptide vaccine based on omps of Klebsiella pneumoniae: An in silico approach. *International Journal of Peptide Research and Therapeutics, 21*(3), 325–341.
38. Farhadi, T., Ovchinnikov, R. S., & Ranjbar, M. M. (2016). In silico designing of some agonists of toll-like receptor 5 as a novel vaccine adjuvant candidates. *Network Modeling Analysis in Health Informatics and Bioinformatics, 5*(1), 31.
39. Dar, H. A., Zaheer, T., Shehroz, M., Ullah, N., Naz, K., Muhammad, S. A., Zhang, T., & Ali, A. (2019). Immunoinformatics-aided design and evaluation of a potential multi-epitope vaccine against Klebsiella Pneumoniae. *Vaccine, 7*(3), 88.
40. Shahbazi, M., Haghkhah, M., Rahbar, M. R., Nezafat, N., & Ghasemi, Y. (2016). In silico sub-unit hexavalent peptide vaccine against an Staphylococcus aureus biofilm-related infection. *International Journal of Peptide Research and Therapeutics, 22*(1), 101–117.
41. Jain, R., Singh, S., Kumar Verma, S., & Jain, A. (2019). Genome-wide prediction of potential vaccine candidates for Campylobacter jejuni using reverse vaccinology. *Interdisciplinary Sciences: Computational Life Sciences, 11*(3), 337–347.
42. Solanki, V., Tiwari, M., & Tiwari, V. (2019). Prioritization of potential vaccine targets using comparative proteomics and designing of the chimeric multi-epitope vaccine against Pseudomonas aeruginosa. *Scientific Reports, 9*(1), 1–19.
43. Sharma, D., Patel, S., Padh, H., & Desai, P. (2016). Immunoinformatic identification of potential epitopes against shigellosis. *International Journal of Peptide Research and Therapeutics, 22*(4), 481–495.
44. Vishnu, U. S., Sankarasubramanian, J., Gunasekaran, P., & Rajendhran, J. (2017). Identification of potential antigens from non-classically secreted proteins and designing novel multitope peptide vaccine candidate against Brucella melitensis through reverse vaccinology and immunoinformatics approach. *Infection, Genetics and Evolution, 55*, 151–158.
45. Monterrubio-López, G. P., & Ribas-Aparicio, R. M. (2015). Identification of novel potential vaccine candidates against tuberculosis based on reverse vaccinology. *BioMed Research International*.
46. Kolesanova, E. F., Sobolev, B. N., Moysa, A. A., Egorova, E. A., & Archakov, A. I. (2015). The way to the peptide vaccine against hepatitis C. *Biochemistry (Moscow) Supplement Series B: Biomedical Chemistry, 9*(3), 217–227.
47. Bruno, L., Cortese, M., Rappuoli, R., & Merola, M. (2015). Lessons from Reverse Vaccinology for viral vaccine design. *Current Opinion in Virology, 11*, 89–97.
48. Hasan, M., Ghosh, P. P., Azim, K. F., Mukta, S., Abir, R. A., Nahar, J., & Khan, M. M. H. (2019). Reverse vaccinology approach to design a novel multi-epitope subunit vaccine against avian influenza A (H7N9) virus. *Microbial Pathogenesis, 130*, 19–37.
49. Ul Qamar, M. T., Bari, A., Adeel, M. M., Maryam, A., Ashfaq, U. A., Du, X., Muneer, I., Ahmad, H. I., & Wang, J. (2018). Peptide vaccine against chikungunya virus: Immunoinformatics combined with molecular docking approach. *Journal of Translational Medicine, 16*(1), 298.
50. Mittal, A., Sasidharan, S., Raj, S., Balaji, S. N., & Saudagar, P. (2020). Exploring the Zika Genome to Design a Potential Multiepitope Vaccine Using an Immunoinformatics Approach. *International Journal of Peptide Research and Therapeutics*, 1–10.

51. Shahid, F., Ashfaq, U. A., Javaid, A., & Khalid, H. (2020). Immunoinformatics guided rational design of a next generation multi epitope based peptide (MEBP) vaccine by exploring Zika virus proteome. *Infection, Genetics and Evolution, 80*, 104199.
52. Florian, D. D., Shawan, A. K., Al Mahmud, H., Hasan, M. M., Parvin, A., Rahman, M. N., & Rahman, S. B. (2014). In silico modeling and immunoinformatics probing disclose the epitope based peptide vaccine against Zika virus envelope glycoprotein. *Indian Journal of Pharmaceutical and Biological Research, 2*(04), 44–57.
53. Saha, C. K., Hasan, M. M., Hossain, M. S., Jahan, M. A., & Azad, A. K. (2017). In silico identification and characterization of common epitope-based peptide vaccine for Nipah and Hendra viruses. *Asian Pacific Journal of Tropical Medicine, 10*(6), 529–538.
54. Ravichandran, L., Venkatesan, A., & Febin Prabhu Dass, J. (2019). Epitope-based immunoinformatics approach on RNA-dependent RNA polymerase (RdRp) protein complex of Nipah virus (NiV). *Journal of Cellular Biochemistry, 120*(5), 7082–7095.
55. Ojha, R., Pareek, A., Pandey, R. K., Prusty, D., & Prajapati, V. K. (2019). Strategic development of a next-generation multi-epitope vaccine to prevent Nipah virus zoonotic infection. *ACS Omega, 4*(8), 13069–13079.
56. Abdulla, F., Adhikari, U. K., & Uddin, M. K. (2019). Exploring T & B-cell epitopes and designing multi-epitope subunit vaccine targeting integration step of HIV-1 lifecycle using immunoinformatics approach. *Microbial Pathogenesis, 137*, 103791.
57. Azim, K. F., Hasan, M., Hossain, M. N., Somana, S. R., Hoque, S. F., Bappy, M. N. I., Chowdhury, A. T., & Lasker, T. (2019). Immunoinformatics approaches for designing a novel multi epitope peptide vaccine against human norovirus (Norwalk virus). *Infection, Genetics and Evolution, 74*, 103936.
58. Sayed, S. B., Nain, Z., Khan, M. S. A., Abdulla, F., Tasmin, R., & Adhikari, U. K. (2020). Exploring Lassa Virus Proteome to Design a Multi-epitope Vaccine Through Immunoinformatics and Immune Simulation Analyses. *International Journal of Peptide Research and Therapeutics*, 1–19.
59. Ahmad, B., Ashfaq, U. A., Rahman, M. U., Masoud, M. S., & Yousaf, M. Z. (2019). Conserved B and T cell epitopes prediction of ebola virus glycoprotein for vaccine development: An immuno-informatics approach. *Microbial Pathogenesis, 132*, 243–253.
60. Ali, M., Pandey, R. K., Khatoon, N., Narula, A., Mishra, A., & Prajapati, V. K. (2017). Exploring dengue genome to construct a multi-epitope based subunit vaccine by utilizing immunoinformatics approach to battle against dengue infection. *Scientific Reports, 7*(1), 1–13.
61. Yong, C. Y., Ong, H. K., Yeap, S. K., Ho, K. L., & Tan, W. S. (2019). Recent advances in the vaccine development against Middle East respiratory syndrome-coronavirus. *Frontiers in Microbiology, 10*, 1781.
62. Srivastava, S., Kamthania, M., Singh, S., Saxena, A. K., & Sharma, N. (2018). Structural basis of development of multi-epitope vaccine against middle east respiratory syndrome using in silico approach. *Infection and drug resistance, 11*, 2377.
63. Ul Qamar, M. T., Saleem, S., Ashfaq, U. A., Bari, A., Anwar, F., & Alqahtani, S. (2019). Epitope-based peptide vaccine design and target site depiction against Middle East Respiratory Syndrome Coronavirus: An immune-informatics study. *Journal of Translational Medicine, 17*(1), 362.
64. Khatoon, N., Pandey, R. K., & Prajapati, V. K. (2017). Exploring Leishmania secretory proteins to design B and T cell multi-epitope subunit vaccine using immunoinformatics approach. *Scientific Reports, 7*(1), 1–12.
65. Pandey, R. K., Bhatt, T. K., & Prajapati, V. K. (2018). Novel immunoinformatics approaches to design multi-epitope subunit vaccine for malaria by investigating anopheles salivary protein. *Scientific Reports, 8*(1), 1–11.
66. Pritam, M., Singh, G., Swaroop, S., Singh, A. K., & Singh, S. P. (2019). Exploitation of reverse vaccinology and immunoinformatics as promising platform for genome-wide screening of new effective vaccine candidates against Plasmodium falciparum. *BMC Bioinformatics, 19*(13), 468.

67. Jakhar, R., Kumar, P., Sehrawat, N., & Gakhar, S. K. (2019). A comprehensive analysis of amino-peptidase N1 protein (APN) from Anopheles culicifacies for epitope design using Immuno-informatics models. *Bioinformation, 15*(8), 600.
68. Zahroh, H., Ma'rup, A., Tambunan, U. S. F., & Parikesit, A. (2016). Immunoinformatics approach in designing epitope-based vaccine against meningitis-inducing bacteria (Streptococcus pneumoniae, Neisseria meningitidis, and Haemophilus influenzae type b). *Drug Target Insights, 10*, DTI-S38458.
69. Moradi, J., Tabrizi, M., Izad, M., Mosavari, N., & Feizabadi, M. M. (2017). Designing a novel multi-epitope DNA-based vaccine against tuberculosis: in silico approach. *Jundishapur Journal of Microbiology, 10*(3).
70. Chauhan, N., Khatri, V., Banerjee, P., & Kalyanasundaram, R. (2018). Evaluating the vaccine potential of a tetravalent fusion protein (rBmHAXT) vaccine antigen against lymphatic filariasis in a mouse model. *Frontiers in Immunology, 9*, 1520.
71. Chauhan, V., Rungta, T., Goyal, K., & Singh, M. P. (2019). Designing a multi-epitope based vaccine to combat Kaposi Sarcoma utilizing immunoinformatics approach. *Scientific Reports, 9*(1), 1–15.
72. Sarkar, B., Ullah, M. A., Johora, F. T., Taniya, M. A., & Araf, Y. (2020). Immunoinformatics-guided designing of epitope-based subunit vaccine against the SARS Coronavirus-2 (SARS-CoV-2). *Immunobiology*, 151955.
73. Ojha, R., Gupta, N., Naik, B., Singh, S., Verma, V. K., Prusty, D., & Prajapati, V. K. (2020). High throughput and comprehensive approach to develop multiepitope vaccine against minacious COVID-19. *European Journal of Pharmaceutical Sciences, 105375*.
74. Srivastava, S., Verma, S., Kamthania, M., Kaur, R., Badyal, R. K., Saxena, A. K., Shin, H. J., Kolbe, M., & Pandey, K. (2020). Structural basis to design multi-epitope vaccines against Novel Coronavirus 19 (COVID19) infection, the ongoing pandemic emergency: An in silico approach. *JMIR Bioinformatics and Biotechnology, 1*(1), e19371.
75. Tazehkand, M. N., & Hajipour, O. (2020). Evaluating the vaccine potential of a tetravalent fusion protein against coronavirus (COVID-19). *Journal of Vaccines Vaccination, 2*, 411–416.
76. Enayatkhani, M., Hasaniazad, M., Faezi, S., Guklani, H., Davoodian, P., Ahmadi, N., Einakian, M. A., Karmostaji, A., & Ahmadi, K. (2020). Reverse vaccinology approach to design a novel multi-epitope vaccine candidate against COVID-19: an in silico study. *Journal of Biomolecular Structure and Dynamics*, 1–16.
77. Jakhar, R., Kaushik, S., & Gakhar, S. K. (2020). 3CL Hydrolase Based Multi Epitope Peptide Vaccine Against Sars-CoV-2 Using Immunoinformatics. *Journal of Medical Virology*, 1–10.
78. Peele, K. A., Srihansa, T., Krupanidhi, S., Sai, A. V., & Venkateswarulu, T. C. (2020). Design of multi-epitope vaccine candidate against SARS-CoV-2: an in-silico study. *Journal of Biomolecular Structure & Dynamics*, 1.
79. Ka, T., Narsaria, U., Basak, S., De, D., Castiglion, F., Mueller, D. M., & Srivastava, A. P. (2020). A Ceandidate multi-epitope vaccine against SARS-CoV-2.
80. Gupta, A. K., Khan, M., Choudhury, S., Mukhopadhyay, A., Rastogi, A., Thakur, A., Kumari, P., Kaur, M., Saini, C., Sapehia, V., Patel, P. K., & Corona, V. R. (2020). A computational resource and analysis of epitopes and therapeutics for severe acute respiratory syndrome coronavirus-2. *Frontiers in Microbiology, 11*, 1858.
81. Yadav, P. D., Potdar, V. A., Choudhary, M. L., Nyayanit, D. A., Agrawal, M., Jadhav, S. M., Majumdar, T. D., Shete-Aich, A., Basu, A., Abraham, P., & Cherian, S. S. (2020). Full-genome sequences of the first two SARS-CoV-2 viruses from India. *The Indian Journal of Medical Research, 151*(2–3), 200.
82. Naz, A., Shahid, F., Butt, T. T., Awan, F. M., Ali, A., & Malik, A. (2020). Designing multi-epitope vaccines to combat emerging coronavirus disease 2019 (COVID-19) by employing immuno-informatics approach. *Frontiers in Immunology, 11*, 1663.
83. Norizadehtazehkand, M., & Hajipour, O. (2020). In silico recombinant vaccine candidate against coronavirus (2019-nCoV). *Acta Scientific Microbiology, 3*(4), 17–23.

84. Mukherjee, S., Tworowski, D., Detroja, R., Mukherjee, S. B., & Frenkel-Morgenstern, M. (2020). Immunoinformatics and structural analysis for identification of immunodominant epitopes in SARS-CoV-2 as potential vaccine targets. *Vaccine, 8*(2), 290.
85. Abdelmageed, M. I., Abdelmoneim, A. H., Mustafa, M. I., Elfadol, N. M., Murshed, N. S., Shantier, S. W., & Makhawi, A. M. (2020). Design of a multiepitope-based peptide vaccine against the E protein of human COVID-19: An immunoinformatics approach. *BioMed Research International*.
86. Bency, J., & Helen, M. (2020). Novel epitope based peptides for vaccine against SARS-CoV-2 virus: Immunoinformatics with docking approach. *International Journal of Research in Medical Sciences, 8*(7), 2385.
87. Zhou, G., & Zhao, Q. (2020). Perspectives on therapeutic neutralizing antibodies against the Novel Coronavirus SARS-CoV-2. *International Journal of Biological Sciences, 16*(10), 1718.
88. Dhama, K., Sharun, K., Tiwari, R., Sircar, S., Bhat, S., Malik, Y. S., Singh, K. P., Chaicumpa, W., Bonilla-Aldana, D. K., & Rodriguez-Morales, A. J.. (2020). Coronavirus disease 2019–COVID-19.
89. Dangi, M., Kumari, R., Singh, B., & Chhillar, A. K. (2018). Advanced In Silico Tools for Designing of Antigenic Epitope as Potential Vaccine Candidates Against Coronavirus. In *Bioinformatics: Sequences, Structures, Phylogeny* (pp. 329–357). Singapore: Springer.
90. Golosova, O., Henderson, R., Vaskin, Y., Gabrielian, A., Grekhov, G., Nagarajan, V., Oler, A. J., Quinones, M., Hurt, D., Fursov, M., & Huyen, Y. (2014). Unipro UGENE NGS pipelines and components for variant calling, RNA-seq and ChIP-seq data analyses. *PeerJ, 2*, e644.
91. Okonechnikov, K., Golosova, O., Fursov, M., & Ugene Team. (2012). Unipro UGENE: a unified bioinformatics toolkit. *Bioinformatics, 28*(8), 1166–1167.
92. Doytchinova, I. A., & Flower, D. R. (2007). VaxiJen: A server for prediction of protective antigens, tumour antigens and subunit vaccines. *BMC Bioinformatics, 8*(1), 4.
93. Dimitrov, I., Bangov, I., Flower, D. R., & Doytchinova, I. (2014). AllerTOP v. 2—a server for in silico prediction of allergens. *Journal of Molecular Modeling, 20*(6), 2278.
94. Saha, S., & Raghava, G. P. S. (2006). AlgPred: prediction of allergenic proteins and mapping of IgE epitopes. *Nucleic Acids Research, 34*(suppl_2), W202–W209.
95. Gupta, S., Kapoor, P., Chaudhary, K., Gautam, A., Kumar, R., Raghava, G. P., & Open Source Drug Discovery Consortium. (2013). In silico approach for predicting toxicity of peptides and proteins. *PloS One, 8*(9), e73957.
96. Geourjon, C., & Deleage, G. (1995). SOPMA: Significant improvements in protein secondary structure prediction by consensus prediction from multiple alignments. *Bioinformatics, 11*(6), 681–684.
97. Gasteiger, E., Hoogland, C., Gattiker, A., Wilkins, M. R., Appel, R. D., & Bairoch, A. (2005). Protein identification and analysis tools on the ExPASy server. In *The proteomics protocols handbook* (pp. 571–607). Humana Press.
98. Magnan, C. N., Randall, A., & Baldi, P. (2009). SOLpro: Accurate sequence-based prediction of protein solubility. *Bioinformatics, 25*(17), 2200–2207.
99. Sachdeva, G., Kumar, K., Jain, P., & Ramachandran, S. (2005). SPAAN: A software program for prediction of adhesins and adhesin-like proteins using neural networks. *Bioinformatics, 21*(4), 483–491.
100. Shen, H. B., & Chou, K. C. (2010). Virus-mPLoc: A fusion classifier for viral protein subcellular location prediction by incorporating multiple sites. *Journal of Biomolecular Structure and Dynamics, 28*(2), 175–186.
101. Krogh, A., Larsson, B., Von Heijne, G., & Sonnhammer, E. L. (2001). Predicting transmembrane protein topology with a hidden Markov model: Application to complete genomes. *Journal of Molecular Biology, 305*(3), 567–580.
102. Frank, K., & Sippl, M. J. (2008). High-performance signal peptide prediction based on sequence alignment techniques. *Bioinformatics, 24*(19), 2172–2176.

103. Marchler-Bauer, A., Bo, Y., Han, L., He, J., Lanczycki, C. J., Lu, S., Chitsaz, F., Derbyshire, M. K., Geer, R. C., Gonzales, N. R., & Gwadz, M. (2017). CDD/SPARCLE: Functional classification of proteins via subfamily domain architectures. *Nucleic Acids Research, 45*(D1), D200–D203.
104. Schaeffer, R. D., Liao, Y., Cheng, H., & Grishin, N. V. (2017). ECOD: New developments in the evolutionary classification of domains. *Nucleic Acids Research, 45*(D1), D296–D302.
105. Finn, R. D., Attwood, T. K., Babbitt, P. C., Bateman, A., Bork, P., Bridge, A. J., Chang, H. Y., Dosztányi, Z., El-Gebali, S., Fraser, M., & Gough, J. (2017). InterPro in 2017—Beyond protein family and domain annotations. *Nucleic Acids Research, 45*(D1), D190–D199.
106. Larsen, J. E. P., Lund, O., & Nielsen, M. (2006). Improved method for predicting linear B-cell epitopes. *Immunome Research, 2*(1), 1–7.
107. Ponomarenko, J., Bui, H. H., Li, W., Fusseder, N., Bourne, P. E., Sette, A., & Peters, B. (2008). ElliPro: A new structure-based tool for the prediction of antibody epitopes. *BMC Bioinformatics, 9*(1), 514.
108. Tomar, N., & De, R. K. (2010). Immunoinformatics: An integrated scenario. *Immunology, 131*(2), 153–168.
109. Soria-Guerra, R. E., Nieto-Gomez, R., Govea-Alonso, D. O., & Rosales-Mendoza, S. (2015). An overview of bioinformatics tools for epitope prediction: Implications on vaccine development. *Journal of Biomedical Informatics, 53*, 405–414.
110. Vita, R., Overton, J. A., Greenbaum, J. A., Ponomarenko, J., Clark, J. D., Cantrell, J. R., Wheeler, D. K., Gabbard, J. L., Hix, D., Sette, A., & Peters, B. (2015). The immune epitope database (IEDB) 3.0. *Nucleic Acids Research, 43*(D1), D405–D412.
111. Larsen, M. V., Lundegaard, C., Lamberth, K., Buus, S., Lund, O., & Nielsen, M. (2007). Large-scale validation of methods for cytotoxic T-lymphocyte epitope prediction. *BMC Bioinformatics, 8*(1), 424.
112. Calis, J. J., Maybeno, M., Greenbaum, J. A., Weiskopf, D., De Silva, A. D., Sette, A., Keşmir, C., & Peters, B. (2013). Properties of MHC class I presented peptides that enhance immunogenicity. *PLoS Computational Biology, 9*(10), e1003266.
113. Karosiene, E., Rasmussen, M., Blicher, T., Lund, O., Buus, S., & Nielsen, M. (2013). NetMHCIIpan-3.0, a common pan-specific MHC class II prediction method including all three human MHC class II isotypes, HLA-DR, HLA-DP and HLA-DQ. *Immunogenetics, 65*(10), 711–724.
114. Dhanda, S. K., Vir, P., & Raghava, G. P. (2013). Designing of interferon-gamma inducing MHC class-II binders. *Biology Direct, 8*(1), 30.
115. Singh, H., & Raghava, G. P. S. (2003). ProPred1: Prediction of promiscuous MHC class-I binding sites. *Bioinformatics, 19*(8), 1009–1014.
116. Bui, H. H., Sidney, J., Li, W., Fusseder, N., & Sette, A. (2007). Development of an epitope conservancy analysis tool to facilitate the design of epitope-based diagnostics and vaccines. *BMC Bioinformatics, 8*(1), 361.
117. Bui, H. H., Sidney, J., Dinh, K., Southwood, S., Newman, M. J., & Sette, A. (2006). Predicting population coverage of T-cell epitope-based diagnostics and vaccines. *BMC Bioinformatics, 7*(1), 1–5.
118. María, R. R., Arturo, C. J., Alicia, J. A., Paulina, M. G., & Gerardo, A. O. (2017). The impact of bioinformatics on vaccine design and development. In *Vaccines*. Rijeka, Croatia: InTech.
119. Berman, H. M., Westbrook, J., Feng, Z., Iype, L., Schneider, B., & Zardecki, C. (2003). The nucleic acid database. *Methods of Biochemical Analysis, 44*, 199–216.
120. Waterhouse, A., Bertoni, M., Bienert, S., Studer, G., Tauriello, G., Gumienny, R., Heer, F. T., de Beer, T. A. P., Rempfer, C., Bordoli, L., & Lepore, R. (2018). SWISS-MODEL: Homology modelling of protein structures and complexes. *Nucleic Acids Research, 46*(W1), W296–W303.
121. Källberg, M., Wang, H., Wang, S., Peng, J., Wang, Z., Lu, H., & Xu, J. (2012). Template-based protein structure modeling using the RaptorX web server. *Nature Protocols, 7*, 1511.

122. Yang, J., Yan, R., Roy, A., Xu, D., Poisson, J., & Zhang, Y. (2015). The I-TASSER Suite: Protein structure and function prediction. *Nature Methods, 12*(1), 7–8.
123. Kim, D. E., Chivian, D., & Baker, D. (2004). Protein structure prediction and analysis using the Robetta server. *Nucleic Acids Research, 32*(suppl_2), W526–W531.
124. Pettersen, E. F., Goddard, T. D., Huang, C. C., Couch, G. S., Greenblatt, D. M., Meng, E. C., & Ferrin, T. E. (2004). UCSF Chimera—A visualization system for exploratory research and analysis. *Journal of Computational Chemistry, 25*(13), 1605–1612.
125. Johansson, M. U., Zoete, V., Michielin, O., & Guex, N. (2012). Defining and searching for structural motifs using DeepView/Swiss-PdbViewer. *BMC Bioinformatics, 13*(1), 173.
126. Wang, W., Xia, M., Chen, J., Deng, F., Yuan, R., Zhang, X., & Shen, F. (2016). Data set for phylogenetic tree and RAMPAGE Ramachandran plot analysis of SODs in Gossypium raimondii and G. arboreum. *Data in Brief, 9*, 345–348.
127. Wiederstein, M., & Sippl, M. J. (2007). ProSA-web: Interactive web service for the recognition of errors in three-dimensional structures of proteins. *Nucleic Acids Research, 35*(suppl_2), W407–W410.
128. Benkert, P., Künzli, M., & Schwede, T. (2009). QMEAN server for protein model quality estimation. *Nucleic Acids Research, 37*(suppl_2), W510–W514.
129. Thevenet, P., Shen, Y., Maupetit, J., Guyon, F., Derreumaux, P., & Tuffery, P. (2012). PEP-FOLD: An updated de novo structure prediction server for both linear and disulfide bonded cyclic peptides. *Nucleic Acids Research, 40*(W1), W288–W293.
130. Trott, O., & Olson, A. J. (2010). AutoDock Vina: Improving the speed and accuracy of docking with a new scoring function, efficient optimization, and multithreading. *Journal of Computational Chemistry, 31*(2), 455–461.
131. Comeau, S. R., Gatchell, D. W., Vajda, S., & Camacho, C. J. (2004). ClusPro: a fully automated algorithm for protein–protein docking. *Nucleic Acids Research, 32*(suppl_2), W96–W99.
132. Schneidman-Duhovny, D., Inbar, Y., Nussinov, R., & Wolfson, H. J. (2005). PatchDock and SymmDock: servers for rigid and symmetric docking. *Nucleic Acids Research, 33*(suppl_2), W363–W367.
133. Weng, G., Wang, E., Wang, Z., Liu, H., Zhu, F., Li, D., & Hou, T. (2019). HawkDock: A web server to predict and analyze the protein–protein complex based on computational docking and MM/GBSA. *Nucleic Acids Research, 47*(W1), W322–W330.
134. Yan, Y., Zhang, D., Zhou, P., Li, B., & Huang, S. Y. (2017). HDOCK: A web server for protein–protein and protein–DNA/RNA docking based on a hybrid strategy. *Nucleic Acids Research, 45*(W1), W365–W373.
135. Macindoe, G., Mavridis, L., Venkatraman, V., Devignes, M. D., & Ritchie, D. W. (2010). HexServer: an FFT-based protein docking server powered by graphics processors. *Nucleic Acids Research, 38*(suppl_2), W445–W449.
136. De Vries, S. J., Van Dijk, M., & Bonvin, A. M. (2010). The HADDOCK web server for data-driven biomolecular docking. *Nature Protocols, 5*(5), 883.
137. Wallace, A. C., Laskowski, R. A., & Thornton, J. M. (1995). LIGPLOT: A program to generate schematic diagrams of protein-ligand interactions. *Protein Engineering, Design and Selection, 8*(2), 127–134.
138. Hu, W., Li, F., Yang, X., Li, Z., Xia, H., Li, G., Wang, Y., & Zhang, Z. (2004). A flexible peptide linker enhances the immunoreactivity of two copies HBsAg preS1 (21–47) fusion protein. *Journal of Biotechnology, 107*(1), 83–90.
139. Heo, L., Park, H., & Seok, C. (2013). GalaxyRefine: Protein structure refinement driven by side-chain repacking. *Nucleic Acids Research, 41*(W1), W384–W388.
140. Van Der Spoel, D., Lindahl, E., Hess, B., Groenhof, G., Mark, A. E., & Berendsen, H. J. (2005). GROMACS: Fast, flexible, and free. *Journal of Computational Chemistry, 26*(16), 1701–1718.

141. Rapin, N., Lund, O., Bernaschi, M., & Castiglione, F. (2010). Computational immunology meets bioinformatics: The use of prediction tools for molecular binding in the simulation of the immune system. *PLoS One, 5*(4), e9862.
142. Kroger, A. T. (2003). *General Recommendations on Immunization; US Department of Health and Human Services*. Atlanta, GA: Public Health Servic, Centers for Disease Control.
143. Castiglione, F., Mantile, F., De Berardinis, P., & Prisco, A. (2012). How the interval between prime and boost injection affects the immune response in a computational model of the immune system. *Computational and Mathematical Methods in Medicine, 2012*, 842329.
144. Grote, A., Hiller, K., Scheer, M., Münch, R., Nörtemann, B., Hempel, D. C., & Jahn, D. (2005). JCat: a novel tool to adapt codon usage of a target gene to its potential expression host. *Nucleic Acids Research, 33*(suppl_2), W526–W531.
145. Wu, X., Wu, S., Li, D., Zhang, J., Hou, L., Ma, J., Liu, W., Ren, D., Zhu, Y., & He, F. (2010). Computational identification of rare codons of Escherichia coli based on codon pairs preference. *BMC Bioinformatics, 11*(1), 61.

**Dr. Renu Jakhar** She completed her Ph.D. degree in Medical Biotechnology from M.D. University Rohtak (Haryana). She attended many national and international conferences and has various publications in reputed national and international journal. She worked in DBT-IPLS project, and her area of interest lies in the field of molecular biology, culture techniques, immunoinformatics, and structural chemistry.

**Dr. Neelam Sehrawat** She is an Assistant Professor in the Department of Genetics, Maharshi Dayanand University, Rohtak, Haryana, India. She has completed her Ph.D. (Biotechnology) in 2012 at the Centre for Biotechnology, Maharshi Dayanand University, Rohtak, Haryana, India. Her main thrust areas are malaria vector genetics, immunoinformatics, and transmission-blocking vaccine. Dr. Neelam Sehrawat has published 16 research papers in reputed international/national journals and conferences. She has completed three research projects sanctioned by the Department of Biotechnology, New Delhi; University Grants Commission, New Delhi; and Maharshi Dayanand University, Rohtak. She is a professional member in Faculty of Life Sciences, PGBOS, Departmental Research Committee, etc.

**Prof. S. K. Gakhar** He is an eminent Genetic Engineer and Immunologist; his teaching and research career spans over 35 years. He is currently working as Vice-Chancellor of IGU, Meerpur, Rewari (Haryana). He worked as Biotechnology National Associate at All India Institute of Medical Sciences, New Delhi, and Visiting Scientist at the University of California, Irvine, USA, and also at Cold Spring Harbor Laboratory, NY, USA. He has been Vice-Chancellor of CBLU, Bhiwani. He was the Dean Faculty of Life Sciences at M.D. University, Rohtak. He contributed in Academic Growth of the Department as Director and Coordinator, Bioinformatics Centre (DBT – sponsored), DST-FIST, UGC SAP, DBT-HRD Project, and Life Sciences Builders Grant, DBT, Govt. of India. He has to his credit more than 100 research publications in refereed and impact factor journals and 2 edited books. He has completed 15 Extra Mural Major Research Projects funded by DST, CSIR, ICMR, UGC, DBT, etc. He has also been a member of various national and international committees and forums.

# Chapter 10
# Big Data Analytics for Modeling COVID-19 and Comorbidities: An Unmet Need

**Sushil K. Shakyawar, Sahil Sethi, Siddesh Southekal, Nitish K. Mishra, and Chittibabu Guda**

## 10.1 Multi-organ Association of COVID-19

The novel coronavirus disease 2019 (COVID-19) is associated with multi-organ responses, causing severe illness or even death. Pneumonia, one of the most serious and frequent symptoms of COVID-19, has been observed in many patients. In a recent study, 17% of the infected patients exhibited acute respiratory distress syndrome (ARDS), and 65% of those died due to worsening conditions, especially from multi-organ failure [1–3]. Similarly, another study revealed that ARDS is heavily associated with age groups over 65 years [4]. Higher susceptibility and mortality of elderly patients were also correlated with reduced functioning of organs such as the lungs, kidney, and liver, causing serious illness [5].

COVID-19 progression is also affected by existing cardiovascular diseases as well as other conditions like hypertension and diabetes, as shown by the study performed on 46,248 COVID-19 patients [6]. In a similar context, Zhou and co-workers also concluded a higher association of an existing cardiovascular disease with COVID-19-related mortality [7]. Another previous study also showed that COVID-19-infected patients suffered kidney dysfunction by developing acute kidney injury (AKI) or mild-to-moderate proteinuria; however, the mechanism of disease progression is poorly understood [8]. Molecular-level studies to understand the expression of angiotensin-converting enzyme 2 (ACE2), an infection promoting enzyme in kidney cell, suggested its direct association with COVID-19 [9, 10]. Another study also mentioned the association of gastrointestinal symptoms like nausea, diarrhea, and abdominal pain in COVID-19 patients [11]. These associations were further clarified with a metagenomic-level study which confirmed higher

S. K. Shakyawar · S. Sethi · S. Southekal · N. K. Mishra · C. Guda (✉)
Department of Genetics, Cell Biology and Anatomy, University of Nebraska Medical Center, Omaha, NE, USA
e-mail: babu.guda@unmc.edu



S. Kautish et al. (eds.), *Computational Intelligence Techniques for Combating COVID-19*, EAI/Springer Innovations in Communication and Computing,
https://doi.org/10.1007/978-3-030-68936-0_10

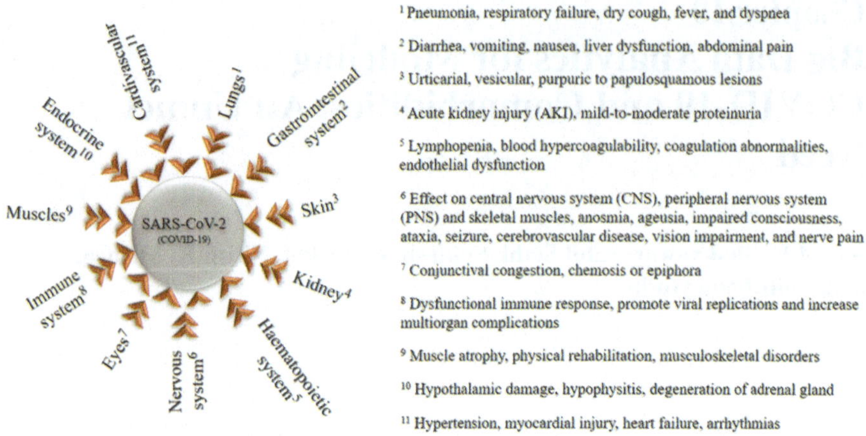


**Fig. 10.1** A pictorial representation of the association of COVID-19 with different organs and biological systems with their clinical manifestations in human body

expression of ACE2 in the gastrointestinal tract [12]. Later, it was concluded that COVID-19 can cause liver damage, as interpreted by elevation in the expression of liver enzymes like alanine aminotransferases and aspartate aminotransferases [11].

The nervous system is another biological system that could be affected by SARS-CoV-2 causing neurological diseases like encephalopathy, neuralgia, and unconsciousness [13, 14] as well as injuries to skeletal muscles [15]. Figure 10.1 shows a pictorial representation of various organs affected by COVID-19 in humans. In the same context, disseminated intravascular coagulation (DIC) is another associated phenotype in COVID-19 patients [16, 17]. Another study showed that rhabdomyolysis, the breakdown of muscles, is also found to be associated with COVID-19, which may cause severe injuries to skeletal muscles and can be life-threatening [18]. Several other severe symptoms are related to other organs or biological systems including the heart, blood vessels, and intestine, according to previous studies [19–21].

## 10.2 Crowdsourcing and Data Collection

From the point of view of computational modeling, reliable and high-quality data collection is particularly important to understand comorbidities and their patterns in association with COVID-19. Data related to omics, geographic location, demographics, mobility, clinics, and so on will be useful in this regard. The different data types and COVID-19 resources have been briefly described in Table 10.1. Although a variety of online databases and web-based tools are available to retrieve this information, we also want to emphasize text mining-based approaches to extract meaningful information. Text mining algorithms can be used to extract useful information on SARS-CoV-2 from unstructured, quantitative, or qualitative data. In this

**Table 10.1** COVID-19-related data resources available and studies using big data analyses

| S. no | Category | Data type | Brief description | Data sources |
|---|---|---|---|---|
| 1 | Epidemiological data | Geographic data | Represents the distribution of COVID-19 cases, deaths, and recoveries over the countries worldwide | Worldometers coronavirus, WHO, ECDC |
| | | Demographic data | Shows the distribution of death rate among different groups: age, sex, and comorbidities | Worldometers coronavirus demographics, CDC, World meters demographics, World meters demographics by country |
| | | Mobility data | Shows the movement patterns of populations indicating how strictly lockdowns have been enforced in different countries | Facebook data for good, Google Mobility data |
| 2 | Molecular data | Viral genomic data | Describes SARS-CoV-2 genomic sequences, annotations, and genomic expression data | NCBI SARS-CoV-2 resources, COVID-19, Pandemic Resources at UCSC, GISAID |
| | | Host genomic data | Describes host genetic variants that contribute to susceptibility, the severity of infection, and outcomes | The COVID-19 host genetics initiative |
| | | Other omics data (e.g., proteomics, metabolomics, epigenetics, glycomics, etc.) | Describes the involvement of molecules like RNA, proteins, metabolites, etc. in COVID-19 infection | RDA-COVID-19-Omics. EMBL-EBT's COVID-19 Data Portal |
| | | Chemical compounds and targets | Includes the biochemical activity, drug screens, and potential viral targets to reduce or end the viral infection | PubChem, CAS COVID-19 antiviral candidate compounds dataset, COVID-19 Molecular Structure. Therapeutics Hub |

(continued)

**Table 10.1** continued

| S. no | Category | Data type | Brief description | Data sources |
|---|---|---|---|---|
| 3 | Clinical data | Patient data and clinical trials | Includes the mechanisms and causes of pathogenesis, and information on how and why patients die or recover from the infections | ClinicalTrials.gov COVID-19 related studies. UCSF COVID-19 Clinical Data, LEOSS, UC Health Clinical Data Warehouse |
| | | Symptoms and diagnostics | Includes information related to symptoms of COVID-19 self-reported by patients, imaging data, and blood tests from health professionals | COVID-19 CT segmentation dataset, GitHub COVID-CT set, GitHub ieee8023/ covid-chestxray-dataset, Open-Source-COVID-19 |
| 4 | Morbidity data | Comorbidities | Describes existing health conditions causing serious injuries to the organs in COVID-19 patients | CDC, HealthData.gov, IARS |

context, LitCovid provides downloadable literature data that was annotated by PubTator [22]. Also, crowdsourcing can be used for collecting COVID-19 symptoms that patients or potential patients can self-report using online applications and can be used later to create ML-based models for predicting COVID-19 symptoms for enabling authorities to forecast potential hotspots. Open-Source-COVID-19 includes crowdsourced data obtained by patient self-reported COVID-19 symptoms (http://open-source-covid-19.weileizeng.com/world). A very comprehensive list of online resources for data related to COVID-19 is also provided by the National Institute of Health (NIH) portal (https://datascience.nih.gov/covid-19-open-access-resources).

## 10.3 Big Data Modeling for Personalized Treatment

In an era of high-throughput technologies, a massive amount of data are being generated every day. The healthcare systems, mostly in developed and developing countries, have already established robust systems for capturing and storing health-related patient data. For this purpose, different data collection tools like Enterprise Data Warehouses (EDWs) and Oracle Healthcare Data Repository (https://www.oracle.com/industries/healthcare/data-repository.html) play important roles by providing platforms for managing clinical information, electronic medical records (EMRs), personal health records (PHRs), etc.

At the same time, high-throughput technologies such as next-generation sequencing (NGS) and mass spectrometry (MS) have revolutionized the molecular-level profiling of patient samples to empower the use of multidimensional data for integrative analysis and correlation, to better understand the biological processes in diseased/normal conditions. Using multi-omics data is more effective if analyzed in an integrative fashion. Moreover, molecular data, when conjugated with healthcare analytics, provide synergistic opportunities to devise personalized treatment strategies.

The current COVID-19 pandemic, with limited information on disease dynamics and progression, requires an integrative approach in terms of analyzing data from various domains, as illustrated in Fig. 10.2. SARS-CoV-2 affects multiple organs; hence, transcriptomic- and metabolomic-level experiments will provide insights into disease progression across biological systems. Moreover, organ-specific studies should be emphasized in a sophisticated way to make sense of large-scale data. Table 10.1 lists different repositories for providing multidimensional data on COVID-19. Examples of managing health-related data using software like Hadoop [23] and Apache Shark [24] are explained well in a previous review [25].

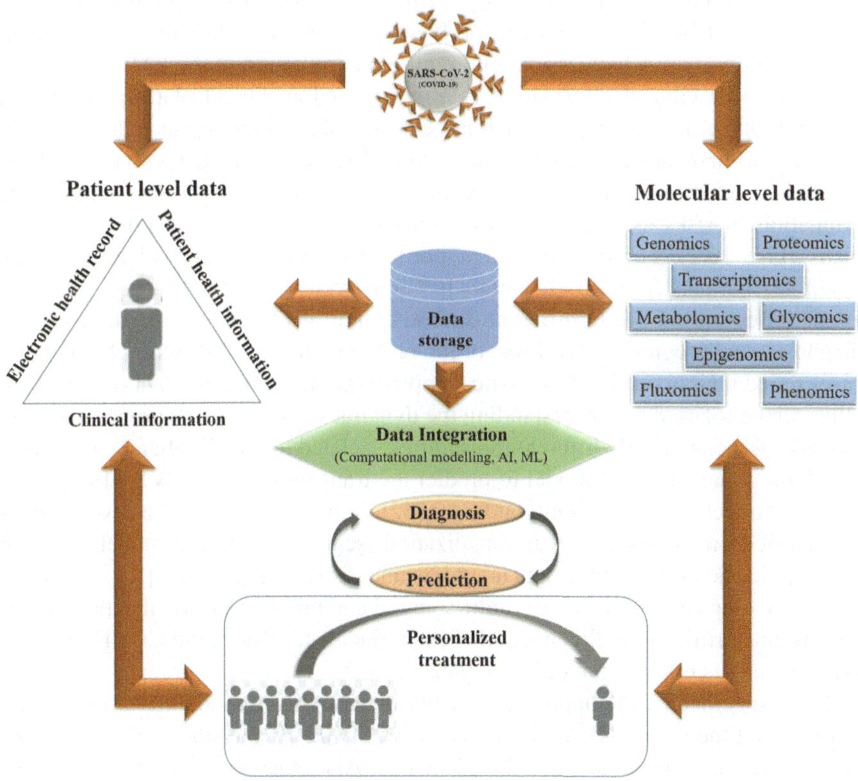


**Fig. 10.2** A strategical workflow for integrating multi-scale data from different domains to develop clinically viable solutions for personalized treatment of COVID-19 patients

## 10.4 Big Data Analysis and Integration: Modeling Data on Comorbidities

### *10.4.1 The Need for Comorbidity Data Integration*

Based on the clinical manifestation, it has been clearly understood that people with underlying health conditions are at higher risk of being infected with COVID-19. According to the Centers for Disease Control and Prevention (CDC), health conditions such as sickle cell disease, kidney diseases, obstructive pulmonary disease, immunocompromization from an organ transplant, and serious heart problems (like heart failure or cardiomyopathies) are more likely to cause serious illness in patients infected by COVID-19. Recent findings suggested that hypertension, diabetes, and obesity are highly associated comorbidities [26, 27]. Having considered these vulnerable characteristics, COVID-19 treatments are required to focus on comorbidities in patients, as these may cause serious illness, which sometimes leads to death, as reported in several previous studies [28–30]. According to the news report, around 94% of hospitalized COVID-19-infected patients had comorbidities (https://www.the-scientist.com/news-opinion/nearly-all-nyc-area-covid-19-hospitalizations-had-comorbidities-67476). To tackle this problem, accurate evaluation of comorbid conditions is important, which essentially require incorporation of the EMR, PHR, and access to other clinical information. A sophisticated analytical platform would be helpful to integrate and analyze such large-scale data from multiple sources to provide easy-to-understand outcomes due to comorbidities associated with COVID-19.

Studies generating an enormous amount of multidimensional data support the evaluation of risks associated with comorbid phenotypes and specific treatment plans (Fig. 10.2). For example, in a pre-COVID study, statistical analyses on 8,572,137 patients from 453 hospitals in China were carried out to determine the effects of comorbidities in different disease conditions to understand disease risk, diagnosis, and prognosis [31]. Most of the previous studies on different human diseases relied mainly on simple statistical approaches; however, big data-driven modeling can be focused for understanding the dynamics of COVID-19 progression and the risks associated with different morbidities. Related to this, Kucharski and members built a mathematical model to predict the transmission of COVID-19 by considering "traveling" as an important factor [32]. Similarly, a comprehensive analysis was carried out by focusing on visualization, segmentation, and modeling using geographic and demographic data to understand disease progression [33]. The same study also emphasized the use of multi-sourced and multidimensional data in building ML and artificial intelligence (AI)-based models to understand COVID-19 progression and its effects on multiple organs.

More specifically, the application of big data analytics to identify comorbidity patterns and their complex associations with COVID-19 can substantially contribute to advance understanding of the pandemic. Also, the co-occurrence of comorbidities, as observed in many patients [34, 35], needs to be targeted more in COVID-19 treatment strategies. As highlighted in Xtelligent Healthcare Media (https://healthitanalytics.com/news/forecasting-covid-19-with-predictive-analytics-big-data-tools), the predictive tools based on ML and AI are on high demand to determine risk, severity, progression, and outcomes of COVID-19 comorbidities. For conducting such analyses, collection of relevant data, application of the right analytics, and interpretation of the results are crucial parts of the analytical strategy. As mentioned in Table 10.1, morbidity-specific data can be utilized to model comorbidity correlations in association with COVID-19, which can provide a deeper understanding of shared molecular mechanisms of co-occurring diseases and help design specific treatment plans for COVID-19 patients. Multi-sourced data is even more powerful for building models for long-term forecasting of COVID-19 outcomes. Here, we propose a strategy to incorporate morbidity-specific data, demographic data, genotypic data, and other clinical information to understand the comorbidity network of diseases in the context of COVID-19 (Fig. 10.3). An earlier study by Chen et al. (2016) helps understand the comorbidities of diabetes in adults [36] and serves as an example of such approaches. The same study used longitudinal clinical and disease-related data spanning across 12 years (2002 to 2013) to understand comorbidity networks and help with accurate diagnosis. These approaches can also provide correlational perspectives of comorbidities. Understanding the patterns of co-occurrence of multiple comorbidities can be an advanced feature that can be evaluated using large-scale data from multiple sources. Furthermore, the comorbidity-specific networks or sub-networks can be used to understand the effects of COVID-19 treatment on multiple organs, which further can help minimizing the severe injuries to organs. Circumstances might vary based on an individual's existing health conditions, and thus, these types of approaches should be considered on a more personalized basis, and the decisions especially for treating COVID-19 symptoms should be taken carefully.

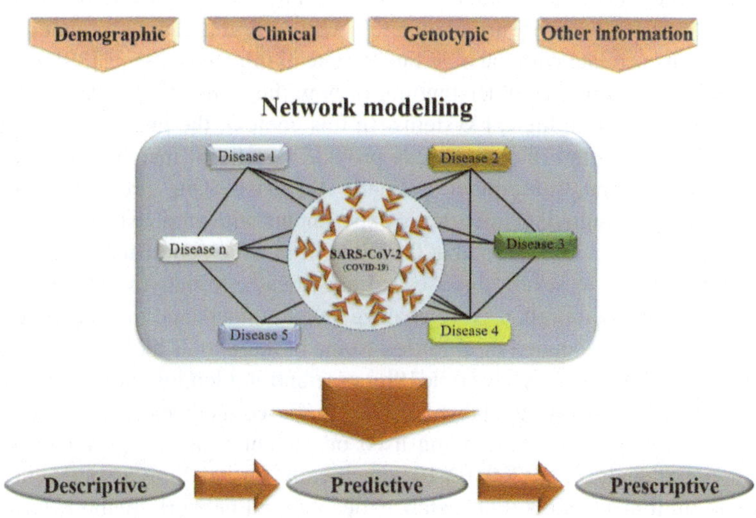


**Fig. 10.3** Comorbidity network modeling using big and multi-scale data for predictive and prescriptive outcomes

### 10.4.2 Omics Data on COVID-19 and Associated Comorbidities

Multi-omics approaches involve integration and analysis of various "omics" data such as genomics, epigenetics and proteomics, and metabolomics. The advantages of using multi-omics data as opposed to relying on single "omics" data have been evident from previous reports on various diseases [37]. Identifying the molecular mechanisms that promote the progression of the COVID-19 disease and its influences on different organs is critical. Multi-omics-based molecular data, pertaining to COVID-19, are being generated at a rapid rate; however, the complexity of integrating, storing, managing, and analyzing such high-dimensional datasets continues to be challenging. Since the beginning of the COVID-19 pandemic, around 75,000 viral genomic sequences have been generated by various laboratories around the world and made available to the public on the GISAID website as of July 30, 2020 (Table 10.1). These datasets have been extensively used by researchers around the world to track the movement of the virus across different regions of the world, and identify different strains and their mutation patterns, to understand the evolution of viral genomes and the virulence of different viral strains, design antigens and viroids for laboratory testing, etc. Viral sequence information is also essential to develop and evaluate diagnostic tests and to identify potential intervention options. The UCSC Genome Browser (Table 10.1) provides access to information on the mutations of SARS-CoV-2 genomes that are deposited in GISAID and other international nucleotide sequencing databases, enabling phylogenetic analysis of viral genomes. Availability of and easy accessibility to such data resources would promote extensive future research on COVID-19.

Of late, integrated comparative genomics and ML techniques are being used to identify protein features that are unique to SARS-CoV-2 and the associated comorbidities which correlate with the high fatality rate of infected patients [38]. However, there is a large gap in our understanding of how the virus affects the functions of different organs and biological systems. In this context, the integration of genetic and clinical information of patients can provide significant insights into the viral-host interaction and subsequent patient's response. Our proposed approach (Fig. 10.3) helps design data integration experiments with emphasis on comorbidity networks and associations to combat COVID-19, in which clinical symptoms range from asymptomatic to severe disease and even death. Initiatives are underway to collect, share, and comprehensively analyze data to understand the genetic makeup of COVID-19 and associated morbidities. Some of these tools including COVID-19 Host Genetics Initiative (www.covid19hg.org) and epidemiological, comorbidity, and outcome data are now available [2, 39]. ML-based methods such as deep learning architectures [75] are now being used on patient data as a powerful tool for prediction and analysis of COVID-19, specifically for handling associated comorbidities to minimize deaths. For instance, deep neural network methods have been developed for the diagnosis of COVID-19 using raw chest X-ray images and computed tomography (CT) images [40, 41]. Similarly, the taxonomic classification of

COVID-19 genomes has been done using ML approaches [42]. Some of the recent review articles provide a comprehensive overview of the application of ML strategies to understand prioritized genetic variants of COVID-19, identification of potential vaccine candidates and drug targets, predicting the spread of diseases, and forecasting the next pandemic [43–45].

## 10.5 Drug Repurposing: Treating COVID-19 and Comorbidities

Currently, there are no effective drugs targeting SARS-CoV-2, and only symptomatic treatment is given to patients. Other direct therapeutic approaches to treat COVID-19 patients include the use of repurposed drugs such as hydroxychloroquine, camostat, and nafamostat and viral RNA-dependent RNA polymerase (RdRp)-targeted drugs like remdesivir and favipiravir to mitigate associated comorbid conditions [46]. Given their targeted and anti-inflammatory effects, many anticancer agents are also being investigated as potential drug repurposing molecules. Some of the approved anticancer agents being tested on COVID-19 patients include interleukin (IL) inhibitors (e.g., tocilizumab, siltuximab), corticosteroid (e.g., prednisolone, dexamethasone, hydrocortisone), and checkpoint inhibitors (e.g., nivolumab, pembrolizumab) [47, 48]. The Global Coronavirus COVID-19 Clinical Trial Tracker (https://covid-trials.org) has identified about 1890 clinical trials as of July 30, 2020. The most common treatments include (hydroxy)chloroquine, plasma-based therapy, lopinavir/ritonavir, azithromycin, and alternative therapy.

Drug repositioning, which essentially reuses existing drugs for exploring new therapeutics, makes it more efficient, less time-consuming, and cost-effective [49]. To make a rational and effective choice, other viable strategies such as integration of existing and published multi-omics and patient clinical data from experimental and translational research, and incorporation of the existing library of FDA-approved or clinically investigated drugs are used, which help in discovering potential drug candidates and accelerating the drug discovery process [50]. Omics datasets can be used for computational repurposing of drugs through the incorporation of structures and/or signatures of the molecule(s) from public databases [51]. Zheng and colleagues used an integrative approach for prioritizing and repurposing 353 drug targets which may potentially interact with SARS-CoV-2 [52]. Similarly, in another study, the expression of 26 SARS-CoV-2 proteins in human cells helped to identify the physical association between the host and viral proteins using mass spectrometry. These analyses were helpful in identifying 332 protein-protein interactions (PPIs) between SARS-CoV-2 and human proteins with high confidence. Among the identified, 66 are druggable proteins showing potential interactions with 69 compounds, of which 29 are FDA-approved drugs, whereas 12 and 28 are in clinical and preclinical trials, respectively [53]. The challenges to incorporate comorbidity-related data in such analyses still exist. Other methods include data-driven drug repurposing approaches such as network-based approach, quantification of the interplay among the viral-host interactome, and potential drug targets in PPI network [54]. Approaches to improve the drug discovery process also include making data more accessible to researchers. COVID-19 Drug and Gene Set Library (https://amp.pharm.mssm.edu/covid19/) is one such data source which provides COVID-19-related drugs and gene sets. Network-based approaches have also used strategies to identify disease comorbidity networks to rapidly detect drug repurposing candidates. For instance, Gysi et al. (2020) overlapped PPI networks between the proteins associated with each of the 299 diseases and the targets of SARS-CoV-2 and observed comorbidities associated with cardiovascular diseases and cancer, which are known to be associated with COVID-19 [55]. In a similar context, a network-based integrative model built by incorporating different connections among drugs, disease-causing proteins/genes, diseases and associated pathways, and expressions was successfully used to identify repurposable drugs for COVID-19 [56]. Another deep neural network-based model was developed to perform screening of chemical libraries for the repurposing of drug molecules against the 3CLpro (3C-like protease) and PLpro (papain-like protease) of COVID-19 [57]. In conclusion, computational drug repurposing methods can further be improved by using advanced AI- and ML-based methods coupled with increased computational power [58]. Collectively, these datasets can be therapeutically exploited for the treatment of COVID-19 and associated life-threatening comorbidities.

## 10.6 Data Analytics for ACE2 Inhibitors: A Common Link in COVID-19 Comorbidity Network

Previous studies showed different levels of expression of ACE2 in various organs like the brain, heart, kidney, small intestine, stomach, thymus, and lungs [59]. Single-cell RNA-seq data further classified the lungs, esophagus, ileum, bladder, and kidney as high-risk organs having higher than 1% proportion of ACE2-positive cells [60]. Given the interactions of key amino acids (Lys31 and Lys353) on the ACE2 receptor with the spike RNA-binding domain (S-RBD) motif of the viral protein, the cells with ACE2 expression may be targeted to provide a promising therapeutic intervention to COVID-19. In silico screening of large compound libraries followed by molecular docking studies identified RS504393, GNF-5, TNP [N2-(m-Trifluorobenzyl), N6-(p-nitrobenzyl)purine], and eptifibatide acetate as potential inhibitors of the virus entry step by blocking SARS-CoV-2-ACE-2 receptor interface [61]. While the virus uses ACE2 as the primary cellular receptor, a membrane serine protease, TMPRSS2, catalyzes in stabilizing the process of entry and fusion of the viral protein with the cell membrane. An AI-based approach interrogating the potential of 2657 FDA-approved drugs identified beta-lactam antibiotic, fosamprenavir, emricasan, and glutathione, which showed interactions with ACE-2 and TMPRSS2 [62]. Another study employed molecular mechanics-assisted structure-based virtual screening (SBVS) of 7173 ligands which were clinically approved. These ligands were screened for their ability to bind to ACE-2 and prevent recognition by the virus. This resulted in the identification of lividomycin, burixafor, quisinostat, fluprofylline, pemetrexed, spirofylline, edotecarin, and diniprofylline as promising repurposable candidate drugs [63]. Moreover, the comprehensive integration of docking simulations combined with supervised and steered molecular dynamic simulations identified simeprevir and lumacaftor that could inhibit the viral spike protein-ACE-2 interactions with high affinity [64]. Further, ML and ensemble-based docking methods have been used to screen possible ligand molecules for two systems, namely, isolated SARS-CoV-2 S-protein at its host receptor region and the S-protein-ACE2 interface complex [65]. These studies highlighted the importance of AI-based systems approach to identify potential therapeutic targets for SARS-CoV-2, which were predicted to hamper the virus-receptor interaction in multiple organs. Since these drugs are readily available, further validation studies can be rapidly performed on these candidate drug targets for activity against SARS-CoV-2.

## 10.7 Artificial Intelligence (AI) and COVID-19

The rapid and exponential growth in the number of COVID-19 patients has exposed the limitations of the diagnostic infrastructure of many developed nations around the world. It also offers an opportunity to learn and be prepared for a potential future pandemic of similar or worse magnitude. In this context, the development of automated AI-based computer-aided diagnostic tools is warranted. The treasure of increasing amount of data related to COVID-19 can be used to speed up the research for understanding, controlling, and eradicating the pandemic using AI-driven approaches (Fig. 10.2). For example, crowdsourcing can be used in collecting COVID-19 data such as symptoms that patients or potential patients can self-report using online tools, and this data can be fed to create ML-based models that can make an early forecast of regional hotspots and alert authorities to take preventive measures to contain the spread of the disease. Moreover, curve fitting models can use geographic and demographic epidemiological data to predict growth and death rates of COVID-19 pandemic, since the growth curve of SARS-CoV-2 generally follows Gaussian or exponential distribution. One of the most common prediction models used in pandemics is the susceptible-infected-recovered (SIR) model, which predicts the number of infected, recovered, and dead individuals overtime by utilizing ordinary differential equations (ODEs) [66]. Also, regression models can be used in identifying the effects of multiple variables like genetic variants, immunity status, gender, and age on the severity and susceptibility of COVID-19 infections and outcomes by utilizing the viral and host genomic and molecular data and the demographic and epidemiological data [67].

ML-based methods such as support vector machines (SVMs) can be used to predict potential COVID-19 infections by utilizing information on self-reported symptoms, susceptibility of host genetic variants, viral proteomic and genomic data, immunogenicity of new vaccines in combination with host's immunology data, and data from biochemical activities of viral proteins [67]. Additionally, stochastic models like hidden Markov chains can use viral genomic, phylogenomic, and protein data to predict future changes in the viral antigens to develop new vaccines before the virus mutates into a new strain and in forecasting new COVID-19 cases.

Deep learning, another popular AI technique that is widely used to handle and analyze large volumes of patient data, is also applicable to COVID-19 data. Recent studies used deep learning for the diagnosis and prognosis of COVID-19 [41, 68]. Deep learning approaches can predict the level of disease severity based on CT images [41, 68]. Deep neural network models can also separate COVID-19 patients from other pneumonia and viral pneumonia patients with high accuracy, as previously reported [41, 69, 70]. Moreover, these methodologies can also predict the risk of COVID-19 patients developing critical illnesses based on clinical characteristics and comorbidity information [71]. Random forest (RF) model boosted by the AdaBoost algorithm, and using COVID-19 patients' geographic, travel, health, and demographic data, has predicted the severity of the cases, possible outcomes, recovery, or death [72]. In another study using worldwide patient data with clinical and comorbidity information, machine learning algorithms such as SVM, artificial neural networks, RF, decision tree, logistic regression, and K-nearest neighbor were used to predict the mortality rate in patients with COVID-19 [73]. Similarly, supervised XGBoost classifier-based interpretable decision tree model was developed based on the patients' clinical data to predict the mortality of COVID-19 patients [74].

## 10.8 Conclusions

The infectivity, the rate of spread, the severity of disease, and a high fatality rate all warrant the scientific community to find strategic and effective solutions to combat the current as well as potential future pandemics. Although minimal data are available, it is clear that existing health issues such as hypertension, obesity, cardiovascular diseases, lung diseases, and several others are linked to more deteriorating and fatal cases of COVID-19 infections. This chapter focuses on big data analysis and integration approaches to understand associated comorbidities and their patterns in COVID-19 infections. We emphasized that integrative analysis of multidimensional data from different domains such as genetic, molecular, clinical, demographic, and epidemiological studies using ML and AI tools would be extremely powerful to develop disease management strategies from forecasting to diagnosis and treatment. Also, our proposed approach can provide insights to better understand the association between comorbidities and COVID-19 and design a more effective strategy for personalized treatment. However, more concerted experimental work along with computational analysis is needed to understand the mechanistic aspects of disease progression, host-viral interactions, and comorbidity associations.

**Acknowledgments** This work has been supported by the startup funds to CG from the University of Nebraska Medical Center. The authors would like to thank the Bioinformatics and Systems Biology Core (BSBC) at UNMC for providing the computational infrastructure. BSBC is partly supported by multiple NIH awards [5P20GM103427, 5P30CA036727, 5P30MH062261].

## References

1. Chen, J., Qi, T., Liu, L., et al. (2020). Clinical progression of patients with COVID-19 in Shanghai, China. *The Journal of Infection*. https://dx.doi.org/10.1016/j.jinf.2020.03.004.
2. Chen, N., Zhou, M., Dong, X., et al. (2020). Epidemiological and clinical characteristics of 99 cases of 2019 novel coronavirus pneumonia in Wuhan, China: A descriptive study. *Lancet*. https://doi.org/10.1016/S0140-6736(20)30211-7.
3. Wang, Y., Lu, X., Li, Y., et al. (2020). Clinical course and outcomes of 344 intensive care patients with COVID-19. *American Journal of Respiratory and Critical Care Medicine*. https://doi.org/10.1164/rccm.202003-0736le.
4. Wu, C., Chen, X., Cai, Y., et al. (2020). Risk factors associated with acute respiratory distress syndrome and death in patients with coronavirus disease 2019 pneumonia in Wuhan, China. *JAMA Internal Medicine*. https://doi.org/10.1001/jamainternmed.2020.0994.
5. Liu, K., Chen, Y., Lin, R., & Han, K. (2020). Clinical features of COVID-19 in elderly patients: A comparison with young and middle-aged patients. *The Journal of Infection*. https://doi.org/10.1016/j.jinf.2020.03.005.
6. Baradaran, A., Ebrahimzadeh, M. H., Baradaran, A., & Kachooei, A. R. (2020). Prevalence of comorbidities in COVID-19 patients: A systematic review and meta-analysis. *The Archives of Bone and Joint Surgery*. https://doi.org/10.22038/abjs.2020.47754.2346.
7. Zhou, F., Yu, T., Du, R., et al. (2020). Clinical course and risk factors for mortality of adult inpatients with COVID-19 in Wuhan, China: A retrospective cohort study. *Lancet*. https://doi.org/10.1016/S0140-6736(20)30566-3.
8. Mclntosh, K. (2020). Coronavirus disease 2019 (COVID-19): Epidemiology, virology, clinical features, diagnosis, and prevention. *Journal of Chemical Information and Modeling*. https://doi.org/10.1017/CBO9781107415324.004.
9. Xu, X. W., Wu, X. X., Jiang, X. G., et al. (2020). Clinical findings in a group of patients infected with the 2019 novel coronavirus (SARS-Cov-2) outside of Wuhan, China: Retrospective case series. *BMJ*. https://doi.org/10.1136/bmj.m606.
10. Naicker, S., Yang, C. W., Hwang, S. J., et al. (2020). The novel coronavirus 2019 epidemic and kidneys. *Kidney International*. https://doi.org/10.1016/j.kint.2020.03.001.
11. Wong, S. H., Lui, R. N. S., & Sung, J. J. Y. (2020). Covid-19 and the digestive system. *Journal of Gastroenterology and Hepatology*. https://doi.org/10.1111/jgh.15047.
12. Holshue, M. L., DeBolt, C., Lindquist, S., et al. (2020). First case of 2019 novel coronavirus in the United States. *The New England Journal of Medicine*. https://doi.org/10.1056/NEJMoa2001191.
13. Hageman, J. R. (2020). The coronavirus disease 2019 (COVID-19). *Pediatric Annals*. https://doi.org/10.3928/19382359-20200219-01.
14. Li, Y. C., Bai, W. Z., & Hashikawa, T. (2020). The neuroinvasive potential of SARS-CoV2 may play a role in the respiratory failure of COVID-19 patients. *Journal of Medical Virology*. https://dx.doi.org/10.1002/jmv.25728.
15. Mao, L., Wang, M., Chen, S., et al. (2020). Neurological manifestations of hospitalized patients with COVID-19 in Wuhan, China: A retrospective case series study. *SSRN Electronic Journal*. https://doi.org/10.2139/ssrn.3544840.
16. Tang, N., Li, D., Wang, X., & Sun, Z. (2020). Abnormal coagulation parameters are associated with poor prognosis in patients with novel coronavirus pneumonia. *Journal of Thrombosis and Haemostasis*. https://doi.org/10.1111/jth.14768.

17. Lillicrap, D. (2020). Disseminated intravascular coagulation in patients with 2019-nCoV pneumonia. *Journal of Thrombosis and Haemostasis*. https://doi.org/10.1111/jth.14781.
18. Jin, M., & Tong, Q. (2020). Rhabdomyolysis as potential late complication associated with COVID-19. *Emerging Infectious Diseases*. https://doi.org/10.3201/eid2607.200445.
19. Guzik, T. J., Mohiddin, S. A., Dimarco, A., et al. (2020). COVID-19 and the cardiovascular system: Implications for risk assessment, diagnosis, and treatment options. *Cardiovascular Research*. https://doi.org/10.1093/cvr/cvaa106.
20. Ng, S. C., & Tilg, H. (2020). COVID-19 and the gastrointestinal tract: More than meets the eye. *Gut*. https://doi.org/10.1136/gutjnl-2020-321195.
21. Bao, Y., Lin, S. Y., Cheng, Z. H., et al. (2020). Clinical features of COVID-19 in a young man with massive cerebral hemorrhage—Case report. *SN Comprehensive Clinical Medicine*. https://doi.org/10.1007/s42399-020-00315-y.
22. Chen, Q., Allot, A., & Lu, Z. (2020). Keep up with the latest coronavirus research. *Nature*. https://doi.org/10.1038/d41586-020-00694-1.
23. Shvachko, K., Kuang, H., Radia, S., & Chansler, R. (2010). The Hadoop distributed file system. In *2010 IEEE 26th symposium on mass storage systems and technologies, MSST2010*. https://doi.org/10.1109/MSST.2010.5496972.
24. Zaharia, M., Xin, R. S., Wendell, P., et al. (2016). Apache spark: A unified engine for big data processing. *Communications of the ACM*. https://doi.org/10.1145/2934664.
25. Dash, S., Shakyawar, S. K., Sharma, M., & Kaushik, S. (2019). Big data in healthcare: Management, analysis and future prospects. *Journal of Big Data*. https://doi.org/10.1186/s40537-019-0217-0.
26. Singh, A. K., Gupta, R., Ghosh, A., & Misra, A. (2020). Diabetes in COVID-19: Prevalence, pathophysiology, prognosis and practical considerations. *Diabetes and Metabolic Syndrome: Clinical Research & Reviews*. https://doi.org/10.1016/j.dsx.2020.04.004.
27. Garg, S., Kim, L., Whitaker, M., et al. (2020). Hospitalization rates and characteristics of patients hospitalized with laboratory-confirmed coronavirus disease 2019 — Covid-net, 14 states, March 1–30, 2020. *Morbidity and Mortality Weekly Report*. https://doi.org/10.15585/mmwr.mm6915e3.
28. Guan, W. J., Liang, W. H., Zhao, Y., et al. (2020). Comorbidity and its impact on 1,590 patients with Covid-19 in China: A nationwide analysis. *The European Respiratory Journal*. https://doi.org/10.1183/13993003.00547-2020.
29. Xu, P. P., Tian, R. H., Luo, S., et al. (2020). Risk factors for adverse clinical outcomes with COVID-19 in China: A multicenter, retrospective, observational study. *Theranostics*. https://doi.org/10.7150/thno.46833.
30. Liang, W. H., Guan, W. J., Li, C. C., et al. (2020). Clinical characteristics and outcomes of hospitalised patients with COVID-19 treated in Hubei (epicentre) and outside Hubei (non-epicentre): A nationwide analysis of China. *The European Respiratory Journal*. https://doi.org/10.1183/13993003.00562-2020.
31. Guo, M., Yu, Y., Wen, T., et al. (2019). Analysis of disease comorbidity patterns in a large-scale China population. *BMC Medical Genomics*. https://doi.org/10.1186/s12920-019-0629-x.
32. Kucharski, A. J., Russell, T. W., Diamond, C., et al. (2020). Early dynamics of transmission and control of COVID-19: A mathematical modelling study. *The Lancet Infectious Diseases*. https://doi.org/10.1016/S1473-3099(20)30144-4.
33. Zhou, C., Su, F., Pei, T., et al. (2020). COVID-19: Challenges to GIS with Big Data. *Geography and Sustainability*. https://doi.org/10.1016/j.geosus.2020.03.005.
34. Jiang, F., Deng, L., Zhang, L., et al. (2020). Review of the clinical characteristics of coronavirus disease 2019 (COVID-19). *Journal of General Internal Medicine*. https://doi.org/10.1007/s11606-020-05762-w.
35. Shiau, S., Krause, K. D., Valera, P., et al. (2020). The burden of COVID-19 in people living with HIV: A syndemic perspective. *AIDS and Behavior*. https://dx.doi.org/10.1007/s10461-020-02871-9.
36. Chen, H., Zhang, Y., Wu, D., et al. (2016). Comorbidity in adult patients hospitalized with type 2 diabetes in Northeast China: An analysis of hospital discharge data from 2002 to 2013. *BioMed Research International*. https://doi.org/10.1155/2016/1671965.

37. Hasin, Y., Seldin, M., & Lusis, A. (2017). Multi-omics approaches to disease. *Genome Biology*. https://doi.org/10.1186/s13059-017-1215-1.
38. Gussow, A. B., Auslander, N., Faure, G., et al. (2020). Genomic determinants of pathogenicity in SARS-CoV-2 and other human coronaviruses. *Proceedings of the National Academy of Sciences*. https://doi.org/10.1073/pnas.2008176117.
39. Richardson, S., Hirsch, J. S., Narasimhan, M., et al. (2020). Presenting characteristics, comorbidities, and outcomes among 5700 patients hospitalized with COVID-19 in the New York City area. *JAMA – Journal of American Medical Association*. https://doi.org/10.1001/jama.2020.6775.
40. Ozturk, T., Talo, M., Yildirim, E. A., et al. (2020). Automated detection of COVID-19 cases using deep neural networks with X-ray images. *Computers in Biology and Medicine*. https://doi.org/10.1016/j.compbiomed.2020.103792.
41. Wang, S., Zha, Y., Li, W., et al. (2020). A fully automatic deep learning system for COVID-19 diagnostic and prognostic analysis. *The European Respiratory Journal*. https://doi.org/10.1183/13993003.00775-2020.
42. Randhawa, G. S., Soltysiak, M. P. M., El Roz, H., et al. (2020). Machine learning using intrinsic genomic signatures for rapid classification of novel pathogens: COVID-19 case study. *PLoS One*. https://doi.org/10.1371/journal.pone.0232391.
43. Tárnok, A. (2020). Machine learning, COVID-19 (2019-nCoV), and multi-OMICS. *Cytometry. Part A*. https://doi.org/10.1002/cyto.a.23990.
44. Alimadadi, A., Aryal, S., Manandhar, I., et al. (2020). Artificial intelligence and machine learning to fight covid-19. *Physiological Genomics*. https://doi.org/10.1152/physiolgenomics.00029.2020.
45. Albahri, A. S., Hamid, R. A., Alwan, J. K., et al. (2020). Role of biological data mining and machine learning techniques in detecting and diagnosing the novel coronavirus (COVID-19): A systematic review. *Journal of Medical Systems*. https://dx.doi.org/10.1007/s10916-020-01582-x.
46. Kiplin Guy, R., DiPaola, R. S., Romanelli, F., & Dutch, R. E. (2020). Rapid repurposing of drugs for COVID-19. *Science*. https://doi.org/10.1126/science.abb9332.
47. Saini, K. S., Lanza, C., Romano, M., et al. (2020). Repurposing anticancer drugs for COVID-19-induced inflammation, immune dysfunction, and coagulopathy. *British Journal of Cancer*. https://dx.doi.org/10.1038/s41416-020-0948-x.
48. Ciliberto, G., Mancini, R., & Paggi, M. G. (2020). Drug repurposing against COVID-19: Focus on anticancer agents. *Journal of Experimental & Clinical Cancer Research*. https://dx.doi.org/10.1186/s13046-020-01590-2.
49. Xue, H., Li, J., Xie, H., & Wang, Y. (2018). Review of drug repositioning approaches and resources. *International Journal of Biological Sciences*. https://dx.doi.org/10.7150/ijbs.24612.
50. Xing, J., Shankar, R., Drelich, A., et al. (2020). Analysis of infected host gene expression reveals repurposed drug candidates and time-dependent host response dynamics for COVID-19. *bioRxiv*. https://doi.org/10.1101/2020.04.07.030734.
51. Shukla, R., Henkel, N., Alganem, K., et al. (2020). Integrative omics for informed drug repurposing: Targeting CNS disorders. *bioRxiv*. https://doi.org/10.1101/2020.04.24.060392.
52. Zheng, J., Zhang, Y., Liu, Y., et al. (2020). Multi-omics study revealing tissue-dependent putative mechanisms of SARS-CoV-2 drug targets on viral infections and complex diseases. *medRxiv*. https://doi.org/10.1101/2020.05.07.20093286.
53. Gordon, D. E., Jang, G. M., Bouhaddou, M., et al. (2020). A SARS-CoV-2 protein interaction map reveals targets for drug repurposing. *Nature*. https://doi.org/10.1038/s41586-020-2286-9.
54. Zhou, Y., Hou, Y., Shen, J., et al. (2020). Network-based drug repurposing for novel coronavirus 2019-nCoV/SARS-CoV-2. *Cell Discovery*. https://doi.org/10.1038/s41421-020-0153-3.
55. Gysi, D. M., Do Valle, Í., Zitnik, M., et al. (2020). Network medicine framework for identifying drug repurposing opportunities for COVID-19. *ArXiv*. arXiv:2004.07229v1. Preprint.
56. Zeng, X., Song, X., Ma, T., et al. (2020). Repurpose open data to discover therapeutics for COVID-19 using deep learning. *Journal of Proteome Research*. https://doi.org/10.1021/acs.jproteome.0c00316.

57. Hofmarcher, M., Mayr, A., Rumetshofer, E., et al. (2020). Large-scale ligand-based virtual screening for SARS-CoV-2 inhibitors using deep neural networks. *SSRN Electronic Journal*. https://doi.org/10.2139/ssrn.3561442.
58. Lalmuanawma, S., Hussain, J., & Chhakchhuak, L. (2020). Applications of machine learning and artificial intelligence for Covid-19 (SARS-CoV-2) pandemic: A review. *Chaos, Solitons and Fractals*. https://doi.org/10.1016/j.chaos.2020.110059.
59. Hamming, I., Timens, W., Bulthuis, M. L. C., et al. (2004). Tissue distribution of ACE2 protein, the functional receptor for SARS coronavirus. A first step in understanding SARS pathogenesis. *The Journal of Pathology, 203*, 631–637. https://doi.org/10.1002/path.1570.
60. Zou, X., Chen, K., Zou, J., et al. (2020). Single-cell RNA-seq data analysis on the receptor ACE2 expression reveals the potential risk of different human organs vulnerable to 2019-nCoV infection. *Frontiers in Medicine, 14*, 185–192. https://doi.org/10.1007/s11684-020-0754-0.
61. Choudhary, S., Malik, Y. S., & Tomar, S. (2020). Identification of SARS-CoV-2 cell entry inhibitors by drug repurposing using in silico structure-based virtual screening approach. *Frontiers in Immunology*. https://doi.org/10.3389/fimmu.2020.01664.
62. Kim, J., Zhang, J., Cha, Y., et al. (2020). Advanced bioinformatics rapidly identifies existing therapeutics for patients with coronavirus disease-2019 (COVID-19). *Journal of Translational Medicine*. https://doi.org/10.1186/s12967-020-02430-9.
63. Teralı, K., Baddal, B., & Gülcan, H. O. (2020). Prioritizing potential ACE2 inhibitors in the COVID-19 pandemic: Insights from a molecular mechanics-assisted structure-based virtual screening experiment. *Journal of Molecular Graphics & Modelling*. https://doi.org/10.1016/j.jmgm.2020.107697.
64. Trezza, A., Iovinelli, D., Santucci, A., et al. (2020). An integrated drug repurposing strategy for the rapid identification of potential SARS-CoV-2 viral inhibitors. *Scientific Reports*. https://doi.org/10.1038/s41598-020-70863-9.
65. Batra, R., Chan, H., Kamath, G., et al. (2020). Screening of therapeutic agents for COVID-19 using machine learning and ensemble docking studies. *Journal of Physical Chemistry Letters*. https://doi.org/10.1021/acs.jpclett.0c02278.
66. Tuli, S., Tuli, S., Tuli, R., & Gill, S. S. (2020). Predicting the growth and trend of COVID-19 pandemic using machine learning and cloud computing. *Internet of Things*. https://doi.org/10.1016/j.iot.2020.100222.
67. Gonzalez-Dias, P., Lee, E. K., Sorgi, S., et al. (2020). Methods for predicting vaccine immunogenicity and reactogenicity. *Human Vaccines and Immunotherapeutics, 16*, 269–276. https://doi.org/10.1080/21645515.2019.1697110.
68. Li, Z., Zhong, Z., Li, Y., et al. (2020). From community acquired pneumonia to COVID-19: A deep learning based method for quantitative analysis of COVID-19 on thick-section CT scans. *European Radiology*. https://dx.doi.org/10.1007/s00330-020-07042-x.
69. Mahmud, T., Rahman, M. A., & Fattah, S. A. (2020). CovXNet: A multi-dilation convolutional neural network for automatic COVID-19 and other pneumonia detection from chest X-ray images with transferable multi-receptive feature optimization. *Computers in Biology and Medicine*. https://doi.org/10.1016/j.compbiomed.2020.103869.
70. Albahri, O. S., Zaidan, A. A., Albahri, A. S., et al. (2020). Systematic review of artificial intelligence techniques in the detection and classification of COVID-19 medical images in terms of evaluation and benchmarking: Taxonomy analysis, challenges, future solutions and methodological aspects. *Journal of Infection and Public Health*. https://doi.org/10.1016/j.jiph.2020.06.028.
71. Liang, W., Yao, J., Chen, A., et al. (2020). Early triage of critically ill COVID-19 patients using deep learning. *Nature Communications, 11*, 1–7. https://doi.org/10.1038/s41467-020-17280-8.
72. Iwendi, C., Bashir, A. K., Peshkar, A., et al. (2020). COVID-19 patient health prediction using boosted random Forest algorithm. *Frontiers in Public Health, 8*, 357. https://doi.org/10.3389/fpubh.2020.00357.

73. Pourhomayoun, M., & Shakibi, M. (2020). Predicting mortality risk in patients with COVID-19 using artificial intelligence to help medical decision-making. *medRxiv*. https://doi.org/10.1101/2020.03.30.20047308.
74. Yan, L., Zhang, H.-T., Goncalves, J., et al. (2020). An interpretable mortality prediction model for COVID-19 patients. *Nature Machine Intelligence*. https://doi.org/10.1038/s42256-020-0180-7.
75. Rani, S., & Kautish, S. (2018). Association clustering and time series based data mining in continuous data for diabetes prediction. In *2018 second international conference on intelligent computing and control systems (ICICCS)* (pp. 1209–1214). IEEE.

**Sushil K. Shakyawar** obtained his PhD (supported by European Marie Curie ITN) with specialization in Computational Systems Biology and Metabolic Modelling from the University of Minho (Portugal). He did MRes (Master of Research) in Computational Biology from the University of York (UK) and BTech in Biotechnology from Indian Institute of Technology Guwahati (India). His previous research focused on machine learning applications and metabolic systems biology approaches to understand the infection of human protozoan parasites and prediction of drug-target interactions in human cancer. His current research interests at University of Nebraska Medical Center (UNMC) include machine learning applications, big data (omics) analysis and integration, and computational biology modeling to understand biological networks.

**Sahil Sethi** graduated with a Bachelor's degree in Bioinformatics from Jaypee University of Information Technology (India) and a Master's degree in Biomedical Informatics from the University of Nebraska Omaha. While doing his Master's degree, he worked on the thesis, titled "HLA Expression and HLA Typing in Human Cancer." After graduation, he went on to get some industry experience and then decided to pursue a PhD in Biomedical Informatics from the University of Nebraska Medical Center (UNMC). Currently, he is in the second year of his PhD program.

**Siddesh Southekal** is a PhD student in the Biomedical Informatics Program at the University of Nebraska Medical Center (UNMC). He obtained his MS in Life Science Informatics from the University of Bonn, Germany. His research interest and peer-reviewed publications are in the application of bioinformatics and using machine learning approaches in the area of translational research.

**Nitish K. Mishra** completed his PhD from the Institute of Microbial Technology, Chandigarh, India, and the title of his PhD thesis was "Development of in-silico method for searching for potential drug molecules and targets." In this project, he developed several open-source tools and web servers in the area of computer-aided drug design. He was a postdoctoral fellow at the Samuel Roberts Noble Foundation, Ardmore, OK, before joining UNMC, where he currently works as an instructor. Dr. Mishra's current research is focused on "genomic aberrations in pancreatic ductal adenocarcinoma" to investigate the role of SNP, indel, large-scale structural variation, and DNA methylation in pancreatic cancer.

**Chittibabu Guda** is the assistant dean for Research Development in the College of Medicine and a professor and vice-chair for Bioinformatics Research and Training at the University of Nebraska Medical Center (UNMC). He obtained his PhD in Molecular Biology from Auburn University and postdoctoral training in Computational Biology at the University of California, San Diego. Dr. Guda has published over 100 peer-reviewed research articles mostly on data-intensive research projects related to the development of novel algorithms in bioinformatics, using machine learning approaches to analyze big data, and building data analysis pipelines in the areas of cancer genomics and precision medicine.

# Chapter 11
# AR and VR and AI Allied Technologies and Depression Detection and Control Mechanism

**S. B. Goyal, Pradeep Bedi, and Navin Garg**

## 11.1 Introduction

Virtual reality (VR) is defined as a virtual environment generated by software that simulates reality, whereas augmented reality (AR) integrates the computer graphics to VR with actual reality. AR enables to place a virtual object in the real world. Advancements in virtual reality (VR) and augmented reality (AR) showed the potential to bring revolution in different research areas such as healthcare, commercial, education, communication, fashion world, etc. [1]. The AR/VR provides a user interface that users can place head-mounted display (HMD) which provides a real experience in virtual characters or things. It has a unique power that can make the human mind believe that they are in a real environment [2]. This ability to deliver experiences on demand is where the power of VR lies. AR/VR can be delivered in many ways such as screen-based, 360° videos, interactive AR/VR, etc. Previously, in medical literature, screen-based learning was considered to be as "virtual reality." In this learning, virtual reality creates a sense of presence [3]. In 360° videos, the complete picture was filmed in 360 degrees and viewed using a VR headset. Interactive VR involves a dynamic, adaptive, and interactive virtual world which can be used in highly realistic learning, games, etc. [4]. AR is said to be a combination of real and virtual objects and their environment. Augmented reality is close to the real environment whereas augmented virtuality is near to the virtual environment (Fig. 11.1). In the case of mobile AR, technology adds the digital world to the real environment through a smartphone camera. For example, Pokémon GO is an AR-based mobile game that uses the navigation system and enables users to catch

S. B. Goyal (✉)
City University, Petaling Jaya, Selangor, Malaysia

P. Bedi · N. Garg
Graphic Era Hill University, Clement Town Dehradun, Uttarakhand, India



S. Kautish et al. (eds.), *Computational Intelligence Techniques for Combating COVID-19*, EAI/Springer Innovations in Communication and Computing,
https://doi.org/10.1007/978-3-030-68936-0_11

**Fig. 11.1** Schematic diagram integrating real and virtual environment [8]

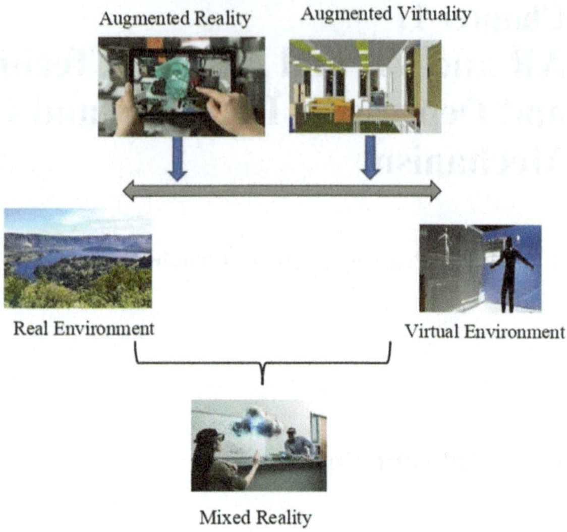


various digital Pokémon creatures around their area [5], whereas virtual reality is different from AR. In VR, the user enters from the real environment to a virtual environment using a VR headset such as Oculus Rift or Samsung Gear VR [6, 7].

## *11.1.1 Applications of AR/VR*

### 11.1.1.1 Gaming/Entertainment

In the game industry, AR/VR provides an interactive environment that provides a real experience of virtual objects. Nowadays there are huge opportunities in the game industry to design and develop portable games augmented with a real environment. With the integration of a 3D virtual environment, the gaming experience will go to the next level, for example, "Pokemon Go" and PubG [7].

### 11.1.1.2 Education

In the educational sector, virtual classroom/laboratories are created to provide students to catch and boost up their knowledge about subjects or topics. This also increases the creativity level of the student as well as teachers. These technologies virtually provide easy real learning. Sometimes it is also difficult for teachers to visualize concepts on the board, and also it is difficult for students to grasp it. AR/VR had evolved as a solution to such conditions. Today, due to the occurrence of COVID-19, all schools, colleges, or universities are taking their class online, which seems to be distributed over the Internet. This had reduced the disciplinary culture of the classroom, so AR/VR can be taken as a solution as it can connect real online distributed classroom to centralized virtual classroom. This means in a real scenario all students are at a different location and all are connected over the Internet, but due to the application of VR, all students and teachers will feel that they are in actual classroom reading together [9].

#### 11.1.1.3 Healthcare

Another sector in which AR/VR is used frequently is healthcare. These technologies benefit in medical surgeries to visualize the inner body parts by simulating in 3D view, especially for doctor's training to level up their surgical skills. In another way, AR/VR also illustrates to give therapies or treatment to different types of phobia or anxieties [10]. For example, social anxiety disorder (SAD) is a situation in which an individual feels social anxiety while having interaction with others. So, in such condition, AR/VR technologies will provide a virtual social environment in which an individual can interact. VR had also shown their contribution in treatment of posttraumatic stress disorder such as world trade center attacks, etc. Augmedics, the world's leading AR supplier, has developed an AR control system called the Xvision Spine System (XVS). This system helps surgeons visualize the three-dimensional anatomy of the spine during surgery. Besides, this AR system accurately determines the position of the surgical instruments used during the operation in real time. Furthermore, augmented reality is used for drug development or the creation of chemical structures. For example, Nottingham scientists are working to discover drugs and create chemical structures using AR. Additionally, the computational chemistry division known as Sygnature Discovery used the VisMol system as part of AR technology to develop a product prototype. Additionally, AR can be used for vein visualization, education, and surgical visualization. For example, AccuVein is a widely used healthcare tool that makes it easy to search or navigate the human body's vein so that medical professionals can easily inject drugs directly into their veins.

#### 11.1.1.4 Tourism

One of the evergreen industries is travel and tourism, as all over the world people like to travel, see different places, experience new cultures, etc. People always want to spend their holidays traveling to different places. It has become a trend to consult travel agencies to organize their entire tour. So, all travel agencies have to care about their customers always to serve best and to expand their business. AR/VR will contribute to this the most. Through the application of AR/VR, they can make customers visualize virtual travel experience [11].

**Table 11.1** Examples of existing AR/VR products

| Product name | Application area | Description | Image | Ref |
|---|---|---|---|---|
| Daydream View | Adventure and entertainment | It is used to watch immersive videos and for experiencing incredible adventures | 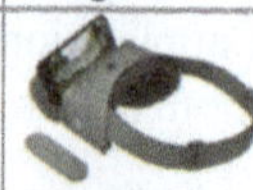 | [13] |
| Hololens | Gaming | Through hololens anyone can create 3D images and can play virtual games also | 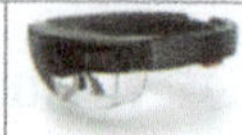 | [14] |
| Google Cardboard | Entertainment | Low-cost system that can encourage development of VR applications | 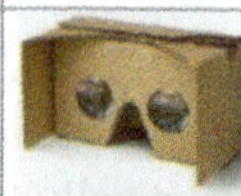 | [13] |
| Google Lens | Education | Sometimes it cannot be described that anyone wants to search. So, to get precise search results, google lens is pointed towards tilings that can be focused and it will help to find it | 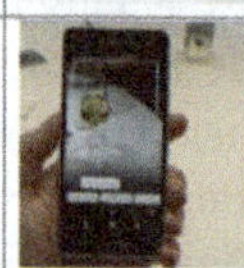 | [15] |
| Live View in Google Maps | Social | In this feature, it can orient anyone quickly to know the direction on the virtual street view | 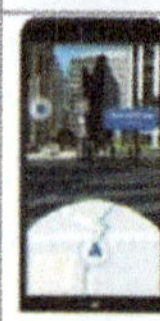 | [16] |
| NeuroVR | Medical | The virtual environments enable medical researchers to learn and to control situations | 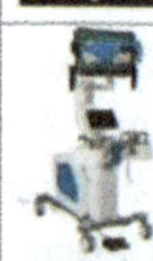 | [17] |
| Real Estate VR | Real estate | The virtual environment is created that can move in 3D to demonstrate the property from all angles and customers can optimize the design accordingly | 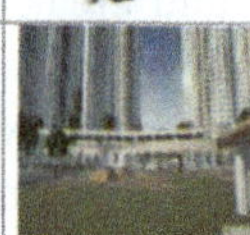 | [18] |
| Virtual B2B Products | | | 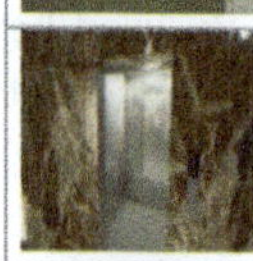 | [18] |
| Amazon Echo (virtual audio) | Entertainment | It is AI-based virtual voice assistant that is capable of voice interaction, music play, organizers, as well as it can control smart devices | 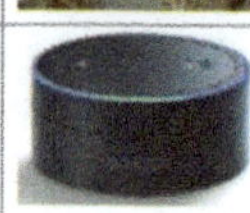 | [19] |

#### 11.1.1.5 Virtual Shopping

The enhancement of technology made us experience virtual shopping without any hustle of crowded shopping malls. It provides us a close-up view in each section of mall that an individual cannot experience. For example, Alibaba, Buy+, IKEA, etc. have started to provide experience of virtual shopping to their customers [12].

Some applications of AR/VR and respective products available in the market are stated below in Table 11.1.

There are many application areas in which AR/VR can be implemented. One of the most important application areas is healthcare, especially for the treatment of depression/anxieties in an individual, as depression is a kind of mental disability that leads to demotivation of an individual. Many research works have been done for the psychological treatment of such depressive conditions by an application of AR/VR to increase the level of presence and interactivity or motivate them [20]. In [21], the author used the application of virtual reality to treat the phobia of an individual by using 3D virtual games. In [22], the researcher had proposed a medical aid by application of augmented reality to take care of elderly people who are suffering from mild Alzheimer's disease. This application has presented an AR interface with an application of speech commands and medicine time reminders, distinguishing between medicine, family members' recognition from photos, etc. In [23], the author focused the research on stress inoculation training virtually by creating a stress-induced environment to evaluate the emotional connection factor of an individual. In [24], the author proposed the diagnosis model for depression assessment by application of virtual reality. In [25], the author studied the impact of augmented reality exposure-based therapy (AR-EBT) for the treatment of an individual that is suffering from specific phobias using VR environments. In [26], the author discussed the application of virtual reality for the treatment of anxiety disorder, especially in youth, by cognitive behavior therapy (CBT).

Previous research works are mainly focused on the application of AR/VR in the treatment of anxiety disorders such as fear of height, flying, water, animals, social interactions, etc. Recently, many research works are focused on the treatment of other disorders such as eating disorders and sexual dysfunctions. The purpose of this chapter is to study the benefits and future scope of AR/VR after the outbreak of COVID-19. The consequences of COVID-19 results in a shortage of resources and had led to an increase in depression levels among people. In this chapter, depression detection is proposed by an application of electroencephalogram (EEG) signal processing along with an AR/VR interface to determine whether the augmented and virtual environments are equally capable of healing depression levels in an individual.

The outline of the chapter is stated as follows: In Sect. 11.2, a brief description of application and working of AR/VR technologies during COVID-19 pandemic is given. In Sect. 11.3, application of AR/VR for psychological support is given. In Sect. 11.4, the impact of AR/VR on mental health is discussed. Section 11.5 discusses about deep learning techniques with advantages, disadvantages, and application. Section 11.6 discusses about the application of deep leaning in mental healthcare, and Sect. 11.7 discusses about the contribution of researcher in the diagnosis of depression from EEG signals. Section 11.8 proposes a deep learning-based model for depression detection and control methodology using AR/VR technologies. Sections 11.9 and 11.10 give a brief discussion and conclusion, respectively.

## 11.2 Working Process of AR/VR for COVID-19

The virtual reality is not a single application; it can be used to provide a bunch of applications in the field of healthcare that attracts many medical practitioners [27]. AR/VR is capable to mitigate the effects of COVID-19 in different ways. Various advantages of these technologies to fight against the COVID-19 pandemic are shown in Fig. 11.2. The proper training of medical staff during COVID-19 pandemic will make them efficient to handle the actual situation during the pandemic. The application of virtual reality offers doctors or medical caretakers to learn more quickly and handle any adverse situation positively. It ultimately utilizes and offers an interactive and immersive experience [28–30].

### *11.2.1 Patient Education*

The virtual reality application is powerful that it not only trains medical caretakers but also provides impressive facilities to the patients. This directly or indirectly provides satisfaction to patients that come to know about the treatment process that what doctors are going to do. The efficiency level of doctors is also increased [31].

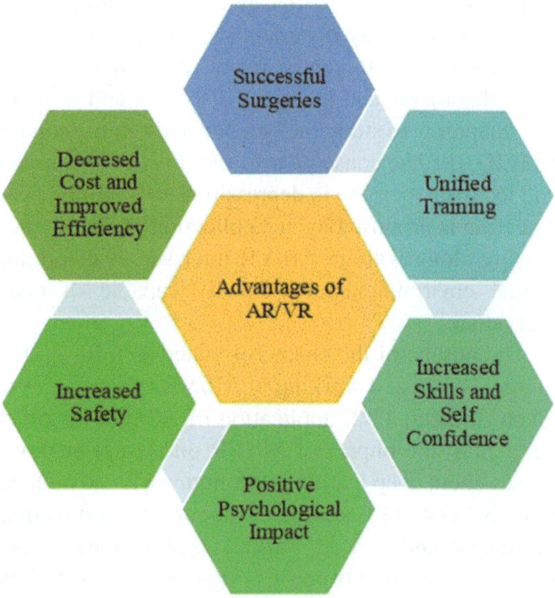
Successful Surgeries
Decresed Cost and Improved Efficiency
Unified Training
Advantages of AR/VR
Increased Safety
Increased Skills and Self Confidence
Positive Psychological Impact

**Fig. 11.2** Advantages of AR/VR during COVID-19 pandemic

### *11.2.2 Physical Therapies*

Apart from surgical treatment, virtual reality technology also effectively worked for physical treatment [32]. The virtual training and learning help the patients to heal up more quickly, as the patient is mentally satisfied and healing which reduces the recovery time of physical injuries.

### *11.2.3 Psychological Treatment*

Psychological treatment is much more difficult than physical treatment. In such an extreme condition, the concept of virtual reality has proved to be an effective tool. For example, Oxford had developed VR-enabled therapy treatment for diagnosis of an individual for acrophobia or fear of heights and achieved a remarkable success in reducing the patient's fear by 70% [33]. This demonstrates the potential of VR technology to address a variety of mental health issues. With the extreme stress level that had occurred in people after a pandemic like COVID-19, some people have gone under psychosomatic disturbances. In such cases, the VR application had become one of the powerful tools to handle such a situation.

## 11.3 COVID-19 and Application of AR/VR for Psychological Support

The coronavirus disease 2019 (COVID-19) pandemic had severely affected the economy, health, and education sectors all over the world. Due to such global crisis, it has impacted the mental health of millions of people worldwide. According to the statistics on October 16, 2020, 216 countries have been affected, with more than 8 million active cases and approximately 1 million deaths [34]. The contrary influence on mental health is not only limited to healthcare workers, but it has also affected millions of people during lockdown or quarantine period. People are social creatures who go out of the house to socialize with other people.

Due to COVID-19, all individuals are confined to their houses who have disconnected socially. This leads to an increase in anxiety/depression levels among the masses. Nowadays people are feeling as if they are like prisoners and they are punished to stay in their homes. Before the outbreak of COVID-19, people go outside their homes to meet and talk to other people and also share their good or bad times. After the outbreak of the pandemic, COVID-19 had turned the entire world upside down. This situation had turned the drastic change in technologies. The application of AR/VR has provided the people to socialize on these platforms.

These platforms are easily available to all. During the lockdown period, most people are adaptable to such technologies and are used to them. Even after the lockdown, until the vaccine doesn't come in the market, people remain socially distant. But AR/VR technologies bring people virtually close. These platforms allow people to run smoothly their jobs/businesses irrespective of challenges faced by social distancing. Many people are working either on smartphones or laptops from their homes. This is the best time to take pandemic as the right time to scale AR/VR technologies [35].

## 11.4 Impact of AR/VR on Mental Health

Such a long duration during the lockdown had developed stress-related psychological symptoms, anxiety, depression, and posttraumatic stress disorder (PTSD). The major reason for such condition was the loss of money, jobs, lack of social interaction, etc. It has affected mostly the lower-income population or middle-income population which leads people to take suicidal steps. This is one side of the impact of COVID-19, but on the other side, many researchers are giving their efforts toward artificial intelligence as well as its application in the field of augmented reality (AR) or virtual reality (VR) [36]. The application of these technologies can help patients with emotional distress to better manage their stress or depression. According to the above discussion, different studies demonstrated that people used to play games or watch movies/videos to get distraction from undesirable anxiety or stress. But such diversion will provide only temporary solutions. There is a need for some permanent solution that is needed to be focused on. For example, In Italy, hospitals have adopted AR/VR to combat the stress level of hospital workers. To improve their psychological and emotional health, the VR used visualization of positive memories or feelings. Additionally, AR/VR games are used as an effective tool to decrease stress, depression, or anxiety in individuals. But it needed to first analyze the reason for depression to determine the level of treatment. So, there is a need to integrate with some other tools with AR/VR for the treatment process.

## 11.5 Overview of Deep Learning

In machine learning, small dataset is required to train the model, whereas a large dataset is required to train the model. Low-end machines are enough for machine learning processing as it requires less time for training, but it requires more computational time for testing. Whereas in deep learning, high processing is required during the training process but takes very little time for testing. So, deep learning is considered to be an emerging part of machine learning that consists of diverse learning and representation learning, as deep learning is a branch of machine learning that has proved its effectiveness over traditional machine learning models (shallow models) in most of the application areas, especially real-life applications.

Some of the difference between shallow models and deep models are stated below in Table 11.2.

Some of the popular deep learning architecture are deep belief networks (DBNs), deep neural networks (DNNs), convolutional neural networks (CNNs), recurrent neural networks (RNNs), deep autoencoders, restricted Boltzmann machines (RBMs), etc. Many researchers are focusing their work toward deep learning since 2015 in different fields such as image processing, big data, digital signal processing, etc. [39–42].

Some of the deep learning methodologies are discussed below.

### 11.5.1 Deep Autoencoder

An autoencoder is designed by combining encoder and decoder type neural network, as shown in Fig. 11.3a. Raw input data is fed into encoder units where features are extracted, and these features are fed into the decoder to reconstruct the data from the extracted features. While training the deep autoencoder model, the divergence of encoder and decoder is reduced gradually. The feature extraction by encoder and reconstruction by the decoder is not supervised information. Different types of deep autoencoder are focused on by researchers such as denoising autoencoders and sparse autoencoders [38].

Advantages of deep autoencoder

- Unsupervised learning

Disadvantages of deep autoencoder

- It is compressive and decompressive. So, sometimes it may be lossy.

Application area of deep autoencoder

- Used especially for feature extraction
- Denoising
- Compression

**Table 11.2** Difference between shallow and deep learning

| Parameters | Shallow learning [37, 38] | Deep learning [39–41] |
|---|---|---|
| Training time | Less | More |
| Testing time | More | Less |
| Learning parameters | Manually set | Calculated automatically |
| Feature representation | Feature vector is taken as input | Raw data is taken as input capabilities to extract features |
| Leaning capacity | Overfilling | Greater fitting |
| Large data volume processing | Slow processing | Faster processing |
| Performance | Good | Better |
| Accuracy | Good | Better |

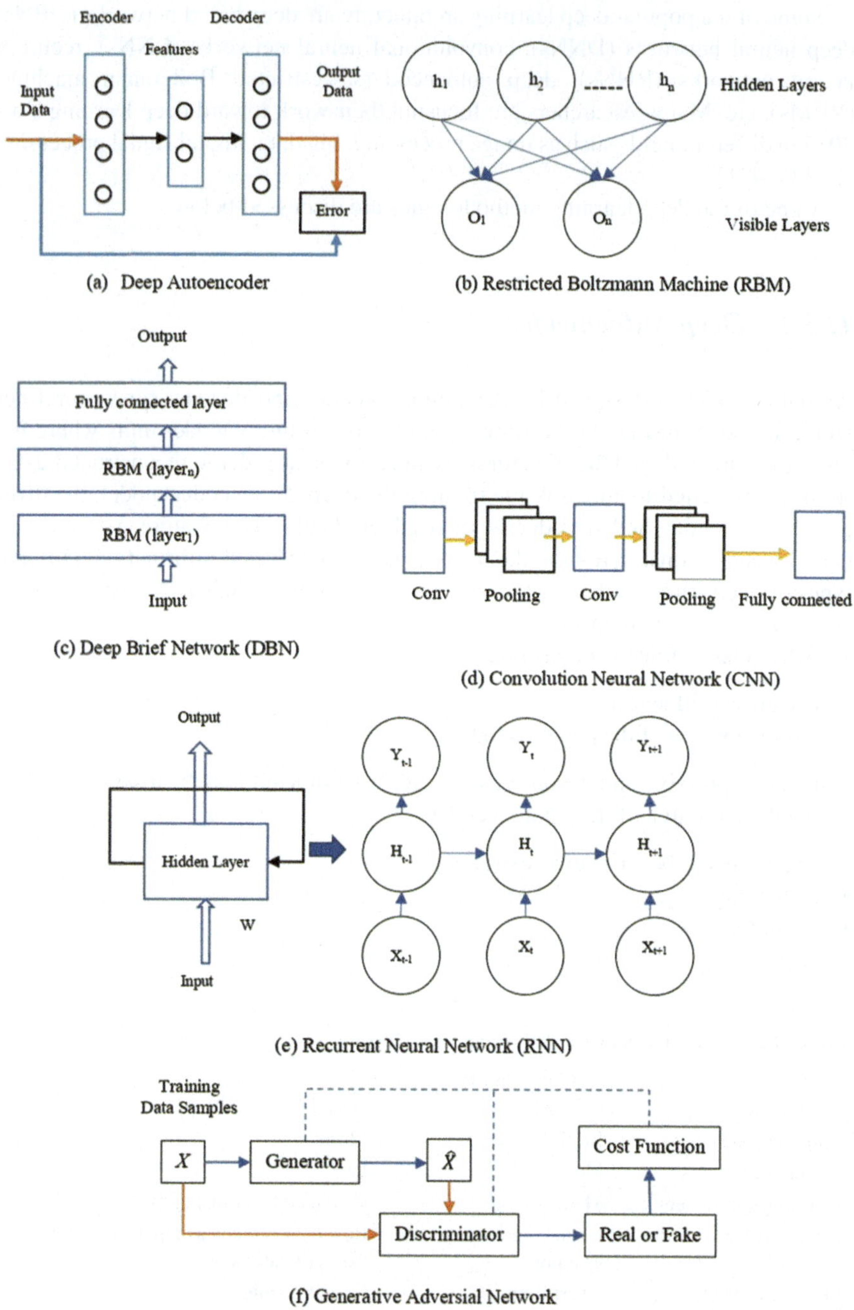


**Fig. 11.3** Examples of deep learning

### 11.5.2 Restricted Boltzmann Machines (RBMs)

Restricted Boltzmann machines (RBMs) are a type of randomized neural network in which Boltzmann distribution is applied on nodes. This deep network is composed of two layers: one is a hidden layer, while the other is a visible layer. The modes in the same layer are not connected, while with other layers nodes are fully connected as depicted in Fig. 11.3c. In the figure, visible layer is represented by $v_i$ and the hidden layer is represented by $h_i$. As this network is not distinguished as a forward or backward network, thus the same weight is taken in both directions. As RBMs are unsupervised trained using contrastive divergence algorithm, they are generally used for feature extraction or denoising [39]. However, in recent research, RBMs are being replaced by generative adversarial networks (GANs).

Advantages of RBMs

- Layer-to-layer pretraining
- Can be trained on unlabeled data
- Better learning generative process

Disadvantages of RBMs

- High computational cost
- Slow training process

Application area of RBMs

- Used especially for feature extraction
- Denoising

### 11.5.3 Deep Belief Networks (DBNs)

Deep belief networks (DBNs) are composed of a stack of different RBM layers where nodes in each layer are connected to other layers as shown in Fig. 11.3d. The training process in DBNs is performed in two stages. Pretraining is unsupervised, while further fine-tuning learning is supervised by using labeled data. So, it is composed of both labeled training layers and unlabeled training layers [39].

Advantages of DBNs

- Performs better than boosting
- Effective in pattern recognition

Disadvantages of DBNs

- High computational cost
- Slow training process

Application area of DBNs

- Natural language processing
- Motion capturing
- Image and video processing

### 11.5.4 Convolutional Neural Networks (CNNs)

Convolutional neural network (CNN) is a type of deep neural network that is designed to interpret similar to the human visual system (HVS). Previously, CNN showed great achievements in the field of computer vision. Recently, it has been applied in other fields also. Many recent human-computer interfaces are designed using CNNs. CNNs show advantages over feed-forward networks because they are capable of finding feature localities. Thus, it is capable to extract features and processes. CNNs can work on two-dimensional (2D) as well as three-dimensional (3D) data in which input data are converted into matrices accordingly [40].

Advantages of CNNs:

- Removes the overfitting problem of traditional neural networks
- High accuracy
- Effective in pattern recognition
- Weight sharing among layers

Disadvantages of CNNs:

- High computational cost
- Slow training process in the absence of GPUs

Application area of CNNs:

- Image recognition and speech recognition and OCR application
- Human-computer interface

### 11.5.5 Recurrent Neural Networks (RNNs)

Recurrent neural network (RNN) is a type of neural network architecture that is designed for sequential data, especially used for time series predictive problems. In such a network output of the previous state is fed into the current state, whereas, in all traditional networks, all inputs and outputs are independent of each other. In RNNs, the hidden state remembers information about the sequence. The structure of an RNN is shown in Fig. 11.3e. The standard RNNs can handle only limited-length sequences. To solve such an issue, a modified version of RNNs has been proposed, termed as long short-term memory (LSTM), gated recurrent unit (GRU), etc. [41].

Advantages of RNNs:

- Store information concerning time
- Remember the previous features

Disadvantages of RNNs:

- Gradient vanishing problem
- Problem in processing long sequences

Application area of RNNs:

- Predictive problems or time series problems
- Image recognition, speech recognition, and OCR application
- Human-computer interface

### *11.5.6 Generative Adversarial Network (GAN)*

A generative adversarial network (GAN) is a type of neural network model that consists of two sub-network units, one is the generator and the other is the discriminator (Fig. 11.5f). The generator generates the fake date corresponding to real data, whereas the discriminator distinguishes between real and fake data. The losses are backpropagated to both generators as well as the discriminator. Thus, the generator and the discriminator improve each other. Currently, GANs are used in recent research works for augmenting data. GANs are generally used where a shortage of dataset exists. During the training process, adversarial learning is performed to improve the accuracy of models [42].

Advantages of GANs:

- Better data distribution.
- Any kind of generator network can be trained.
- Avoiding approximation for calculation.
- Avoid the use Markov chains and reduce the computational cost.

Disadvantages of GANs:

- Without good synchronization between generator and discriminator, it is hard to train the model.
- Missing learning pattern.

Application areas of GANs:

- Computer vision applications such as super resolution
- Text to image synthesis
- Sequential data-based applications such as speech

## 11.6 Application of Deep Learning in Mental Healthcare

Mental illness is considered to be one of the major health issues that change the mental state, emotional state, or behavioral state of an individual that adversely impacts their health directly or indirectly. Mental illness includes depression, schizophrenia, autism spectrum disorder (ASD), etc., which are frequently occurring today, and all over the world, it is estimated that approximately 450 million people, especially adolescents and adults, are suffering from mental issues. So, mental health is considered to be a serious concern worldwide. For example, one of the leading causes of mental disability is depression which had increased the probability of suicidal attempts [43]. According to the World Health Organization (WHO), depression is considered to be one of the major leading causes of death by 2020 which had already influenced millions of people worldwide. The cause of depression can be financial, social, or psychological issues but the fact is that it is quite dangerous for an individual as it not only affects an individual but also influences their families. However, based on the severity of symptoms, an assessment of depression can be performed. Currently, many people suffering from depression do not consult doctors due to fear and shame, and current diagnosis techniques are not that accurate [44–47]. So, finding an appropriate, effective, and accurate diagnosis process that makes the patient comfortable is still a challenging task. Before providing treatment for mental illness, the first thing that is needed to know is about the different symptoms for different types of mental illness. In this chapter, the diagnosis and treatment process for depression is proposed which integrate deep learning with AR/VR technologies. For this deep learning model needed to be trained. For this deep learning model needed to be trained. So, for accurate training, firstly it is needed to identify the symptoms. Some of the symptoms are discussed below in Fig. 11.4.

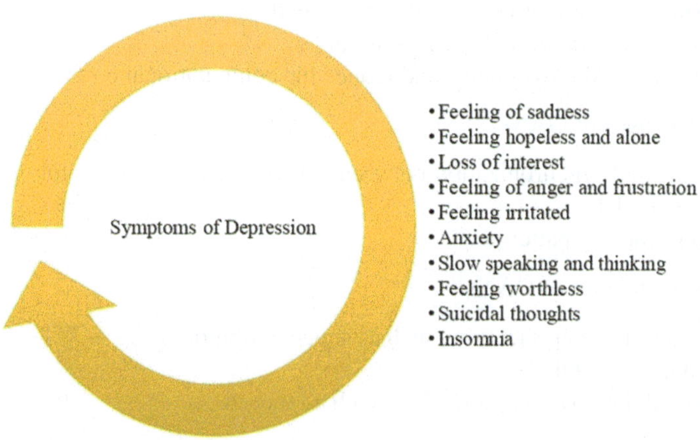


**Fig. 11.4** Symptoms of depression

To better understand the mental condition, it is necessary to detect and address symptoms of mental illness in the early stage. Early-stage detection will result in an accurate diagnosis, and effective treatment can be delivered. As the effect of mental illness will adversely affect family and an individual. Traditional diagnosis and treatment methods used face-to-face interviews and questionnaire session to detect specific emotions or feelings. However, such traditional methods are time-consuming, and many people feel shame to take psychological consultancy. Then, wearable sensors and smartphone applications were developed for diagnosis, but these applications are needed to be monitored over time [48]. Due to increased resource availability, new technologies are emerging to diagnose mental health status, in which machine learning had emerged as the most effective tool that can be used in different forms of treatment and improved clinical decision-making to assist healthcare providers. As one of the latest advances, machine learning is deep learning (DL) technology that has made the complex learning process easy. In different application areas, including the healthcare sector, deep learning technology has proved their superiority over other machine learning algorithms. In recent research works, many researchers had contributed their efforts to survey and develop machine learning or deep learning applications in the medical field, especially in the psychological domain. Existing research assessed the robustness, reliability, and accuracy of algorithms as well as opportunities and challenges faced during their adaptation. To inspect and focus better overview on different application areas of ML in the mental health domain, Shatte et al. [48] conducted a review of the main application domain related to mental health, i.e., detection and diagnosis, prognosis, treatment, and support, public health, and research and administration. They conclude that machine learning had the potential to improve in all four application areas. Sanches et al. [49] designed a human-computer interface (HCI) using machine learning for supporting automated diagnosis and self-tracking. Subhani et al. [50] proposed electroencephalogram (EEG) analysis using a machine learning approach for stressed people. The experimental analysis is performed by inducing stress among people by adopting Montreal Imaging Stress Task. The analysis was performed in three steps; in the first step, features are extracted from EEG signals generated during induced stress, and then feature selection was performed on digital signals, and in the last step, classification of signals is performed using different machine learning approaches such as logistic regression, support vector machine, and naïve Bayes classifiers. To validate the performance of the classifier, tenfold cross-validation was also done. The result obtained from the analysis was measured using parameters such as accuracy and achieved 83.4% accuracy for multiple level identification.

## 11.7 Depression Diagnosis Using EEG Signals

In the current scenario, depression is considered as one of the main health issues worldwide. Problems associated with the diagnosis of depression are lack of patient cooperation, subjective bias, and low effectiveness. So, there is a need for reliable and effective tools that can reach an optimal level. There are several methods to diagnose and treat depression, but the most effective method is electroencephalogram (EEG) signal data [52] that are widely used for depression detection as it is easy to record using a headset and does not need invasion inside the body parts. EEG signals are neurological signals that represent the functional state of mind of any person which gets generated according to the situation. In different stimuli, the human mind generates different signals. For example, if an individual is happy by seeing some relaxing video, then the eye will stimulate the brain, and it generates signals accordingly. So, for proper diagnosis, it is required to distinguish between brain signals generated. So, many researchers focus their research area on EEG signals as it is the most reliable detection method. Mahato et al. [51] used EEG signals for classification of mental state as healthy or depressive by extracting linear features and nonlinear features from brain signals, respectively. The result analysis was also performed using a combination of linear and nonlinear features and achieved the highest accuracy than a single feature. So, it can be concluded that feature selection can also be a criterion for achieving high efficiency. Li [53] used a deep learning approach to detect depression from EEG signals. Family and an individual adversely had affected due to mental illness.

Zhu [54] proposed a context-aware ensemble machine learning approach for depression detection from the EEG signal. In this experiment analysis, both the static and the dynamic scenarios were investigated. For result analysis, the EEG dataset was divided into subsets, and a voting strategy was performed to determine the subject label. The approach was validated on two datasets, EEG and eye movement, for depression identification. This shows the future application for the auxiliary diagnosis of depression. Guo et al. [55] presented a hybrid depression detection technique using linear discriminant analysis (LDA) and particle swarm optimization (PSO). The algorithm was designed with multiple objective subjects to minimize misclassification, minimize the internal distance, and maximize the external distance.

Purnamasari et al. [56] developed an application for minimizing stress levels by the application of meditation using EEG signals. For feature extraction, fast Fourier transform (FFT) was used with k nearest neighbor (k-NN) classifier. It was analyzed that, from brain signals, delta, theta, alpha, and beta waves are the most suitable frequency range to work on. According to the above discussion, depression is considered to be one of the mental disorders that mostly affect a person's thoughts, behaviors, feelings, and sense of well-being. After the outbreak of COVID-19, in 2020, depression had become one of the major life-threatening illnesses. Different studies and research works considered electroencephalogram (EEG) signals as the best tool for physiological treatment or healing process. Shen et al. [57] studied empirical mode decomposition (EMD) feature extraction method for complex and nonlinear EEG signals. However, in the EMD feature extraction method, some special data and the neighboring components extracted through EMD could certainly have sections of data carrying the same frequency at different time durations. This issue was resolved by improved EMD using singular value decomposition (SVD) using feature extraction for depression detection using EEG signals. Similarly,

Zhang et al. [58] designed a convolutional neural network (CNN) for extracting features from EEG signals. In this work, EEG signals were analyzed based on age and gender for depression analysis. This work concluded that the EEG signal is influenced by age and gender which also affected depression diagnosis and treatment process.

## 11.8 Depression Detection and Control Methodology Using AR/VR

Virtual reality (VR) headset provides the feel of real attention, walking into a conference, or watching a product demo. During COVID-19 outbreak, many AR/VR technologies exist such as remote classrooms and conferences. Its popularity has increased during lockdown after the outbreak of COVID-19. The business continuity had taken priority over AR/VR. In this chapter, depression detection is proposed by an application of EEG signal processing along with an AR/VR interface. This research aims to classify different EEG signals generated in an individual to predict either he is depressed or not. If he is depressed, then control audio/visual signals will be generated from the brain-computer interface that is connected to the VR headset. The proposed methodology is performed in four basic steps. In the first step, raw EEG signals will be captured (Fig. 11.5a). In the second step, feature extraction from the EEG signals is performed (Fig. 11.5b). In the third step, classification of EEG signals is performed, and a log is generated in the cloud database (Fig. 11.5b). In the fourth step, control signals are transmitted from the cloud (Fig. 11.5b). The flowchart of the proposed methodology is discussed in Fig. 11.6, respectively.

**Algorithm 1 DDH (Depression Detection and Healing)**

```
procedure DDH (EEG_signal)
Require: i∈N, j∈M, where N,M belongs to number of iterations
result ←Control_signal
for i←0 to N do                                    // Epochs
for j←0 to M do                                    // Iteration
          1D-Conv ← FV; (FV1......., FVn)          // CNN Features
end for
end for
return Control_signal
```

### *11.8.1 Signal Acquisition*

In this step, the raw EEG signals are extracted from the attached EEG headset in the VR headset. Then acquisition signals are taken for feature extraction for further processing.

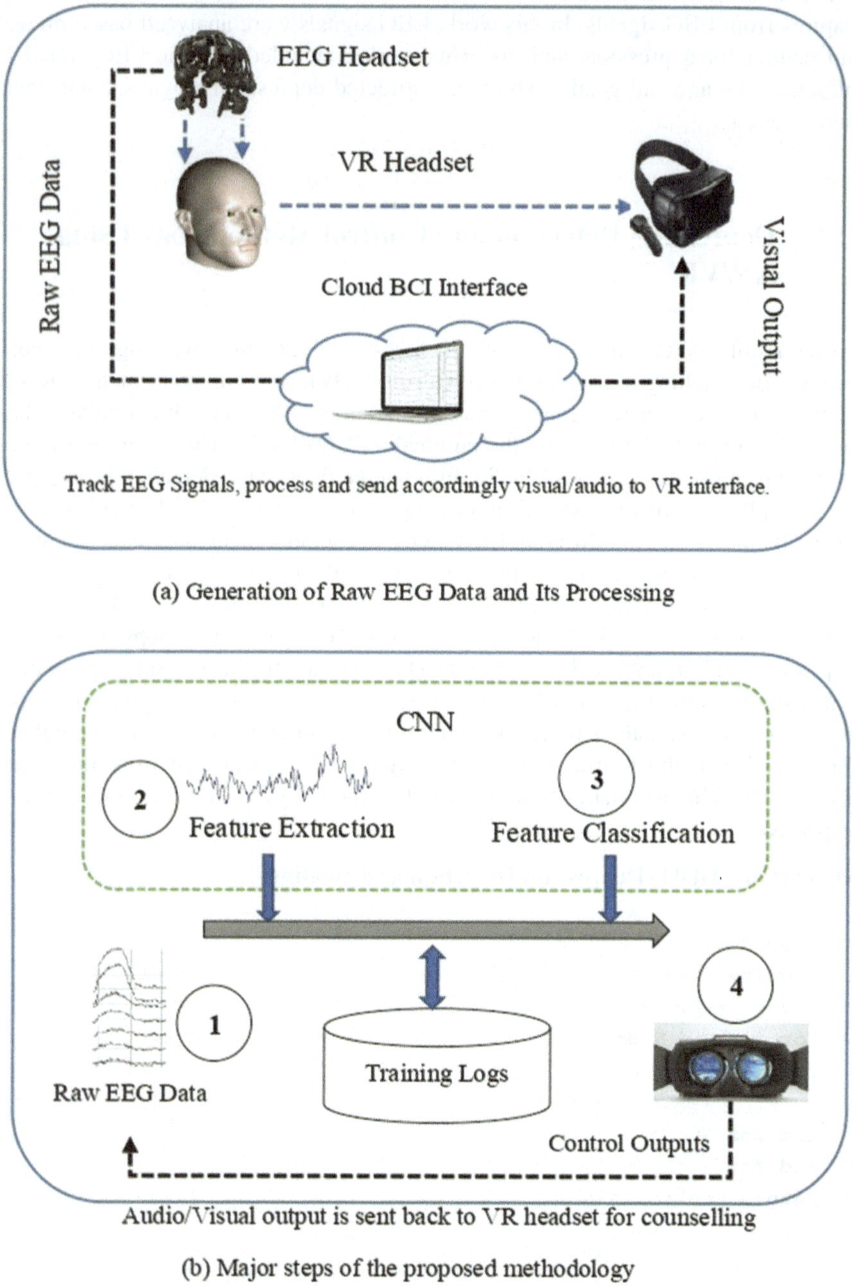


**Fig. 11.5** Depression detection and control mechanism using AR/VR

### *11.8.2 Feature Extraction*

Before feature extraction, noise removal is performed as acquired raw EEG data is usually noisy and contains some artifacts. While recording the EEG signal, it gets mixed with some artifacts such as blinking of the eye, muscle movement, etc. For accurate results, these artifacts are needed to be removed. For the noise removal process, a bandpass filter, Butterworth filter, is applied between 0.5 Hz and 200 Hz [42]. A sample for noise removal is illustrated in Fig. 11.7. After the removal of noise, the signals are sent to a one-dimensional convolutional neural network (CNN). Here the input data is transformed into a representative set of features (features vector). This process is termed as feature extraction. The one-dimensional convolutional architecture is used to extract features and classification as shown in Fig. 11.6.

### *11.8.3 Classification*

After feature extraction, feature vectors are fed into the classifier. In the classifier, it is first trained, and training rules are generated for further classification procedure. In this proposed depression detection model, raw EEG signals induced from the user are fed into the 1D-CNN-RF model for processing and detection of depression. The proposed 1D-CNN-RF model consists of multiple hierarchical layers which

**Fig. 11.6** Flowchart of proposed framework

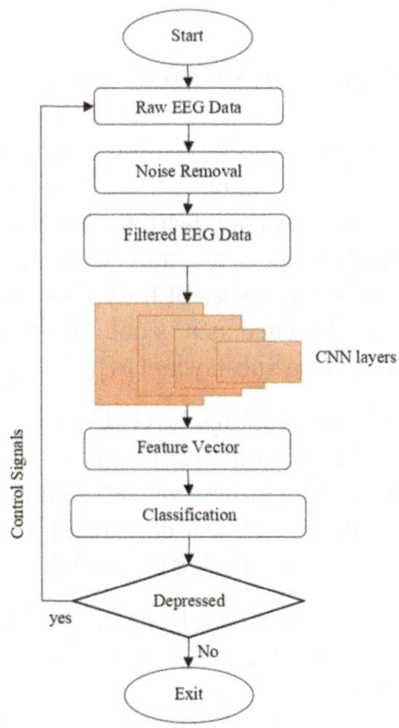

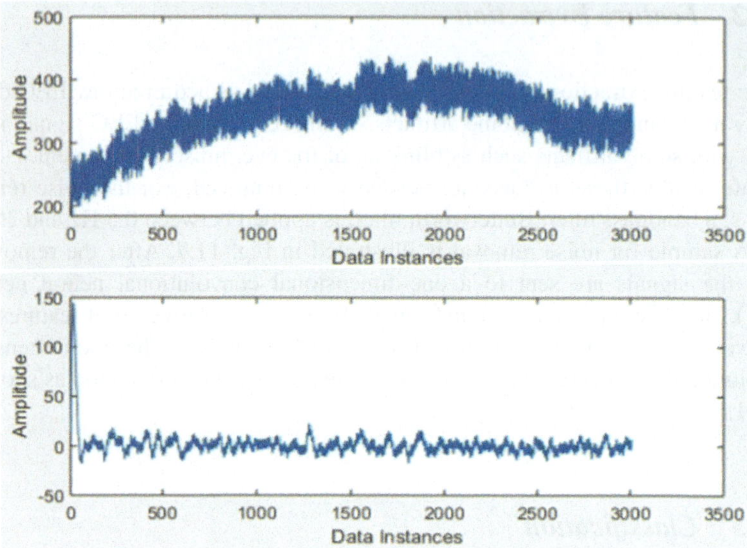


**Fig. 11.7** Sample of noisy and filtered EEG signals

help to extract features from complex EEG signals. This model better identifies normal EEG patterns from depressed patterns. At the end of proposed 1D CNN model, a random forest (RF) classifier is added to classify EEG feature vectors. The proposed system architecture is shown in Fig. 11.8.

#### 11.8.3.1 CNN Architecture

As compared to shallow learning, deep learning effectively solves the real-world problems. Among all available deep learning models, CNN is considered to be one of the best deep learning models that result in high performance level. Most of the CNN models are trained using the backpropagation mechanism. To resolve the overfitting issues of fully connected neural networks, convolutional neural network was designed as it is not a fully connected network. CNN layer is composed of the following sub-layers [14]:

- Convolutional layer (Conv)
- Batch normalization (BN)
- Max pooling layer (MaxPool)
- Rectified linear unit (ReLU)
- Fully connected layer (FC)

Convolutional layer (Conv): The raw data is passed on as input in this layer and generates feature set which is reduced by the convolutional operations.

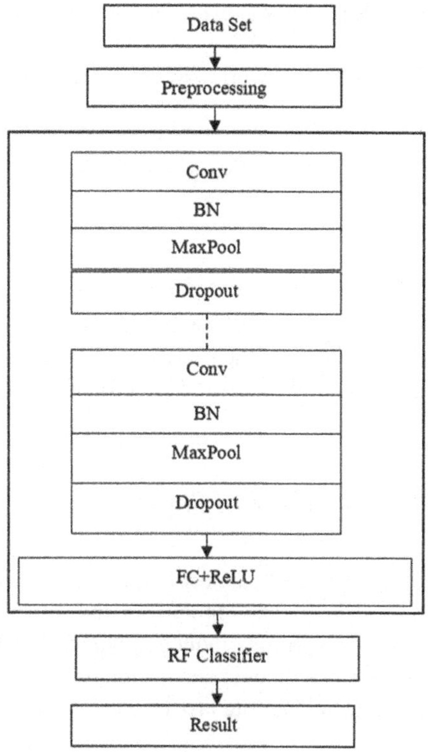


**Fig. 11.8** 1D-CNN-RF block diagram

Batch normalization (BN): For increasing the processing speed of CNN layers, this layer is added.

Max pooling layer (MaxPool): For further reduction in feature vector from previous layer, pooling layer is added. Combination of convolutional layer and pooling layer is performed according to design and dependent on input data size. Otherwise it may cause problem of overfitting due to large processing.

Rectified linear unit (ReLU): This layer is one of the most important layers that determine the efficiency of the network. This layer activates the entire network. Mathematical condition in ReLU activation layer is evaluated as Eq. (11.1):

$$f(x) = \begin{Bmatrix} 0 & \text{for } x < 0 \\ x & \text{for } x \geq 0 \end{Bmatrix} \tag{11.1}$$

According to Eq. (11.1), it is seen that for negative coefficient the returned value is zero. So, some of the internal neurons don't propagate further in network to evaluate output.

#### 11.8.3.2 Propagation in CNN Layers

In each CNN layer, forward propagation is evaluated as in Eq. 11.2 (Fig. 11.9):

$$x_n^p = b_n^p \sum_{i=1}^{N_{p-1}} \text{Conv}\left(w_n^{p-1}, s_i^{p-1}\right) \tag{11.2}$$

where

$x_n^p$ = input
$b_n^p$ = bias of the $n^{\text{th}}$ neuron at layer p
$s_i^{p-1}$ = output of the $i^{\text{th}}$ neuron at layer *p-1*
$w_n^{p-1}$ =kernel from the $i^{\text{th}}$ neuron at layer *p-1* to the $n^{\text{th}}$ neuron at layer *p*

### *11.8.4 Control Signals*

In this stage, the control signals are generated in the form of audio and visual signals. The control signals are fed into VR set for user interaction. The interaction with VR will also induce a change in EEG signals. Again, generated EEG signals are processed, and control signals are generated accordingly. This process continues as a mental healing process.

## 11.9 Discussion

The COVID-19 pandemic has impacted the AR in the healthcare market positively. Despite the COVID-19 pandemic, augmented reality is becoming increasingly important in the healthcare sector due to several technological developments.

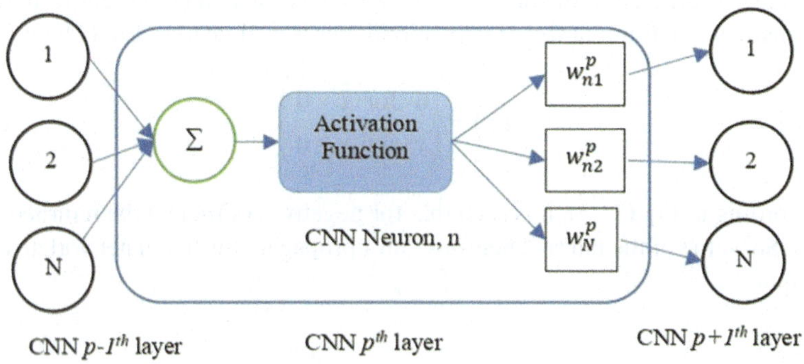


**Fig. 11.9** CNN forward propagation

Several AR apps help project 3D visualization of internal organs so that surgeons have a real view during the operation. The global AR in the healthcare market will witness significant growth in 2020. Many industries focus on product development to cope with the COVID-19 pandemic situation. This chapter is likely to review the benefits of machine learning or deep learning approach that can be successfully applied in the domain of mental health issues that had recently been raised due to the COVID-19 pandemic. A strong human-computer interface can be developed using these technologies for society. This chapter aims to view achieving real-world goals by integrating new emerging technologies for social benefits to realize the successful use of ML in mental health. According to discussions given in the above sections, it is observed that the field of machine learning and AR/VR has revealed exciting advances in the diagnosis and treatment of mental health issues. Research associated with machine learning into other medical applications, including public health, treatment and support, and research and clinical administration, has demonstrated positive results. However, there exist some limitations that currently needed to be focused on. There is a need to work and integrate and use the benefits of different AI techniques in these areas.

### *11.9.1 Positive Impact of AR/VR on Society*

According to above study, in this chapter, augmented reality (AR) and virtual reality (VR) have proved to be effective digital information tools that can be integrated with the physical environment for many applications in different ways. With the occurrence of global pandemic, AR/VR technologies transformed our surroundings in fields of learning, work, healthcare, and entertainment [59]. The AR/VR technologies can do well in three aspects: visualization, annotation, and storytelling. Beyond gaming and entertainment, these technologies are of benefit for the society in commercial aspects, economical aspects, health aspects, etc. This not only provides positive benefits to an individual but also the surrounding society [60]. This chapter also gives an overview on the potential for AR/VR to understand and transform the lifestyle of society. It is vital that the VR industry and our society have to come together to fully leverage the potential of AR/VR for social good such as economic growth, educational growth, resolving health issues, etc. This is the right time to inspire our young generation to use and experiment with such innovative technology.

## 11.10 Conclusion

In the current scenario, all over the world, countries had introduced measures to restrict the movement of people as part of efforts to reduce the number of infected people. Almost all people are making a drastic change to their daily life routines.

The new lifestyle such as working from home, temporary unemployment, home-schooling of children, etc. had impacted the mental state of people a lot. Thus, the situation is somehow getting difficult for people concerning mental health conditions. This chapter discusses technologies that can be used for mental health care and to combat depression during the ongoing COVID-19 pandemic. This chapter discussed the application of augmented reality (AR) and virtual reality (VR) for depression diagnosis and treatment using deep learning techniques and a brief discussion about psychological research using EEG signals to diagnose and treat the depressive state of mind. Using AR/VR along with a deep learning approach will help in mental health healing. The primary focus of this chapter is to use an application of the effectiveness of AR/VR in treating depression or anxiety.

## References


1. Yuan, M. L., Ong, S. K., & Nee, A. Y. C. (2006). Augmented reality for assembly guidance using a virtual interactive tool. *International Journal of Production Research, 46*, 1745.
2. Reinhart, G., & Patron, C. (2003). Integrating augmented reality in the assembly domain - fundamentals, benefits and applications. *CIRP Annals - Manufacturing Technology, 52*, 5–8.
3. Dini, G., Dalle Mura, M. (2015). *Application of augmented reality techniques in through-life engineering services*. International conference on through-life engineering services, procedia CIRP. Vol. 38, pp. 14–23.
4. Azuma, R. T. (1997). A survey of augmented reality. In *Presence: teleoperators and virtual environments* (pp. 55–385).
5. Tseng, J. C. C. (2015). *An interactive healthcare system with personalized diet and exercise guideline recommendation*. Conference on technologies and applications of artificial intelligence (TAAI). pp. 525–532.
6. Papaefthymiou, M. (2017). Gamified AR/VR character rendering and animation-enabling technologies. In M. Ioannides, N. Magnenat-Thalmann, & G. Papagiannakis (Eds.), *Mixed reality and gamification for cultural heritage*. Cham: Springer.
7. McCormack, J., Prine, J., Trowbridge, B., & Rodriguez, A. C., & Integlia, R. (2015). *2D LIDAR as a distributed interaction tool for virtual and augmented reality video games*. IEEE games entertainment media conference (GEM). pp. 1–5.
8. Azuma, R., Baillot, Y., & Behringer, R. (2001). Recent advances in augmented reality. *IEEE Computer Graphics and Applications, 21*, 34–47.
9. Zhan, Z. (2011). The application of virtual reality on distance education. In R. Chen (Ed.), *Intelligent computing and information science. Communications in Computer and Information Science* (Vol. 135).
10. Cacho-Elizondo, S., Lázaro Álvarez, J. D., & Garcia, V. E. (2017). Assessing the opportunities for virtual, augmented, and diminished reality in the healthcare sector. In L. Menvielle, A. F. Audrain-Pontevia, & W. Menvielle (Eds.), *The digitization of healthcare*. London: Palgrave Macmillan.
11. Hsu, C. (2011). *The feasibility of augmented reality on virtual tourism website*. International conference on Ubi-Media computing, Sao Paulo. pp. 253–256.
12. https://www.aumcore.com/blog/2017/07/13/virtual-reality-shopping/#:~:text=It's%20an%20immersive%20experience%20where,new%20way%20to%20consume%20products.
13. https://arvr.google.com/daydream/.
14. https://www.theverge.com/2016/8/2/12358554/microsoft-hololens-augmented-reality-opens-developer-sales.

15. https://www.inputmag.com/tech/google-has-purchased-ar-glasses-company-north.
16. https://arvr.google.com/ar/.
17. Pantelidis, P., Chorti, A., Papagiouvanni, I., Paparoidamis, G., Drosos, C., Panagiotakopoulos, T., Lales, G., & Sideris, M. Virtual and augmented reality in medical education. Medical and surgical education - past, present future, Georgios Tsoulfas. *IntechOpen.* https://doi.org/10.5772/intechopen.71963.
18. http://www.artificialmachines.com/arvr.html.
19. https://www.virtualrealitypulse.com/2020/amazon/.
20. Khan, Y., Xu, Z., & Stigant, M. (2003). *Virtual reality for neuropsychological diagnosis and rehabilitation: A survey.* Proceedings on seventh international conference on information visualization. pp. 158–163.
21. Bouchard, S., Renaud, P., Robillard, G., & St-Jacques, J. (2002). *Applications of virtual reality in clinical psychology: illustrations with the treatment of anxiety disorders.* IEEE International Workshop HAVE Haptic virtual environments and their, Ottawa, Ontario, Canada. pp. 7–11.
22. Kanno, K. M., Lamounier, E. A., Cardoso, A., Lopes, E. J., & Mendes de Lima, G. F. (2018). *Augmented reality system for aiding Mild Alzheimer patients and caregivers*, IEEE conference on virtual reality and 3D user interfaces (VR), Reutlingen. pp. 593–594.
23. Prachyabrued, M., Wattanadhirach, D., Dudrow, R. B., Krairojananan, N., & Fuengfoo, P. (2019). *Toward virtual stress inoculation training of prehospital healthcare personnel: A stress-inducing environment design and investigation of an emotional connection factor.* IEEE conference on virtual reality and 3D user interfaces (VR). pp. 671–679.
24. Liao, D., Shu, L., Huang, Y., Yang, J., & Xu, X. (2018). Scenes design in virtual reality for depression assessment. In J. Chen & G. Fragomeni (Eds.), *Virtual, augmented and mixed reality: Applications in health, cultural heritage, and industry. Lecture notes in computer science.* 10910.
25. Baus, O., & Bouchard, S. (2014). Moving from virtual reality exposure-based therapy to augmented reality exposure-based therapy: A review. *Frontiers in Human Neuroscience, 8.* https://doi.org/10.3389/fnhum.2014.00112.
26. Miller, L. D., Silva, C., Bouchard, S., Bélanger, C., & Taucer-Samson, T. (2012). Using virtual reality and other computer technologies to implement cognitive-behavior therapy for the treatment of anxiety disorders in youth. In T. Davis III, T. Ollendick, & L. G. Öst (Eds.), *Intensive one-session treatment of specific phobias* (Autism and child psychopathology series). New York: Springer.
27. Bohr, A., & Memarzadeh, K. (2020). The rise of artificial intelligence in healthcare applications. Artificial Intelligence in Healthcare. 25–60.
28. Torous, J., Jän Myrick, K., Rauseo-Ricupero, N., & Firth, J. (2020). Digital mental health and COVID-19: Uusing technology today to accelerate the curve on access and quality tomorrow. JMIR Mental Health. 7(3), (2020):e18848, https://mental.jmir.org/2020/3/e18848, https://doi.org/10.2196/18848.
29. Brandão A. F. (2020). *Biomechanics sensor node for virtual reality: A wearable device applied to gait recovery for Neurofunctional rehabilitation.* Computational science and its applications.
30. Antoniou, P., Arfaras, G., Pandria, N., Ntakakis, G., Bambatsikos, E., & Athanasiou, A. (2020). *Real-time affective measurements in medical education, using virtual and mixed reality. Brain function assessment in learning.* Springer.
31. Wen-Han Chang. (2020). A review of vaccine effects on women in light of the COVID-19 pandemic. *Taiwanese Journal of Obstetrics & Gynecology, 59*, 812.
32. Ling, Y., Nefs, H. T., Morina, N., Heynderickx, I., & Brinkman, W.-P. (2014). A meta-analysis on the relationship between self-reported presence and anxiety in virtual reality exposure therapy for anxiety disorders. *PLoS One, 9*(5), 1–12.
33. https://www.med-technews.com/news/five-ways-virtual-reality-is-transforming-mental-health/#:~:text=VR%2Denabled%20therapy%20is%20the,to%20treat%20a%20specific%20ailment.&text=VR%2Denabled%20therapy%20is%20a,lasting%20improvements%20in%20mental%20health.

34. https://www.worldometers.info/coronavirus/.
35. Lee Silvana Trimi, S. M. (2021). Convergence innovation in the digital age and in the COVID-19 pandemic crisis. *Journal of Business Research, 123*, 14–22.
36. https://www.mobihealthnews.com/news/emea/italian-hospital-utilising-vr-combat-clinician-stress-during-covid-19-crisis.
37. Rani, S., & Kautish, S. (2018). *Association clustering and time series based data mining in continuous data for diabetes prediction*. International conference on intelligent computing and control systems. pp. 1209–1214.
38. Sampathkumar, A., Rastogi, R., Arukonda, S., Shankar, A., Kautish, S., & Sivaram, M. (2020). An efficient hybrid methodology for detection of cancer-causing gene using CSC for micro array data. J Ambient Intell Human Comput 11, 4743–4751. https://doi.org/10.1007/s12652-020-01731-7.
39. Lempitsky, V. (2020). Autoencoder. In K. Ikeuchi (Ed.), *Computer vision*. Cham: Springer.
40. Agarwalla, N., Panda, D., & Modi, M. K. (2016). Deep learning using restricted Boltzmann machines. *International Journal of Computer Science and Information Technologies, 7*(3), 1552–1556.
41. Bisong, E. (2019). Recurrent Neural Networks (RNNs). In *Building machine learning and deep learning models on Google cloud platform*. Berkeley: CA Apress.
42. Alqahtani, H., Kavakli-Thorne, M. & Kumar, G. (2021). Applications of Generative Adversarial Networks (GANs): An Updated Review. Arch Computat Methods Eng 28, 525–552. https://doi.org/10.1007/s11831-019-09388-y
43. World Health Organization. (2001). *The World Health report 2001: Mental health: New understanding, new hope*. Geneva: World Health Organization.
44. Marcus, M., Yasamy, M. T., van Ommeren, M., Chisholm, D., & Saxena, S. (2012). *Depression: A global public health concern*. Perth: World Federation of Mental Health, World Health Organisation.
45. Hamilton, M. (1967). Development of a rating scale for primary depressive illness. *The British Journal of Social and Clinical Psychology, 6*, 278–296.
46. Dwyer, D. B., Falkai, P., & Koutsouleris, N. (2018). Machine learning approaches for clinical psychology and psychiatry. *Annual Review of Clinical Psychology, 14*, 91–118.
47. Lovejoy, C. A., Buch, V., & Maruthappu, M. (2019). Technology and mental health: The role of artificial intelligence. *European Psychiatry, 55*, 1–3.
48. Adrian, B., Shatte, R., Hutchinson, D. M., & Teague, S. J. (2019). Machine learning in mental health: A scoping review of methods and applications. *Psychological Medicine, 49*(9), 1426–1448.
49. Sanches, P., Janson, A., Karpashevich, P., Nadal, C., Chengcheng Q., Roquet, C. D., Umair, M., Windlin, C., Doherty, G., Höök, K., & Sas, C. (2019). *HCI and affective health: Taking stock of a decade of studies and charting future research directions*. CHI conference on human factors in computing systems, ACM. pp, 245–262.
50. Subhani, A. R., Mumtaz, W., Saad, M. N. B. M., Kamel, N., & Malik, A. S. (2017). Machine learning framework for the detection of mental stress at multiple levels. *IEEE Access, 5*, 13545–13556.
51. Mahato, S., & Paul, S. (2019). Detection of major depressive disorder using linear and nonlinear features from EEG signals. *Microsystem Technologies, 25*(3), 1065–1076.
52. Ay, B., Yildirim, O., Talo, M., Baloglu, U. B., Aydin, G., Puthankattil, S. D., & Acharya, U. R. (2019). Automated depression detection using deep representation and sequence learning with EEG signals. *Journal of Medical Systems, 43*(7), 205.
53. Li, X., La, R., Wang, Y., Niu, J., Zeng, S., Sun, S., & Zhu, J. (2019). EEG-based mild depression recognition using convolutional neural network. *Medical & Biological Engineering & Computing, 57*(6), 1341–1352.
54. Guo, Y., Zhang, H., & Pang, C. (2017). *EEG-based mild depression detection using multi-objective particle swarm optimization*. Chinese control and decision conference (CCDC). pp. 4980–4984.

55. Zhu, J. (2020). An improved classification model for depression detection using EEG and eye tracking data. *IEEE Transactions on Nanobioscience, 19*(3), 527–537.
56. Purnamasari, P. D., & Fernandya, A. (2019). *Real time EEG-based stress detection and meditation application with K-nearest neighbor*. IEEE R10 humanitarian technology conference. pp. 49–54.
57. J. Shen, X. Zhang, B. Hu, G. Wang, Z. Ding and B. & Hu, B. (2019). An Improved Empirical Mode Decomposition of Electroencephalogram Signals for Depression Detection, in IEEE Transactions on Affective Computing, https://doi.org/10.1109/TAFFC.2019.2934412.
58. Zhang, X. (2020). *EEG-based depression detection using convolutional neural network with demographic attention mechanism*. Annual international conference of the IEEE Engineering in Medicine & Biology Society (EMBC). pp. 128–133.
59. https://www.weforum.org/agenda/2020/04/augmented-reality-covid-19-positive-use/.
60. https://www.themandarin.com.au/131317-three-ways-augmented-reality-can-have-a-positive-impact-on-society/#:~:text=Augmented%20Reality%20(AR)%20enables%20digital,learning%2C%20work%20and%20entertainment%20spaces.

# Chapter 12
# Machine Learning Techniques for the Identification and Diagnosis of COVID-19

**A. Gasmi**

## 12.1 Introduction

Before the present pandemic, ML was previously used to visualize X-ray images and perform image analysis using Manta Ray Foraging optimization, differential evolution (MRFODE), and Fractional Multichannel Exponent Moments (FrMEMS) techniques [46]. The techniques aid chest X-ray image extraction, testing, and training of datasets, while removing irrelevant data and generating solutions with KNN classifier. The KNN classifier trains both datasets and determines the best option to apply in MRFO operators to achieve the exploratory phase [53]. Before the final data execution, the data must be computed to evaluate its fitted value (probability) using differential evolution (DE) [2]. As the pandemic rage uncontrollably, it is significant to project positive results and diagnose in which the success rate of each test depends on data accuracy. Experts ascertained that RNA-based assay with nasopharyngeal swab tests must be conducted, though the test can be discomforting to patients due to the insertion of swab tools inside the lungs and close to the chest. However, chest X-rays might be a better substitute for swab tests and reduce high risks of respiratory disease and pathogen deposits that may compromise patients' health [31].

Over the years, ML has served different interests, which include the identification of diseases by providing imagery and textual data, classification, prediction, and diagnostic options. The global spread indicated with the help of ML diagnostic and prognostic analysis segregates people with ordinary pneumonia infection from those with viral pneumonia and provides visible results with computed tomography images. The computed tomography image machine is a pretrained DL system that

A. Gasmi (✉)
Interuniversity Laboratory of Motor Biology, University of Claude Bernard, Lyon, France

Société Francophone de Nutrithérapie et de Nutrigénétique Appliquée, Villeurbanne, France



S. Kautish et al. (eds.), *Computational Intelligence Techniques for Combating COVID-19*, EAI/Springer Innovations in Communication and Computing,
https://doi.org/10.1007/978-3-030-68936-0_12

comprehends lung reactions to different diseases. The machine discloses patients with gathering infected and other abnormal radiologic findings [14]. Traditionally, the pandemic prompts the utilization of reverse transcription-polymerase chain reactor (RT-PCR) tool previously used for virus diagnosis, though RT-PCR has its limitation due to the rapid spread and screen burden placed on medical experts [101]. Positively, computed tomography (CT) was used to enhance test and diagnose since it has higher sensitivity than RT-PCR and shows bilateral lung lesions, asymptomatic abnormalities, and high risks of potential exposure to the virus [8].

For ML algorithms to perform its task, the use of classic and statistical dataset that records time series that are transformed into regression dataset and trained to perform multilayer perceptron (MLP) and artificial neural network (ANN) [102] is adopted from real model data generated from maximum numbers of patients in different locations. Data extraction can be done with hyper-parameter combinations of patients grouped as deceased, recovered, or infected with COVID-19, evaluating its coefficient of determination (R2) with k-fold algorithms [58].

Zhang [86] explained that ML modeling may help to determine the potential impact of infections and predict the maximum number of people that contracted it and their location. ML algorithms are used to simplify datasets and handle complex models while providing statistical analysis. This report aims to identify ML techniques, predictive parameters, and test accuracy with regression models. It will discuss different approaches utilized to forecast and predict COVID-19 with ML, implore the use of predictive analytics models, and classify methods and dataset descriptions. The report will highlight new feature selections, ML tools, and X-ray data and compare results.

The COVID-19 deep neural network method of detecting viral infection is referred to as "NCOVNET," which helps to analyze lungs through X-rays, to know whether a patient tests positive [103]. It can further be classified with convolutional neural network (CNN), known to be effective in medical imaging and computer vision. CNN offers image mapping data prediction and displays output with confusion matrix and training accuracy. COVID-19 X-rays show 121 layers of convolutional neural network analysis, containing images of frontal view of the lungs and chest, and disclose other possible ailments in the body [104]. To determine whether COVID-19 diagnostic results are accurate, it's significant to either use support vector machine (SVM), random forest, CNN softmax, or K nearest neighbor (KNN) [27]. ReLU-based deep learning image visualization technique shows 86% accuracy rates, in detecting lung infections. Singhal [83] diversified CNN layer clinical ML image scanning device to detect skin lesions, by modeling two binary critical cases of common and deadly skin cancer.

Zhang [86] proposed ML techniques for the classification of tuberculosis in the chest, while Karvekar et al. [73] adopted AI with a 3D ML model for COVID-19 detection. Chimmula and Zhang [28] viewed ML through deep learning LSTM networks that evaluate statistical methods and forecast trends and time series of COVID-19 spread around the globe. Shervin et al. [51] state that CXR image prediction with CNN can be predicted with either ResNet 18 or DenseNet-161 models, whereby CNN four predictive models will subclassify normal images at separate the dataset. Anderson [52] researched to discover how the tuberculosis CXR detecting tool will help the prescreening of viruses while putting to use the CAD system to show visible disease effects and noninfected images of normal patients.

Over time, researchers have used CT scan and chest X-ray images to analyze patients' lungs to spike human protein levels, causing membrane fusion and cellular reception [105]. Coronavirus in most case enters the human respiratory tract through the mouth, eyes, ears, or nose and affects the lungs, causing severe pneumonia and later filling the lungs with inflaming fluid that leads to patches called "ground-glass opacity" (GGO). Asymptomatic carriers will not notice any symptoms at the early stage of contamination unless test kits are introduced to separate and isolate infected patients.

Hence, the quick spread of COVID-19 caused limited test kits, and scientists need to revisit deep learning techniques to capture datasets like chest X-ray and MRI of the brain, which promise better accuracy than test swabs [74].

X-ray radiography (CXR) shows the response and traces of COVID-19, which uses an ML Decision Tree Classifier to reveal viruses. The Decision Tree Classifier consists of three binary tree decisions that are trained with CNN based on Porch image frameworks. CXR images help to distinguish network normal and abnormal results. It was successfully used to disclose early signs of tuberculosis and can also be seen as a prescreening tool that works better than RT-PCR [92].

To overcome COVID-19, fast screening tools that indicate an outbreak will help to limit further contamination, whereas CT scans and CXRs offer rapid results of virus abnormalities featured as peripheral distribution, ground glass, vascular thickening, and fine reticular opacity. However, normal pneumonia shows central-peripheral distributions, lymphadenopathy, and pleural effusion without patches of ground-glass opacity at the early, progressive, and severe phase of the virus [42]. Due to high-diagnostic errors from immature radiographers, Lee et al. [36] proposed CNN three-dimensional ML technique that separates viral pneumonia from ordinary ones, thereby segmenting the infected location and perfecting CT scan accuracy. Chowdhury et al. [60] utilized a prospective UNET ++ architectural system to produce bound boxes of regions affected and regulate the result using image sensitivity [75].

Sethy and Behera [9] researched into CNN models by comparing ResNet and AlexNet machine learning techniques using support vector machine (SVM) to show patients that have positive COVID-19 results. With ResNet, it shows 95.38%, while AlexNet proves less effective with 80%. Shan et al. [21] discovered Inception Net v3, Inception-ResNet-v2, Res-Net50, and classifiers that identify positive CXRs and separate unhealthy patients from healthy ones. The classification reveals lung abnormalities by categorizing the Inception Net v3 model into convolutional layers; max, average, and global pooling layer; and concatenation and Softmax layer [3].

In most scenarios, COVID-19 cases can be illustrated on patches of GGO and consolidation of CXRs, internal pipeline inception model, building of Inception Nets, multiple-size kernels, and spatial resolution. The essence of the inception module is to map the inherent architecture of COVID-19 inputs to the CNN layer that reveals medical image accuracy and performance. Truncated architecture outplayed Inception Net v3 models that only handles ImageNet architectural complexity. Since COVID-19's quick spread overwhelms the initial resolution to use Inception Net v3 model got defeated by demands to conduct intelligent analysis with results [80]. The truncated point model retains the initial three-point inception and I-grid size-reduction block, cascading max pooling, and global pooling layer. The Truncated Inception Net architecture shows visual learning rate, validation losses, and three epochs that reduce the training and processing time of CXR detected for COVID-19 [78].

The aim of facilitating COVID-19 tests using truncate architecture is to generate speed, efficiency, accuracy, and effective computed results [20]. Meanwhile, to perfect Truncated Inception Net protocol, an adaptive learning rate procedure will be needed to control epoch rate and make Truncated Inception Net constant, of high value, and divergent when weighed. Such will minimize errors and loss of functional space, optimize processes, reduce delays, and enable optimization techniques like grid search, particle swarm optimization, and complex genetic algorithms [72].

## 12.2 Identified ML Techniques and Treatment for COVID-19

However, machine learning with its computing infrastructure can support various data mining methods and implement real datasets, using different types of classifiers [17]. These classifiers act as a predictive system that reveals COVID-19 virus possibility and diagnostic options. Albahri et al. [50] mentioned different types of machine learning techniques, such as KNN, decision tree, Naïve Bayes, SVM, logistics regression, latent Dirichlet allocation, Word2Vec, NLP, random forest, Apriori, and Bayesian Belief Network, that can be utilized to control the spread of diseases [80].

Ai et al. [91] explained that KNN, NB, and decision tree algorithms are efficient tools that show traces of infections, since they have been used to predict MERS-COV spread in the Middle East. MERS-COV is referred to as "Middle East Respiratory Syndrome" (MERS)-COV that was first spotted in Saudi Arabia, causing mild/moderate pneumonic cold that can lead to fatal health complications. MERS-COV has symptoms like cough, fever, breath, or nose congestion and possible diarrhea. KNN, NB, and decision tree algorithms offer up to 90% accuracy using cross-validation models. Chan and Yuan [23] explored J48 decision tree and Naïve Bayes, to predict accuracy of infections, and it's re-occurring probability after cure, with an outcome of 53.6–71.58%.

Zhang [86] identified core factors influencing the recovery of COVID-19 using logistics regression, Naïve Bayes, SVM, and J48. Pan et al. [13] analyzed COVID-19 predictive spread and diagnosis with latent Dirichlet allocation, Word2Vec, and NLP.

Zhavoronkov et al. [89] adopted random forest ML tool to diagnose patients with early syndromes of COVID-19 by analyzing using receiver operating characteristics (ROC).

Jang et al. [18] extracted datasets with Apriori algorithms and compare their differences, similarities, and dissimilarities with tenfold positive dataset validation. Pandey et al. [16] achieved its predictive and preventive measures by using global positioning system (GPS) and Bayesian Belief Network to assess risks and propel TP (true-positive) and FP (false-positive) receiver operating characteristics rates. KNN, decision tree, and NB are noted as the best statistical models for multiple classifications of COVID-19 problems. However, SVM classifier provides sigmoid, normal, and polynomial iterations needed to analyze the infection in human body proteins. SVM reveals emotional and behavioral similarities of the cloud-based medical system and offers high accuracy in prediction, prevention, and other attributes that support drug research and organizing of users' medical records [61]. Prediction and diagnosis tools such as neural networks, hybrid classifier, and reinforcement learning are rarely used to handle complex ML analysis because they do not integrate or optimize genetic algorithms and particle swarm optimization [41].

## 12.3 Data Collection

Radiologists and doctors' datasets are gathered to analyze COVID-19 cases based on X-ray tests. Esteva et al. [95] analyze the difference between positive test and negative test results with the COV-NET tool by carrying out volumetric chest CT image scans, after collecting data from ten different medical centers. The collected data were evaluated using the receiver operating characteristic (ROC) curve with diverse inputs to predict class labels of CT images. The receiver operating characteristic curve shows the result of 0.96 chances of COVID-19 cases in medical centers. Huang et al. [62] added a convolutional neural network referred to as "COVID-Net" with two stages of human-machine interaction that uses residual protection expansion protected extension (PEPX) design method. Xu et al. [19] deployed CNN ResNet-18 network-based concatenation to test COVID-19 carriers by observing pulmonary CT images. The same method was utilized during the spread of influenza-A to validate data and demonstrate 86% accuracy [81].

China developed a modifier stacked auto-encoder ML that forecasts COVID-19 confirmed cases. The modifier comes with four latent layers and number nodes which correspond to 8, 32, 4, and 1 respectively [65]. The number node "8" represents 8 days of COVID-19 data collection added to the input, while other latent variables are processed as a single value decomposition method before engaging the clustering algorithms. The cluster algorithms are implored to group COVID-19 cases into regional segments, in turn, to investigate the dynamic range of transmission [82].

The figure below shows "CovNet" architecture model, CT images, and max pooling procedure that combines features from ResNet-50, CNN, and CT slides. The CovNet architecture model combined features in the figure below and computed with probability layers of three classes to indicate whether a patient's data is pneumonia or not.

Stephen et al. [106] proposed a new approach for classifying and separating datasets of patients with pneumonia from patients with COVID-19. The CovNet model trains some sets of data with 12.88% outcome, 95.32% accuracy, 18.30% validation loss, and 92.71% validation accuracy. Ayan and Ünver [107] evaluates pneumonia chest X-ray images with Xception and VGG16, while Kermany et al. [108] reviewed frontal chest images of patients likely to have either ordinary pneumonia or COVID-19. The result shows 85% sensitivity, 86% precision, and 93% recall. Varshni et al. [109] used pretrained CovNet models such as VGG-16, Xception, Res50, and Dense-121 to detect whether pneumonia symptom is normal or abnormal on X-ray images. Cohen, Morrison, and Dao [110] used below tabled COVID-19 datasets with 360 X-ray images and 4 categories to determine whether a patient is free from COVID-19, infected with either bacterial or viral pneumonia (Fig. 12.1).

## 12.4 Data Summary of ML Implementation for COVID-19 Diagnosis Using X-Ray Imaging

Raw datasets are collected from 6 health centers with 5000 chest CT examinations and 4800 patients to perform ordinary pneumonia and COVID-19 test. The proposed datasets were analyzed using 3D convolution ResNet-50, resulting in the

| Dataset/Class | Covid | Normal | Pneumonia_bac | Pneumonia_vir | Total |
|---|---|---|---|---|---|
| Train | 60 | 70 | 70 | 70 | 270 |
| Test | 9 | 9 | 9 | 9 | 36 |
| Total | 69 | 79 | 79 | 79 | 306 |

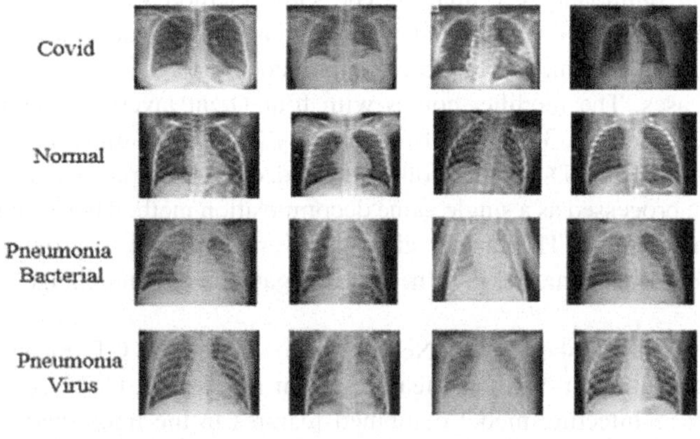


**Fig. 12.1** CovNet architecture model, CT images, and max pooling procedure combining features from ResNet-50, CNN, and CT slides

detection of 0.96 COVID-19 cases. The result proves that about "1885" people have ordinary pneumonia while "1357" test positive for COVID-19 infection [33].

Datasets of 780 CT samples were also collected from 150 COVID-19 patients and 250 CT samples of influenza-A patients and 130 samples of healthy people. The mentioned datasets were analyzed using location-attention network in ResNet-18 architecture, which shows 88.7% accuracy [34].

If the same datasets are implemented as drop weights on Bayesian-based CNN, specifically posterior-anterior chest radiograph to show images of patients with or without COVID-19, the accuracy will exhibit 89.92%. In case the datasets are modified with the inception transfer-learning model, the accuracy rates will drop to 79.3% (approx. 0.83 and 0.67) record sensitivity. Clinically, similar datasets implemented at multilayer perceptron and LSTM algorithms will result in 0.954 accuracies [35].

Suppose 1570 clinical test volumes of more than 500 patients with COVID-19 are compared with a thousand without COVID-19 infection, using 2D deep CNN, it will relate to 94.98% accuracy. Assuming the combination of 3D UNET++ [14] and ResNet-50 are used to determine trained COVID-19 case, the sensitivity rate will start from 0.984 to 0.932 [10].

Meanwhile, machine learning techniques can be helpful in the prescreening process of COVID-19, especially when X-ray images of 50 healthy people and 50 patients with COVID-19 viruses are analyzed using pretrained ResNet-50. The result will demonstrate 98% accuracy while segregating the infected from noninfected patients [25].

AlexNet, ResNet, DenseNet, and SqueezeNet are ML analytical architectural framework that shows up to 98.3% accuracy when separating healthy patients from infected patients. AI dataset implementation shows minimal error due to AI-based systematic satellites projected geographically to collect real-time heterogeneous data in the range of numbers of cases, death rates, demographics and traffic density, and other data from different social media. Social media datasets are confirmed to be limited by Cregan et al. [5], as he further proposed conditional generative adversarial networks (GANs) to observe individual responses to COVID-19 cases.

Zachreson et al. [69] utilized discrete time (AceMod) and stochastic agent-based model to simulate COVID-19 data. The AceMod stands for Australian Census-based Epidemic Model that calculates the spread of COVID-19 within the Australian region. AceMod datasets consist of age, occupation, gender, and records showing immunity to COVID-19 disease and contraction rates. AceMod ML technique was adhered to while observing necessary isolation, social distancing, and travel ban, which resulted in 80% decreases in the rise of COVID-19 cases in Australia.

## 12.5 Methodology

To successfully implement ML algorithms, other AI tools such as IoT, text mining, and NLP models must work correspondently with ML to offer better results. Some machine learning data sets are obtained from smartphones and on-board sensors [7], to further observe and predict collected datasets. El-Sawy et al. [97] explained how IoT tools are used to collect data via temperature fingerprint sensors, in turn, to detect a fever level. Procedures are performed with image or video data collected from phones and cameras.

IoT data can also be collected to detect human fatigue levels in ML.

Lawanont et al. [76] state that smartphones implemented with IoT features can pass through ML prediction, like smartphone videos used to detect or predict nausea symptoms in sick patients. Nemati et al. [77] implored image sensor to measure upper-chest posture and monitor positions and prediction of headaches in patients. IoT and ML algorithms were put together to form audio data to determine cough types and detect its causes [49]. For COVID-19 cases, different data collection methods are explored to preview basic travel history and check locations, to reduce infection risk. Debnath et al. [79] engaged IoT and data sharing protocols to integrate thermal cameras that will help the decision-making of urban health and the implementation of smart cities.

A machine learning approach was once registered as a hybrid AI model to forecast infection rates. The forecast model works perfectly with susceptible-infected-resistant (SIR) model, NLP, and ML tools. The susceptible-infected-resistant technique over the years helped the prediction of infectious diseases. SIR has a mathematical model, where S stands for numbers of susceptible people, I represents numbers of infected patients, and R states numbers of recovered cases. With differential equations characterizing the interrelationship between I, S, and R, the equated model helps to find formulas needed to control the infectious disease [32].

Sometimes, generating accurate data for epidemiological modeling may be difficult due to data scarcity and ongoing data prediction; hence, a susceptible-infected-resistant (SIR) model with a hybrid machine learning approach will help to predict COVID-19 cases [63]. In Hungary, for instance, a hybrid machine learning method of adaptive network holding potential data was implemented on the multilayer perceptron imperialist competitive algorithm (MLP-ICA) and adaptive neuro fuzzy inference system (ANFIS) to predict time-series infection and mortality rate of people with COVID-19 infection. As of May 2020, the result shows substantial results of confirmed accuracy [64]. The susceptible-infected-resistant model displays a high probability of infected class "S," whereby the recovered class "R" and class of infected people "I" will follow basic differential equations written below [40].

$$\frac{ds}{Dt} = -\alpha SI \quad (12.1)$$

Where $I$, $S$, and $\alpha$ stand for infected populations and susceptible population, representing reproduction rates. If the time series "$S$" is analyzed with a differential equation to decrease the time factor, the delay in calculating the spread of the pandemic will be minimized. To calculate the linear increment at the beginning of the pandemic, $S \approx 1$.

Therefore;

$$\frac{ds}{Dt} = \alpha SI \text{ and } \beta I. \tag{12.2}$$

"$\beta$" stands for the parameter of everyday COVID-19 spread, and the susceptible records of patients removed from SIR model will be calculated with class "$R$" as follows:

$$\frac{dR}{Dt} = \beta I \tag{12.3}$$

With the equation mentioned above, it's easier to calculate the unconstrained condition of patients removed from SIR, to discover the SIR model outbreak of the virus. To achieve that:

$$I(t) \approx \text{I0}\exp\{(\alpha - \beta)\} \tag{12.4}$$

In that case, SIR-based model will be evaluated for accuracy using median success function represented as:

$$F = \frac{\text{Prediction}}{\text{True Value}} \tag{12.5}$$

The government of Hungary used the SIR-based model to slow down the pandemic outbreak since the reliance on the SIR model depends on data relevance. To ensure data relevance and use of variable information in demonstrating constant population dynamics with SIR, the data must record numbers of infected patients with susceptible-infected-recovered-deceased (SIRD) model. It's necessary also to make visible the maternally derived-immunity-susceptible-infected-recovered (MSIR) and susceptible-exposed-infected-recovered (SEIR) models. The SIR-based model must include maternally-derived-immunity-susceptible-exposed-infected-recovered-susceptible (MSEIRS) model [38]. The standard models above will enable experts to analyze disease-free equilibrium before encouraging social mixing, which is a critical factor when trying to avoid disease reproduction. To determine the non-stationaries of disease reproductive number Ro, SIR utilized to measure Ro value down to 1 which will help experts to know when to institute lockdowns [39]. In Italy, the COVID-19 outbreak increased tremendously and dropped significantly after they used $F = 1$ performance metrics to determine the lead time of 120 hours while reducing $f = 0.89$ for 144 hours of lead time [11]. They evaluated several data of the infected and separated and integrated with the SIR model, while surveying the environment with CCTVs, creating awareness on social media and mobile apps, and generating data from call data records. To further detect the outbreak, a random forest is used to predict swine fever, H1N1 flu, oyster norovirus, and dengue fever [12].

However, Lopez et al. [100] believed that social media datasets can be interpreted with NLP and text mining tools to be transformed into multilingual data needed to study the regional spread of COVID-19. Vast datasets that constitute ranges of numerical data are acquired to study infection rates and further predict it with radiology images [15]. Data may be sourced from social media handles, Google Search, or raw biological data with the potential of being transformed into numeric time series with NL.

LSTM ML tool is a recurrent neural network predictor that characterizes temperature dynamic behavior and mode infection cases. CNN-based model processes chest X-ray and CT scan images, predicts its high-dimensional data outcome, and represents its visual cortex, in turn, to show receptive fields of human and animal brain neurons, especially the sub-area visual fields and the entire problems in the neuron field [43].

For some machine learning tools to interpret language model inputs, an unstructured text data mining tool like advanced NLP, text summarization, machine translator, and entity recognition tool will need to convert raw data to machine language. It can as well be used to interchange machine language to human interpretable language [16]. Tools such as NLP performs embedding language model task (EIMO) and fine-tune language processing using the Universal Language Model Fine-Tuning (ULMFiT) tool. Alternatively, Google Bidirectional Encoder Representations from Transformer (BERT) and ERNIE multilayer transformer also perform similar tasks. Basic encoding tools like XLNet handle autoregressive pretraining transformer-Xl tasks while supporting complex task and natural language data process [44].

Complex biological data like genomics or proteomic sequence dataset requires hierarchical cluster and density-based spatial clustering of applications with noise (DBSCAN) to demonstrate exposed visible origins of viruses and track its secondary spread and predict its apparent structure using fuzzy logic. Fuzzy logic as a predicting language helps to structure quantitative analysis of the amino-acid properties and backtrace virus causes [47] (Fig. 12.2).

It demonstrates patients' data consisting of different attributes such as patient's ID, age, sex, offset, findings, survival and intubation, ICU (needing supplemental O2), extubated temp, PO2 saturation, leukocyte count, etc. [22].

The validation process demonstrates dataset relevance, whereas the texts are mined and classified before preprocessing to look refined (i.e., to conduct text cleanup like editing for punctuation and lemmatization). Afterward, the preprocessed report will be featured with engineering semantics and probabilistic values using TF/IDF techniques to consider data unigram and bigrams, for the data to correspond with the weight data, input, and ML algorithms. Once the feature engineering is completed, ML tools such as SVM, MNB, logistic regression, decision tree,

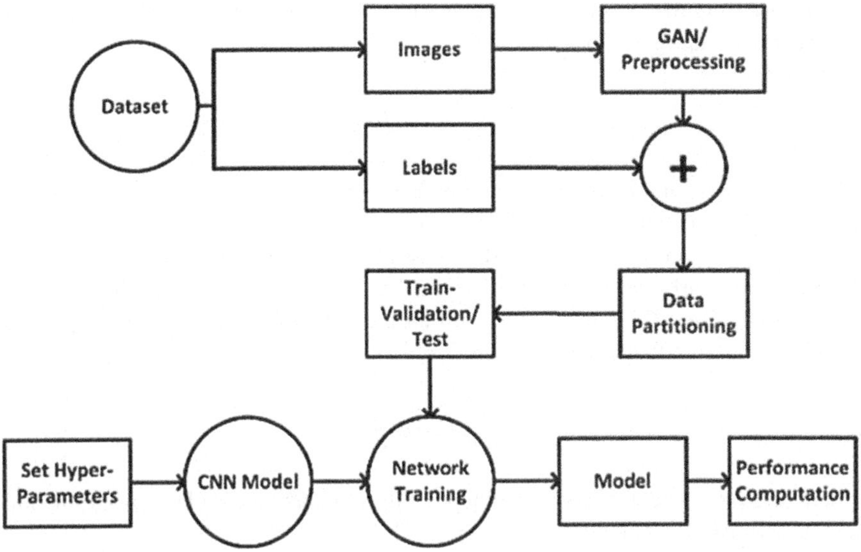


**Fig. 12.2** A proposed CNN, GAN, and image dataset methodology for predicting COVID-19

AdaBoost, etc. will then be used to classify texts into four different types to detect patients with COVID-19, ordinary pneumonia, other kinds of bacteria, and different types of viruses [88].

Logistic regression is another useful ML algorithm used to classify numeric variables that determine the relationship of datasets with data labels. Multinomial Naïve Bayes serves a different purpose, which is to classify computed tests with Bayes rule to determine the probability of data accuracy, based on four classes: $C = 0, 1, 2,$ and 3. Support vector machine (SVM) acts as a supervising ML algorithm that classifies data into diverse categories using unigram and bigram technique, while decision trees separate data input into regions and classify every region differently. AdaBoost observes data equilibrium, strengthens weak learning algorithms, and classifies weak learning coefficients, by handling all misclassified data [48].

## 12.6 Machine Learning Data Molecules for Predicting COVID-19

The epidemiological standards known as susceptible-infected-recovered (SIR) model show reported data of COVID-19 spread through personal contacts. SIR stands for the "*S*" number of non-infected individuals, the "*I*" class represents numbers of people infected, and "*R*" categorizes isolated and immune to COVID-19 patients, and death rate. Lee, Ng, and Khong [8] maintained that class

"*I*" representing the infected people can transmit to noninfected class "*S*," using the differential equations below:

$$\frac{ds}{dt} = -\propto \mathrm{SI}$$

where "*I*" shows numbers of infected people and "*S*" (susceptible fraction) shows the replicating rate of the infection. The data molecule values may decline when the susceptible rates of noninfected individuals are controlled to avoid further spread. The assumed early outbreak can be evaluated as "*S*," whereas the number of the independent class "*I*" is negligible with an incrementing class "*I*" showing linear classification, as equated below:

$$\frac{dI}{dt} \propto SI - \beta I$$

where beta $\beta$ represents daily rate of newly infected class and *R* class excluding non-infected, illustrated below:

$$\frac{dR}{dt} = \beta I$$

The unconstrained group data may show outbreak, if the equation below is used:

$$I(t) \approx Io\exp\{(\propto - \beta)$$

The outbreak equation above was used in different developed countries to model the COVID-19 outbreak before implementing restricting measures. Some countries applied the SIR model to ensure committed quarantine and social distancing. Just like the SEIR model aids the control of Zika outbreak by revealing its incubation period [98]. The SIR model has parameters of social mixing or contact networking for nonstationary control, which the formula Ro estimates lockdown through Ro < 1 equation [45].

## 12.7 ML Time Series Data Molecule Estimation

ML enhances time series modeling through logistics, linear, logarithmic, quadratic, cubic, compound, power, and exponential time series equations. As illustrated in the table below, the used time series model supports ML evolutionary, genetic, and particle swarm optimization (PSO) algorithms [6] (Fig. 12.3).

| Model description | Model name |
|---|---|
| R=A/(1+exp(((4*μ)*(L-x)/A)+2)) | Logistic |
| R=Ax-B | Linear |
| R=A+ Blog(x) | Logarithmic |
| $R=A+Bx+Cx^2$ | Quadratic |
| $R=A+Bx+Cx^2+Dx^3$ | Cubic |
| $R=AB^x$ | Compound |
| $R=Ax^B$ | Power |
| R=AEXP(Bx) | Exponential |

**Fig. 12.3** Time series model supports ML evolutionary, genetic, and particle swarm optimization (PSO) algorithms

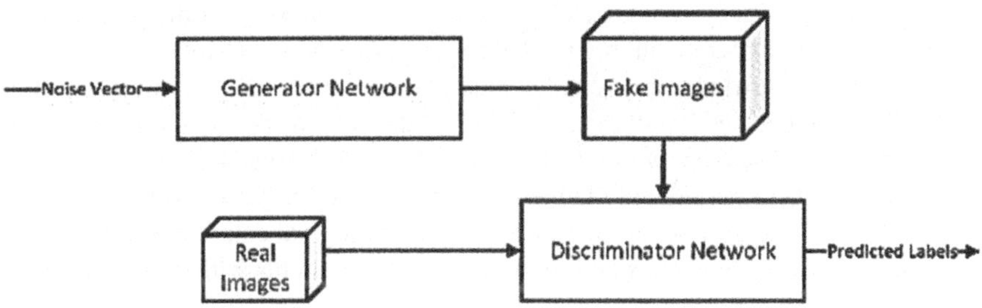


**Fig. 12.4** Illustration of GAN model

## 12.8 Present ML Approach for Identifying and Diagnosing COVID-19 Infection

Science has not approved deep learning models for COVID-19 identification, but prior threats of SRS-CoV-1 and MERS-CoV detection were predicted with the DL image/video classification tool. DL supports algorithm reasoning, simulation, and data mining, which exemplifies input data labels and analyzes hidden data patterns [111]. DL has helped practitioners to perform X-ray recognition, especially the 2009 deep Boltzmann machine that detects a series of infectious diseases [112]. Generative adversarial network (GAN) has two major networks such as generative and discriminative networks. The generative network provides assumed results, while the discriminative offers a distinction between real and fake data analysis [113]. GAN model is illustrated below.

Convolutional neural networks like CovNets and CNN graphics processing units (GPU) enhance visions using MNIST, demonstrated with different languages, Chinese/Arabic characters, and handwritten character recognition [114]. Another novelty tool for achieving image visualization of infected patients with COVID-19 is the imageNet Large Scale Visual Recognition (ILSVR) [115] (Fig. 12.4).

## 12.9 ML Significance in Controlling COVID-19 Cases

Google Deep Mind and AlphaFold tools are known protein structure predictors that assist in predicting COVID-19 cases; hereby the analysis conducted will depend on the amino acid level release when analyzing therapeutic approaches for subduing virus spread. The proposed therapeutic approaches can be achieved with the generative auto-encoder model, GANs, genetic algorithms, or language models [90]. The same therapeutic model experimented with the above-outlined tools can reinforce synthetic testing needed to create drug-like chemicals and possible vaccines.

Goses et al. [59] claimed that COVID-19 taxonomy can be predicted via alignment-free ML, genomic signatures, and decision tree methods, required to classify pathogens and process DNA raw data. It can also support the prediction of genus *Betacoronavirus* taxonomy related to the SARS-Cov-2 family.

Zhou et al. [55] tried to prove subgenius *Sarbecovirus* taxonomy by suggesting his research to the "bat hypothesis." He studied the bat's response to different types of coronavirus diseases; while Nguyen et al. [4] experimented with pangolin genomes that were previously claimed to host the present virus. Randhawa et al. [54] performed a quantitative analysis by mining biological datasets which contribute to the discovery of hydroxychloroquine effect on patients with coronavirus.

## 12.10 Result and Discussion

Sometimes, chest X-ray and CT images permit the identification of abnormalities in viral cases; whereas Gozes et al. [26] proposed localization maps for measuring lung abnormalities. Hu et al. [57] split the map measuring techniques into two 3D subsystems to detect nodule and small opacity with commercial software. The second step involves capturing the lungs "region of interest" (ROI) and extracting the lung segment module (U-Net architecture), by cropping the lung's digital images. The third part of the process involves using deep convolutional neural network model ResNet-50 to identify network activated maps and use Grad-Cam methods to combine outputs of subsystems A and B, while calculating the volumetric summation of the network activation map [93].

Chen et al. [99] utilized deep convolutional neural networks to test 50 X-ray images of infected patients. He divided datasets into training and testing data, while adopting DCNN pretrained models, ResNet-50, and K-fold ($k$ = 5) method to cross-validate values for accuracy obtaining 98% results. Hemdan et al. [24] reviewed COVIDX.NET deep learning classifiers using DCNN architecture to classify 50 X-ray images into positive or negative cases, while showing results of 89–91% with F1 Score.

John et al. [85] used a modified AlexNet model (MAN) and SVM to identify pneumonia images with an accuracy level of 96.8%. Ye et al. [66] also combined MAN and ensemble feature technique (EFT) to enhance performance. He also tried SVM, KNN, and random forest (RF) and obtained better results than the formal analysis.

Jiang et al. [87] examined backbone X-ray using CNN by classifying datasets with $P_{cis}$ classifying score and detected its scalar anomaly with $P_{ano}$ anomaly score, in turn, to attain a calculated threshold T result of 96%.

To assist radiologist's expeditions in classifying automatic annotations of COVID-19 cases, Bai et al. [94] deployed human-in-the-loop (HITL) and VB-Net neural network to evaluate metric volumes and percentage infection in the lungs.

For test results to be accurate, raw data collected after the image input must be preprocessed, before integrating with different ML techniques. Data preprocessing enhances the quality of visual data, eliminates noise in the input images, and deletes low and high frequency, while adjusting image contrast. The process can be attained with intensity normalization and contrast limited adaptive histogram equalization (CLAHE) [30].

Afterward, the preprocessed data will be redirected for pretraining and transferred to either VGG, DenseNet-201, inception-Resnet-v2, or MobileNet-v2 for data classification. These classifiers will help to remove confusing matrices and separate bacteria from viruses [96]. Data augmentation enables data matrix to be segmented into PCN, PCB, PNN, PBB, and PCC, which separates infected from noninfected patients. Patients with ordinary bacteria are denoted as "PBB." Patients with bacteria mistaken for COVID-19 are denoted as "PCB." Patients with other viruses are denoted as PNB. Coronavirus patients are classified as "PCN" and patients without bacteria or viruses are classified as "PNN." Data augmentation aids dataset preprocessing, splitting, and rescaling [67].

Data augmentation increases the number of available samples, multiple preprocessing, and leverage Keras image data generation during training. It has performance metrics, equated as:

$$\text{Accuracy}\left(\text{ACC}\right)=\frac{TP+TN}{N} \tag{12.6}$$

$$\text{Where precision }\left(\text{P}\right)=\frac{TP}{TP+FP} \tag{12.7}$$

To recall data augmented sensitivity, the above equation will be calculated as:

$$\frac{TP}{TP+FN} \tag{12.8}$$

If

$$\text{F1}-\text{score}=2\left(\frac{\text{precision}\times\text{recall}}{\text{precision}+\text{Recall}}\right) \tag{12.9}$$

its specificity will be:

$$\frac{TN}{TN+FP} \tag{12.10}$$

According to the above equations, TP, TN, FP, and FN are known to either show true-positive, false-positive, true-negative, or false-negative samples that classify separate healthy people from patients with COVID and ordinary pneumonia. According to Eq. (12.6), the accuracy can be determined using proportional predicted number of labels. Eq. (12.7) proportionally has correct labels that total the actual number of labels. The Eq. (12.8) called "Recall" recalls eqs. 12.6 and 12.7 by calculating the predicted correct labels to the total number of predicted labels. The "Recall" may show positive sensitivity and true positive rates. Eq. (12.9) conducts harmonic mean precision via recalling specificity of the true negative rate of measured negative proportions to identify the specificity results in Eq. (12.10). Data performance metrics support transfer learning processing in ML while CNNs with two types of transfer learning methods will extract features and fine-tune the extracted data. The fine-tuning process with CNN models will help to identify different classes of data, weight its pretrained images on ImageNet dataset and can categorize them using image recognition tools [29].

The ImageNet database fine-tuning process can be done with VGG16 network architecture, containing 13 convolutional (CONV) layers and Fully Connected (FC)

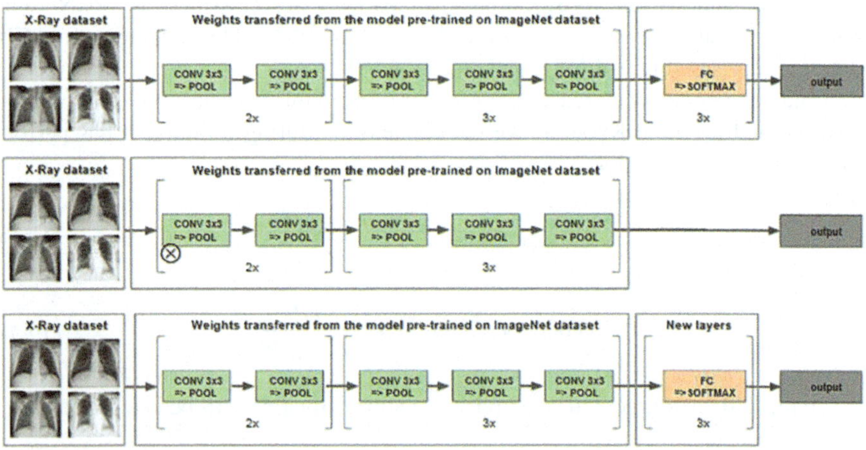


**Fig. 12.5** Weight transfer model with pretraining possibility on ImageNet database after X-ray chest dataset insertion with different classifiers

**Table 12.1** Results of different classifiers used for implementation of X-ray datasets

| Classifiers | Label | Precision | Recall | F1 Score | Specificity | Accuracy (%) |
|---|---|---|---|---|---|---|
| VGG-19 | COVID-19 | 1.01 | 0.92 | 0.99 | 1.01 | 0.9507 |
| VGG-19 | Normal | 0.94 | 1.00 | 0.87 | 0.93 | 0.9507 |
| VGG-19 | Ordinary pneumonia | 0.92 | 1.20 | 0.91 | 0.98 | 0.9507 |
| VGG-16 | COVID-19 | 0.93 | 0.93 | 0.96 | 0.98 | 0.9507 |
| VGG-16 | Normal | 0.91 | 1.01 | 0.92 | 0.96 | 0.9507 |
| VGG-16 | Pneumonia | 0.93 | 0.91 | 0.92 | 0.97 | 0.9507 |
| MobileNetV2 | COVID-19 | 1.01 | o.12 | 0.22 | 1.01 | 0.3432 |
| MobileNetV2 | Normal | 1.00 | 0.09 | 0.17 | 1.02 | 0.3432 |
| MobileNetV2 | Pneumonia | 0.35 | 1.01 | 0.54 | 0.09 | 0.3432 |
| InceptionV3 | COVID-19 | 1.01 | 0.03 | 0.06 | 0.95 | 0.4657 |
| InceptionV3 | Normal | 1.01 | 0.02 | 0.08 | 1.01 | 0.4657 |
| InceptionV3 | Pneumonia | 0.43 | 0.32 | 1.00 | 0.54 | 0.4657 |
| Xception | COVID-19 | 1.00 | 0.64 | 0.72 | 0.67 | 0.6435 |
| Xception | Normal | 0.66 | 0.70 | 0.43 | 0.43 | 0.6435 |
| Xception | Pneumonia | 0.45 | 1.00 | 0.65 | 0.92 | 0.6435 |
| InceptionRestNetV2 | Covid | 1.00 | 0.18 | 0.31 | 1.01 | 0.7654 |
| InceptionRestNetV2 | Normal | 0.21 | 0.31 | 1.00 | 0.98 | 0.7654 |
| InceptionRestNetV2 | Pneumonia | 0.45 | 0.34 | 0.34 | 0.27 | 0.7654 |
| DenseNET201 | COVID-19 | 1.00 | 0.13 | 0.24 | 1.01 | 0.4321 |
| DenseNET201 | Normal | 1.01 | 0.05 | 0.09 | 0.08 | 0.4321 |
| DenseNET201 | Pneumonia | 0.31 | 1.00 | 0.41 | 0.05 | 0.4321 |
| RestNet152V2 | COVID-19 | 1.01 | 0.11 | 0.14 | 0.21 | 0.5432 |
| RestNet152V2 | Normal | 0.54 | 0.43 | 0.34 | 0.12 | 0.5432 |
| RestNet152V2 | Pneumonia | 0.21 | 0.98 | 0.55 | 0.43 | 0.5432 |
| NasNetLarge | COVID-19 | 1.01 | 0.67 | 0.34 | 0.87 | 0.8102 |
| NasNetLarge | Normal | 1.00 | 0.49 | 0.71 | 1.02 | 0.8102 |
| NasNetLarge | Pneumonia | 0.72 | 0.91 | 0.81 | 0.84 | 0.8102 |

layers. The FC layer and Softmax activation function known as "Head", excludes Pooling layer to extract middle figures of the images. However, the FC head layer randomly initiates the process and moves forward to the body of the network and trains, scratches, and randomizes the CONV layer learning feature [68, 84].

The figure below demonstrates a weight transfer model that can be pretrained on ImageNet database; after the X-ray chest test, datasets were inserted. It also shows FC and Softmax integration and data output (Fig. 12.5).

## 12.11 Classification Performance Results from CNN Models of Different Classifiers

Assuming different classifiers are used to implement the X-ray datasets in the figure above, the results will be shown as illustrated in Table 12.1 below.

The above-classified deep transfer precision can be integrated with either python programming language, Keras package, or TensorFlow to obtain the simulated results of chest X-ray CNN detection. While using Keras, you will notice its neural network library built to accommodate TensorFlow model, which can also weigh ImageNet data framework [70]. Some executable CNN networks are configured with Ubuntu 18.04 and accommodate fixed-size images of 224 × 224 pixels. The CNN framework can randomly split 80% training and 20% testing image datasets and conduct 35 epoch fittings at the rate of 1c-3 at batch size of 8. CNN has compiled named "ADAM" for optimizing data and used Rectified Liner Unit (ReLu) to activate convolutional layers [37]. However, it has dropout layers that apply up to 50% of the neuron which are set randomly to zero, during the epoch process. Dropout also regularizes and reinforces network weight placed on small training values. Categorical-Cross-entropy loss functions denoted as P model (y1-C $C_{yi}$) with the probability of the ith and Cth category, the true distribution prediction can easily be demonstrated as a true class. The true class can be represented with hot-encoder vectors modeled with accurate output to lower data losses [56].

## 12.12 Recommendations and the Future of ML in Controlling Viruses

Google Deep Mind is presently partnering with Moorfield Eye Clinic in the UK to create prototypes for technical innovation, precision, and accuracy of optical coherence tomography retinal scans that will address voluminous scan and X-ray images [71]. Microsoft's InnerEye technological radiotherapy planning and heart flow machine learning techniques are developed to achieve 3D coronary modeling for cardiac CT, which will offer clinical coronary angiography [1]. However, the challenge lies in comparing ML algorithms with human performance, especially in addressing COVID-19 parenchymal infection, where radiologists are forced to detect abnormalities with pulmonary nodules/emboli. To get future research accurate, ML algorithms need to be trained to interpret CT spectrum disease images, which can easily be implemented in real life [72].

## 12.13 Conclusion

Machine learning techniques yet to be discussed in this report include random forest classifier and stochastic gradient boosting. For COVID-19 cases, the random forest might be a resourceful tool that works like decision trees but might be different since it acts as a bootstrap aggregator for predicting, modifying, splitting, and featuring a subset of random algorithms. Stochastic gradient boosting handles huge training sample datasets and reduces correlations between trees in gradients boost, iterates sub-sample, and randomly select subsamples for training. To compute datasets, it is important to use windows system with 4GB and 2.3 GHz processor and adopt SCIKET learning tool that handles ML classification for various libraries like NLTK, stop words, etc.

Since the COVID-19 vaccine is unavailable to mitigate the infection, therapeutic or technology alternatives need to be developed to minimize the spread of the COVID-19. This report has examined different algorithms and mentioned how to utilize classifiers to control the spread of COVID-19. It also discussed data detection, precision percentage, and other relevant tools that aid data accuracy. COVID-19 comes with pneumonic symptoms that can simply be controlled with a 2D deep learning framework if the X-ray images separate and show data of infected patients from ordinary pneumonia patients.

The future analysis includes a personalized protective method, using human angiotensin-converting enzyme 2 (ACE2) to express epithelial cells of the lungs, heart, kidneys, and small intestines and spike glycoprotein of patients showing symptoms of COVID-19.

Experts explained how ACE2 stimulants for treating hypertension and diabetes could affect patients' ability to recuperate, but ACE2 may help immune-variant approach of classifying and predicting people vulnerable to contract COVID-19. Recent implementation of machine learning in healthcare helped to control the spread of COVID-19, specifically the predicting of data accuracy and performing of screening to separate the infected from noninfected patients. The development of "MYCIN" for countering SARS-CoV, MERS-CoV, SARS-CoV2, Ebola, and other types of viruses helped to reduce its further spread. Machine learning significantly reduces dataset errors, supports cross-validation, and improves screening, detecting, and diagnosing accuracy. Researchers emphasize that ML techniques can help the control of COVID-19 since ML helps experts to perform computational epidemiology, introduce early detection and diagnosis, and subdue disease progression.

## References

1. Douglas, P. S., De Bruyne, B., Pontone, G., et al. (2020). 1-year outcomes of FFRCT-guided care in patients with suspected coronary disease: the PLATFORM study. *Journal of the American College of Cardiology, 68*, 435–445.

2. Li, L., Qin, L., Xu, Z., et al. (2020). Artificial intelligence distinguishes COVID-19 from community-acquired pneumonia on chest CT. *Radiology*; published online March 19. https://doi.org/10.1148/radiol.2020200905.
3. Apostolopoulos, I. D., & Mpesiana, T. A. (2020). Covid-19: automatic detection from x-ray images utilizing transfer learning with convolutional neural networks. *Physical and Engineering Sciences in Medicine*, 1.
4. Nguyen, L. D., Lin, D., Lin, Z., & Cao, J. (2018). Deep CNNs for microscopic image classification by exploiting transfer learning and feature concatenation. In *IEEE International Symposium on Circuits and Systems (ISCAS)* (pp. 1–5).
5. Ciregan, D., Meier, U., & Schmidhuber, J. (2012). Multi-column deep neural networks for image classification. In *Proceedings of the 2012 IEEE Conference on Computer Vision and Pattern Recognition, Providence, RI, USA* (Vol. 16–21, pp. 3642–3649).
6. Back, T. (1996). *Evolutionary algorithms in theory and practice: Evolution strategies, evolutionary programming, genetic algorithms*. Oxford university press.
7. El-Sawy, A., & EL-Bakry, H.; Loey, M. (2016). CNN for Handwritten Arabic Digits Recognition Based on LeNet-5 BT. In *Proceedings of the International Conference on Advanced Intelligent Systems and Informatics 2016, Cairo, Egypt, 24–26*.
8. Lee, E. Y., Ng, M. Y., & Khong, P. L. (2020). COVID-19 pneumonia, what has CT taught us? *The Lancet Infectious Diseases, 20*(4), 384–385.
9. Sethy, P. K., & Behera, S. K. (2020). Detection of coronavirus disease (COVID-19) based on deep features and support vector machine. *International Journal of Mathematical, Engineering and Management Sciences, 5*(4), 643–651.
10. Phan, L. T., Nguyen, T. V., Luong, Q. C., Nguyen, T. V., Nguyen, H. T., Le, H. Q., & Pham, Q. D. (2020). Importation and human-to-human transmission of a novel coronavirus in Vietnam. *The New England Journal of Medicine, 382*(9), 872–874.
11. Maier, B. F., & Brockmann, D. (2020). Effective containment explains sub-exponential growth in confirmed cases of recent COVID-19 outbreak in Mainland China. *medRxiv*.
12. Koike, F., & Morimoto, N. (2018). Supervised forecasting of the range expansion of novel non-indigenous organisms: alien pest organisms and the H1N1 flu pandemic. *Global Ecology and Biogeography, 27*, 991–1000.
13. Pan, J. R., Huang, Z. Q., & Chen, K. (2012). Evaluation of the effect of varicella outbreak control measures through a discrete-time delay SEIR model. *Chinese Journal of Preventive Medicine, 46*, 343–347.
14. Randhawa, G. S., Soltysiak, M. P., El Roz, H., de Souza, C. P., Hill, K. A., & Kari, L. (2020). Machine learning using intrinsic genomic signatures for rapid classification of novel pathogens: a COVID-19 case study. *bioRxiv*.
15. Barstugan, M., Ozkaya, U., & Ozturk, S. (2020). Coronavirus (COVID-19) classification using ct images by machine learning methods. *arXiv*, arXiv:2003.09424.
16. Pandey, G., Chaudhary, P., Gupta, R., & Pal, S. (2020). SEIR, and Regression Model-based COVID-19 outbreak predictions in India. *arXiv*, arXiv:2004.00958.
17. AlMoammar, A., AlHenaki, L., & Kurdi, H. (2018). Selecting accurate classifier models for a MERS-CoV dataset. *Advances in Intelligent Systems and Computing, 868*, 1070–1084.
18. Jang, S., Lee, S., Choi, S., Seo, J., Choi, H., & Yoon, T. (2016). Comparison between SARS CoV and MERS CoV Using Apriori Algorithm, Decision Tree, SVM. *MATEC Web Conferences, 49*, 08001. https://doi.org/10.1051/matecconf/20164908001.
19. Xu, X., Jiang, X., Ma, C., Du, P., Li, X., LV, S., Yu, L., Chen, Y., Su, J., Lang, G., et al. (2020). Deep learning system to screen coronavirus disease 2019 pneumonia. *arXiv preprint*.
20. Christian, S., Vincent, V., Sergey, I., Jon, S., & Zbigniew, W. (2016). Rethinking the inception architecture for computer vision. In *Proceedings of the IEEE conference on computer vision and pattern recognition* (pp. 2818–2826).
21. Shan, F., Gao, Y., Wang, J., Shi, W., Shi, N., Han, M., Xue, Z., Shen, D., & Shi, Y. (2020). Lung infection quantification of COVID-19 in ct images with deep learning. *arXiv preprint*, arXiv:2003.04655.

22. Zhao, W., Zhong, Z., Xie, X., Yu, Q., & Liu, J. (2020). The relation between chest CT findings and clinical conditions of coronavirus disease (COVID-19) pneumonia: a multicenter study. *American Journal of Roent-Genology, 1*, –6.
23. Chan, J. F. W., Yuan, S., et al. (2020). A familial cluster of Pneumonia associated with the 2019 novel coronavirus indicating person-to-person transmission: A study of a family cluster. *The Lancet, 395*(10223), 514–523.
24. Hemdan, E. E. D., Shouman, M. A., & Karar, M. E. (2020). COVIDX-Net: a framework of deep learning classifiers to diagnose COVID-19 in x-ray images. *arXiv preprint*, arXiv:2003.11055.
25. Song, Y., Zheng, S., Li, L., Zhang, X., Zhang, X., Huang, Z., & Chong, Y. (2020). Deep learning enables accurate diagnosis of novel coronavirus (COVID-19) with CT images. *medRxiv*.
26. Gozes, O., Frid-Adar, M., Greenspan, H., Browning, P. D., Zhang, H., Ji, W., Bernheim, A., & Siegel, E. (2020). Rapid AI development cycle for the coronavirus (COVID-19) pandemic: initial results for automated detection & patient monitoring using deep learning CT image analysis. *arXiv:2003.05037*.
27. Alqudah, A., Qazan, S., & Alqudah, A. (2020). Automated systems for detection of COVID-19 using chest x-ray images and lightweight convolutional neural networks. *Research Square*.
28. Chimmula, V. K. R., & Zhang, L. (2020, 2020). Time series forecasting of COVID-19 transmission in Canada using LSTM networks. *Chaos Solitons Fractals*, 109864.
29. Deng, J., Dong, W., Socher, R., Li, L., Li, K., & Fei-Fei, L. (2009). A large-scale hierarchical image database. In *2009 IEEE Conference on Computer Vision and Pattern Recognition* (pp. 248–255).
30. El Asnaoui, K., Chawki, Y., & Idri, A. (2020). Automated methods for detection and classification pneumonia based on X-ray images using deep learning. *arXiv: 2003.14363*.
31. Lawrence, S., Giles, C. L., Tsoi, A. C., & Back, A. D. (1997). Face recognition a convolutional neural-network approach. *IEEE Transactions on Neural Networks, 8*(1), 98–113.
32. Chang, L., Yan, Y., & Wang, L. (2020). Coronavirus disease 2019; Coronaviruses and blood safety. *Transfusion Medicine Reviews, 34*(2).
33. Shereen, M. A., Khan, S., Kazmi, A., Bashir, N., & Siddique, R. (2020). COVID-19 infection; origin, transmission, and characteristics of human coronaviruses. *Journal of Advanced Research, 24*, 91–98.
34. Lam, T. T.-Y., Shum, M. H.-H., Zhu, H.-C., Tong, Y.-G., Ni, X.-B., Liao, Y.-S., Wei, W., Cheung, W. Y.-M., Li, W.-J., Li, L.-F., et al. (2020). Identifying SARS-CoV-2 related coronaviruses in Malayan pangolins. *Nature*, 1–6.
35. Bastola, A., Sah, R., Rodriguez-Morales, A. J., Lal, B. K., Jha, R., Ojha, H. C., Shrestha, B., Chu, D. K. W., Poon, L. L. M., Costello, A., et al. (2020). The first 2019 novel coronavirus case in Nepal. *The Lancet Infectious Diseases, 20*, 279–280.
36. Li, Y., Yao, L., Li, J., Chen, L., Song, Y., Cai, Z., et al. (2020). Stability issues of RT-PCR testing of SARS-CoV-2 for hospitalized patients clinically diagnosed with COVID-19. *Journal of Medical Virology, 92*(7), 903–908.
37. Kingma, D. P., Ba, & Adam, J. L. (2015). A method for stochastic optimization. In *2015 Presented at 3rd International Conference for Learning Representations*. San Diego, CA.
38. Abadi, M., Agarwal, A., Barham, P., Bravo, E., Chen, Z., Citro, C., Corrado, G. S., Davis, A., Dean, J., Devin, M., Ghemawat, S., Goodfellow, I., Harp, A., Irving, G., Isard, M., Jia, Y., Jozefowicz, R., Kaiser, L., Kudlur, M., Levenberg, J., Mané, D., Monga, R., Moore, S., Murray, D., Olah, C., Schuster, M., Shlens, J., Steiner, B., Sutskever, I., Talwar, K., Tucker, P., Vanhoucke, V., Vasudevan, V., Viégas, F., Vinyals, O., Warden, P., Wattenberg, M., Wicke, M., Yu, Y., & Zheng, X. (2016). TensorFlow: large-scale machine learning on heterogeneous systems. *arXiv:1603.04467*.
39. Gorbalenya, A. E., Baker, S. C., Baric, R. S., de Groot Raoul, J., Drosten, C., Gulyaeva, A. A., Haagmans, B. L., Lauber, C., Leontovich, A. M., & Neuman, B. W. (2020). The species severe acute respiratory syndrome-related coronavirus: Classifying 2019-nCoV and naming it SARS-CoV-2. *Nature Microbiology, 5*, 536–544.

40. Dallas, T. A., Carlson, C. J., & Poisot, T. (2019). Testing predictability of disease outbreaks with a simple model of pathogen biogeography. *Royal Society Open Science*.
41. Choi, S., Lee, J., Kang, M. G., Min, H., Chang, Y. S., & Yoon, S. (2017). Large-scale machine learning of media outlets for understanding public reactions to nation-wide viral infection outbreaks. *Methods, 129*, 50–59. https://doi.org/10.1016/j.ymeth.2017.07.027.
42. Gross, A., Thiemig, D., Koch, F. W., Schwarz, M., Gläser, S., & Albrecht, T. (2020). CT appearance of severe, laboratory-proven coronavirus disease 2019 (covid-19) in a caucasian patient in Berlin, Germany. In *RöFo-Fortschritte auf dem Gebiet der Röntgenstrahlen und der bildgebenden Verfahren*. Georg Thieme Verlag KG.
43. Li, M., Lei, P., Zeng, B., Li, Z., Peng, Y., Fan, B., Wang, C., Li, Z., Zhou, J., Shaobo, H., et al. (2020). Coronavirus disease (COVID-19); spectrum of ct findings and temporal progression of the disease. *Academic Radiology, 27*, 603.
44. Bishnu, W., Ji, G. Z., & Cai, Shen, X. (2020). Analysis clinical features of COVID-19 infection in the secondary epidemic area and report potential biomarkers in evaluation. *medRxiv.*
45. Maier, B. F., & Brockmann, D. (2020). Effective containment explains sub-exponential growth in confirmed cases of recent COVID-19 outbreak in Mainland China. *medRxiv*. https://doi.org/10.1101/2020.02.18.20024414.
46. Elsayed, A. E., Aziz, M., Hosny, K., Salah, A., Darwish, M., Lu, S., & Talaat, A. (2020). New machine learning method for image- based diagnosis of COVID-19. *PLOS One, 15*. https://doi.org/10.1371/journal.pone.0235187.
47. Allam, Z., & Jones, D. S. (2020). On the coronavirus (COVID-19) outbreak and the smart city network: Universal data sharing standards coupled with artificial intelligence (AI) to benefit urban health monitoring and management. *Health, 8*(1), 46.
48. Lawanont, W., Inoue, M., Mongkolnam, P., & Nukoolkit, C. (2018). Neck posture monitoring system based on image detection and smart-phone sensors using the prolonged usage classification concept. *IEEJ Transactions on Electrical and Electronic Engineering, 13*(10), 1501–1510.
49. Vhaduri, S., Van Kessel, T., Ko, B., Wood, D., Wang, S., & Brunschwiler, T. (2019). Nocturnal cough and snore detection in noisy environments using smartphone-microphones. In *IEEE*.
50. Albahri, S., Hamid, R. A., Alwan, J. K., Al-qays, Z. T., Zaidan, A. A., Zaidan, B. B., Albahri, A. O. S., AlAmoodi, A. H., Khalaf, J. M., Almahdi, E. M., Thabet, E., Hadi, S. M., Mohammed, K. I., Alsalem, M. A., Al-Obaidi, J. R., & Madhloom, H. T. (2020). Role of biological Data Mining and Machine Learning Techniques in Detecting and Diagnosing the Novel Coronavirus (COVID-19): A Systematic Review. *Journal of Medical Systems, 44*, 122.
51. Shervin, M., Saeedizadeh, N., Kafieh, R., Yazdani, S., & Sonka, M. (2020). COVID TV-UNet; segmenting COVID-19 chest CT images using connectivity imposed U-net. *arXiv.*
52. Anderson, R. M., Heesterbeek, H., Klinkenberg, D., & Hollingsworth, T. D. (2015). How will country-based mitigation measures influence the course of the COVID-19 epidemic? *The Lancet, 395*(10228), 931–934.
53. Cunningham, P., & Delany, S. (2007). k-Nearest neighbour classifiers. *Multiple Classification System*.
54. Randhawa, G. S., Soltysiak, M. P., El Roz, H., de Souza, C. P., Hill, K. A., & Kari, L. (2020). Machine learning using intrinsic genomic signatures for rapid classification of novel pathogens: A COVID-19 case study. *bioRxiv*. https://doi.org/10.1101/2020.02.03.932350.
55. Zhou, P., Yang, X. L., Wang, X. G., Hu, B., Zhang, L., Zhang, W., et al. (2020). A pneumonia outbreak associated with a new coronavirus of probable bat origin. *Nature, 579*(7798), 270–273.
56. Hawkins, & Douglas. (2004). The Problem of Overfitting. *Journal of Chemical Information and Computer Sciences, 44*, 1–12. https://doi.org/10.1021/ci0342472.
57. Hu, Z., Song, C., Xu, C., Jin, G., Chen, Y., Xu, X., Ma, H. C., Lin, W., Zheng, Y., et al. (2020). *Clinical characteristics of 24 asymptomatic infections with COVID-19 screened among close contacts in Nanjing, China* (pp. 1–6). Science China Life Sciences.

58. Hui, Z., Song, C., Xu, C., Jin, G., Chen, Y., Xu, X., Ma, H., Chen, W., Lin, Y., Zheng, Y., et al. (2019). *Clinical characteristics of 24 asymptomatic infections with COVID-19 screened among close contacts in Nanjing, China* (pp. 1–6). Science China Life Sciences.
59. Gozes, O., Frid-Adar, M., Greenspan, H., Browning, P. D., Zhang, H., Ji, W., & Siegel, E. (2020). Rapid AI development cycle for the coronavirus (COVID-19) pandemic: initial results for automated detection and patient monitoring using deep learning CT image analysis. *arXiv preprint arXiv:2003.05037*.
60. Chowdhury, M. E., Rahman, T., Khandakar, A., Mazhar, R., Kadir, M. A., Mahbub, Z. B., & Reaz, M. B. I. (2020). Can AI help in screening viral and COVID-19 pneumonia? *arXiv preprint arXiv:2003.13145*.
61. Maghdid, H. S., Asaad, A. T., Ghafoor, K. Z., Sadiq, A. S., & Khan, M. K. (2020). Diagnosing COVID-19 pneumonia from X-ray and CT images using deep learning and transfer learning algorithms. *arXiv preprint arXiv:2004.00038*.
62. Huang, G., Liu, Z., Van Der Maaten, L., & Weinberger, K. Q. (2017). Densely connected convolutional networks. In *Proceedings of the IEEE Conference on Computer Vision and Pattern Recognition* (pp. 4700–4708).
63. Xie, S., Girshick, R., Dollar, P., Tu, Z., & He, K. (2017). Aggregated residual transformations for deep neural networks. In *Proceedings of the IEEE Conference on Computer Vision and Pattern Recognition* (pp. 1492–1500).
64. Iandola, F. N., Han, S., Moskewicz, M. W., Ashraf, K., Dally, W. J., & Keutzer, K. (2016). SqueezeNet, AlexNet-level accuracy with 50x fewer parameters and <0.5MB model size. *arXiv preprint arXiv:1602.07360*.
65. Hu, Z., Ge, Q., Jin, L., & Xiong, M. (2016). Artificial intelligence forecasting of Covid-19 in China. *arXiv preprint arXiv:2002.07112*.
66. Ye, Y., Hou, S., Fan, Y., Qian, Y., Zhang, Y., Sun, S., & Laparo, K. (2020). An AI-driven system and benchmark datasets for hierarchical community-level risk assessment to help combat COVID-19. *arXiv preprint arXiv:2003.12232*.
67. Mirza, M., & Osindero, S. (2014). Conditional generative adversarialnets. *arXiv preprint arXiv:1411.1784*.
68. Chang, S. L., Harding, N., Zachreson, C., Cliff, O. M., & Prokopenko, M. (2020). Modeling transmission and control of the COVID-19 pandemic in Australia. *arXiv preprint arXiv:2003.10218*.
69. Zachreson, C., Fair, K. M., Cliff, O. M., Harding, N., Piraveenan, M., & Prokopenko, M. (2018). Urbanization affects peak timing, prevalence, and bimodality of influenza pandemics in Australia: results of a census-calibrated model. *Science Advances, 4*(12), eaau5294.
70. Cliff, O. M., Harding, N., Piraveenan, M., Erten, E. Y., Gambhir, M., & Prokopenko, M. (2018). Investigating spatiotemporal dynamics and synchrony of influenza epidemics in Australia: An agent-based modeling approach. *Simulation Modelling Practice and Theory, 87*, 412–431.
71. Maghdid, H. S., Ghafoor, K. Z., Sadiq, A. S., Curran, K., & Rabie, K. (2020). A novel AI-enabled framework to diagnose coronavirus COVID-19 using smartphone embedded sensors: design study. *arXiv preprint arXiv:2003.07434*.
72. Maddah, E., & Beigzadeh, B. (2020). Use of a smartphone thermometer to monitor thermal conductivity changes in diabetic foot ulcers: A pilot study. *Journal of Wound Care, 29*(1), 61–66.
73. Karvekar, S. B. (2020). *Smartphone-based human fatigue detection in an industrial environment using gait analysis*. Available at: https://scholarworks.rit.edu/theses/10275/. Accessed on 1 Feb 2020.
74. Roldan Jimenez, C., Bennett, P., Ortiz Garcia, A., & Cuesta Vargas, A. I. (2019). Fatigue detection during the sit-to-stand test based on surface electromyography and acceleration: A case study. *Sensors, 19*(19), 4202.
75. Story, A., Aldridge, R. W., Smith, C. M., Garber, E., Hall, J., Fernando, G., et al. (2019). Smartphone-enabled video-observed versus directly observed treatment for tuberculo-

sis: a multicentre, analyst-blinded, randomized, controlled superiority trial. *The Lancet, 393*(10177), 1216–1224.
76. Lawanont, W., Inoue, M., Mongkolnam, P., & Nukoolkit, C. (2018). Neck posture monitoring system based on image detection and smart-phone sensors using the prolonged usage classification concept. *IEEJ Transactions on Electrical and Electronic Engineering, 13*(10), 1501–1510.
77. Nemati, E., Rahman, M. M., Nathan, V., Vatanparvar, K., & Kuang, J. (2019). A comprehensive approach for cough type detection. In *2019 IEEE/ACM International Conference on Connected Health: Applications, Systems and Engineering Technologies (CHASE)* (pp. 15–16). IEEE.
78. Vhaduri, S., Van Kessel, T., Ko, B., Wood, D., Wang, S., & Brunschwiler, T. (2019). Nocturnal cough and snore detection in noisy environments using smartphone-microphones. In *2019 IEEE*.
79. Debnath, S., Barnaby, D., Coppa, K., Makhnevich, A., Kim, E., Ji, C., Saurav, T., Viktor, L., Todd, P., Marc, C., Stuart, H., Jamie, Z., Theodoros, B., Lance, C., Jennifer, D., Karina, D., Andrew, F., Louise, M., Thomas, M., & Jazmin, O. (2020). Machine learning to assist clinical decision-making during the COVID-19 pandemic. *Bioelectronic Medicine, 6*, 14. https://doi.org/10.1186/s42234-020-00050-8.
80. Al-Turaiki, I., Alshahrani, M., & Almutairi, T. (2016). Building predictive models for MERS-CoV infections using data mining techniques. *Journal of Infection and Public Health, 9*(6), 744–748. https://doi.org/10.1016/j.jiph.2016.09.007.
81. Khanday, A. M. U. D., Rabani, S. T., Khan, Q. R., et al. (2020). Machine learning based approaches for detecting COVID-19 using clinical text data. *International Journal of Information Technology*. https://doi.org/10.1007/s41870-020-00495-9.
82. Eraslan, G., Avsec, Ž., Gagneur, J., & Theis, F. J. (2019). Deep learning: new computational modeling techniques for genomics. *Nature Reviews Genetics, 20*, 389–403.
83. Singhal, T. (2020). A review of coronavirus disease-2019 (COVID-19). *The Indian Journal of Pediatrics, 87*, 281–286.
84. Bhandary, A., Prabhu, G. A., Rajinikanth, V., Thanaraj, K. P., Satapathy, S. C., Robbins, D. E., Shasky, C., Zhang, Y.-D., Tavares, J. M. R. S., & Raja, N. S. M. (2020). The deep-learning framework to detect lung abnormality—A study with chest X-Ray and lung CT scan images. *Pattern Recognition Letters, 129*, 271–278. https://doi.org/10.1016/j.patrec.2019.11.013.
85. John, C., et al. (2017). TX-CNN: Detecting tuberculosis in chest X-ray images using convolutional neural network. In *2017 IEEE International Conference on Image Processing (ICIP)* (pp. 2314–2318). Beijing. https://doi.org/10.1109/ICIP.2017.8296695.
86. Zhang, L. J. (2020). Coronavirus disease 2019 (COVID-19): A perspective from China. *Radiology*, 200490.
87. Jiang, X., Coffee, M., Bari, A., Wang, J., Jiang, X., Huang, J., Shi, J., Dai, J., Cai, J., Zhang, T., Wu, Z., He, G., & Huang, Y. (2020). Towards an artificial intelligence framework for data-driven prediction of coronavirus clinical severity. *Computers, Materials and Continua, 63*(1), 537–551.
88. Abdullah, M., Altheyab, M. S., Lattas, A. M. A., & Algashmari, W. F. (2017). MERS-CoV disease estimation (MDE) A study to estimate a MERS-CoV by classification algorithms. In *Communication, Management, and Information Technology – Proceedings of the International Conference on Communication, Management and Information Technology, ICCMIT* (Vol. 2016, pp. 633–638).
89. Zhavoronkov, A., Aladinskiy, V., Zhebrak, A., Zagribelnyy, B., Terentiev, V., Bezrukov, D. S., & Yan, Y. (2020). Potential COVID-2019 3C-like protease inhibitors designed us-ing generative deep learning approaches. *ChemRxiv Preprint*. https://doi.org/10.26434/chemrxiv.11829102.v2.
90. Almansour, N., Kurdia, H., Almansour, N., & Kurdia, H. (2018). Identifying accurate classifier models for a text-based MERS-CoV dataset. In *2017 Intelligent Systems Conference, IntelliSys* (Vol. 2018, pp. 430–435).

91. Ai, T., Yang, Z., Hou, H., Zhan, C., Chen, C., Lv, W., et al. (2020). Correlation of Chest CT 460 and RT-PCR Testing in Coronavirus Disease 2019 (COVID-19) in China: A 461 Report of 1014 Cases [published online ahead of print 26]. *462 Radiology, 2020*, 200642.
92. Vynnycky, E., & White, R. (2010). *An Introduction to Infectious Disease Modelling*. OUP Oxford.
93. Zhang, J., Xie, Y., Li, Y., Shen, C., & Xia, Y. (2020). Covid-19 screening on chest x-ray images using deep learning-based anomaly detection. *arXiv preprint ar X iv:2003.12338*.
94. Bai, H. X., & Hsieh, B. (2020). Performance of radiologists in differentiating COVID-19 from viral pneumonia on chest CT. *Radiology*. https://doi.org/10.1148/radiol.2020200823.
95. Esteva, A., Kuprel, B., & Novoa, R. A. (2017). Dermatologist-level classification of skin cancer with deep neural networks. *Nature, 542*(7639), 115–118. https://doi.org/10.1038/nature21056.
96. Makris, A., Kontopoulos, I., & Tserpes, K. COVID-19 detection from chest X-Ray images using Deep Learning and Convolutional Neural Networks. *medRxiv*. https://doi.org/10.1101/2020.05.22.20110817.
97. El-Sawy, A., Loey, M., & EL-Bakry, H. (2020). Arabic handwritten characters recognition using convolutional neural network. *WSEAS Transactions on Computer Research, 2017*(5), 11–19.
98. Pan, J. R., Huang, Z. Q., & Chen, K. (2012). Evaluation of the effect of varicella outbreak control measures through a discrete time delay SEIR model. *Zhonghua Yu Fang Yi Xue Za Zhi, 46*, 343–347.
99. Chen, J., Wu, L., Zhang, J., Liang, Z., Gong, D., Zhao, Y., Hu, S., Wang, Y., Hu, X., Zheng, B., Zhang, K., Wu, H., Dong, Z., Xu, Y., Zhu, Y., Chen, X., Yu, L., & Yu, H. (2020). Deep learning-based model for detecting 2019 novel coronavirus pneumonia on high-resolution computed tomography: A prospective study. *MedRxiv*.
100. Lopez, B. E., Magliocca, N. R., & Crooks, A. T. (2019). Challenges and opportunities of social media data for socio-environmental systems research. *Land, 8*, 107.
101. Yiqun, M., Rong, W., & Qunwei, Z. (2016). Application of Reverse Transcription-PCR and Real-Time PCR in Nanotoxicity Research. *Methods in Molecular Biology*. Author manuscript; available in PMC.
102. Shiruru, K. (2016). An introduction to artificial neural network. *International Journal of Advance Research and Innovative Ideas in Education, 1*, 27–30.
103. Panwar, H., Gupta, P., Siddiqui, M., Khubeb, M.-M., Ruben, S., & Vaishnavi. (2020). *Application of deep learning for fast detection of COVID-19 in X-Rays using nCOVnet*. Chaos, Solitons & Fractals.
104. Albawi, S., Abed, M., Tareq, A., & Saad. (2017). Understanding of a convolutional neural network. In *Proceedings of the 2017 IEEE International Conference on Engineering and Technology, Antalya, Turkey*.
105. Ebrahim, A. O., Fatemeh, M., Farhad, F., Iraj, K., & Heidar, T. (2020). Diagnosis and treatment of coronavirus disease 2019 (COVID-19), laboratory, PCR, and chest CT imaging findings. *International Journal of Surgery, 79*, 143–153.
106. Stephen, O., Sain, M., Maduh, U. J., & Jeong, D.-U. (2019). An efficient deep learning approach to Pneumonia classification in healthcare. *Journal of Healthcare Engineering, 2019*, 4180949.
107. Ayan, E., & Ünver, H. M. (2019). Diagnosis of Pneumonia from Chest X-ray Images Using Deep Learning. In *Proceedingsof the 2019 Scientific Meeting on Electrical-Electronics & Biomedical Engineering and Computer Science (EBBT), Istanbul, Turkey, 24–26 April* (pp. 1–5).
108. Kermany, D. S., Goldbaum, M., Cai, W., Valentim, C. C. S., Liang, H., Baxter, S. L., McKeown, A., Yang, G., Wu, X., Yan, F., et al. (2018). Identifying medical diagnoses and treatable diseases by image-based deep learning. *Cell, 172*, 1122–1131.
109. Varshni, D., Thakral, K., Agarwal, L., Nijhawan, R., & Mittal, A. (2019). Pneumonia Detection Using CNN based Feature Extraction. In *Proceedings of the 2019 IEEE*

*International Conference on Electrical, Computer and Communication Technologies (ICECCT), Coimbatore, India, 20–22 February* (pp. 1–7).

110. Cohen, J. P., Morrison, P., & Dao, L. COVID-19 Image Data Collection.arXiv2020. *arXiv:2003.11597.*
111. Riordon, J., Sovilj, D., Sanner, S., Sinton, D., & Young, E. W. K. (2019). Deep learning with microfluidics for biotechnology. *Trends in Biotechnology, 37*, 310–324.
112. Goodfellow, I. J., Pouget-Abadie, J., Mirza, M., Xu, B., Warde-Farley, D., Ozair, S., Courville, A., & Bengio, Y. (2014). Generative Adversarial Nets. In *Proceedings of the 27th International Conference on Neural Information Processing Systems—Volume 2, Montreal, QC, Canada, 8–13 December 2014* (pp. 2672–2680). Cambridge, MA: MIT Press.
113. Cao, Y., Jia, L., Chen, Y., Lin, N., Yang, C., Zhang, B., Liu, Z., Li, X., & Dai, H. (2019). Recent Advances of Generative Adversarial Networks in Computer Vision. *IEEE Access, 7*, 14985.
114. El-Sawy, A., Loey, M., & EL-Bakry, H. (2017). Arabic handwritten characters recognition using convolutional neural network. *WSEAS Transactions on Computer Research, 5*, 11–19.
115. Deng, J., Dong, W., Socher, R., Li, L., Kai, L., & Li, F.-F. (2009). ImageNet: a large-scale hierarchical image database. In *Proceedings of the 2009 IEEE Conference on Computer Vision and Pattern Recognition, Miami, FL, USA, 20–25 June* (pp. 248–255).

# Chapter 13
# Factors Associated with COVID-19 and Predictive Modelling of Spread Across Five Urban Metropolises in the World

**Arvind Chandra Pandey, Bikash Ranjan Parida, Shubham Bhattacharjee, Tannu Priya Wasim, Munizzah Salim, and Rahul Kashyap**

## 13.1 Introduction

Severe acute respiratory coronavirus 2 (SARS-COV-2) was identified in Wuhan, China, in late December 2019 and caused an outbreak of the pandemic from the beginning of the year 2020 [1]. The novel coronavirus COVID-19 spread rapidly to 188 countries in the early months of 2020, and WHO declared Public Health Emergency of International Concern (PHEIC) on the 30th of January 2020 [2]. As of 5 October 2020, more than 35 million cases and 1.03 million deaths have been reported across the world [3]. The most affected countries concerning the number of COVID-19 cases were the USA, Brazil, Russia, India, the United Kingdom, Spain, Italy, France, and Germany [2]. To control the spread of novel coronavirus, the government has undertaken rigorous containment measures mostly in early and late March 2020, and such actions were partial to total lockdowns of economic activities and citizen mobility. The break of economic activities has led to a decline in the burning of fossil fuels and fumes from sclerotic traffic across the world. These measures have led to the reduction of atmospheric pollution and at the same time improvement of air quality index across the world [4–6]. The lockdown measures have led to a decline in the spread of infections over majorly affected countries but not to end the epidemic. The whole world is eager to know its end. Thereby, the influence of weather variability, built-up city patterns, and population density is of major interest on the spread of novel coronavirus across cities.

The outbreak has caused a healthcare crisis globally. The government in many countries has adopted various steps to reduce the transmission and to relieve the pressure on the healthcare system. According to researches on China and South

A. C. Pandey (✉) · B. R. Parida · S. Bhattacharjee · T. P. Wasim · M. Salim · R. Kashyap
Department of Geoinformatics, School of Natural Resource Management, Central University of Jharkhand, Ranchi, India
e-mail: arvind.pandey@cuj.ac.in; bikash.parida@cuj.ac.in



S. Kautish et al. (eds.), *Computational Intelligence Techniques for Combating COVID-19*, EAI/Springer Innovations in Communication and Computing,
https://doi.org/10.1007/978-3-030-68936-0_13

Korea, it was observed that governments' action and population support could minimize the uncontrolled spread of the virus [7]. The government adopted two different strategies to suppress COVID-19 effect, i.e., mitigation and suppression [8]. Mitigation aims to lower the healthcare demand by reducing the transmission rate, whereas suppression aims to adopt restrictive measures to lower the infection. One of the common approaches adopted by the government all over the world is lockdown policies [9]. Physical distancing is also in the limelight, and it has gained increased support in balancing healthcare and economy of a country. Various applications have also been launched to reduce the risk of transmission of COVID-19 like Aarogya Setu in India.

In hot seasons when the temperature is at its peak, it leads to slowing down the activity of the virus, and this results in weak transmission. In contrast, moderate hot temperature or cold temperature supports the transmission by making the virus active [10]. It has also been observed that COVID-19 was restricted in an area which lies in between temperature range, i.e., highest temperature >40 °C and the lowest temperature <4 °C [10]. Earlier researchers gave us the view that COVID-19 is highly active in tropical regions between 30 and 50 °north due to high temperature and spreads rapidly from east to west direction. In contrast, temperate regions are least affected because of seasonal variations. Rise in infection rate was high in between low and moderate temperature range, i.e., from <19 °C to <10 °C [11]. According to [12] infection rate is higher in areas with low humidity. It was stated that low temperature and low humidity support the suspended matter in the environment and provide them with an ideal condition to grow, which makes a virus chain and causes transmission [10, 12]. However, high temperature dries out the mucous membrane and makes the virus inactive. Combination of low temperatures and low humidity increases the timespan of virus suspension in the air, and it gives suitable conditions for the virus to grow rapidly. It also makes the nasal prone to small particles which create an opportunity for viruses for transmission [13].

In the light of the above discussion, it is pertinent to infuse scientific understanding about the spread and possible end of this epidemic. Moreover, the influence of social, urban, climatic, and environmental factors on the spread of novel coronavirus across cities of the world is of major interest. Therefore, the present study is envisaged with the following objectives: (1) to study COVID-19 temporal spread across five select cities till July 2020, (2) to investigate the association of climatic variables and urban population density with the spread of COVID-19 cases, and (3) to use predictive modelling for the number of infections across select cities from August to 15 November 2020.

## 13.2 Data Used and Methods

The present study was carried out on five select cities of different countries, namely, New Delhi, Lombardy, Madrid, New York, and New Jersey. The data adopted for accomplishing the research objective are COVID-19 statistical data for detecting the number of infections and mortality. The city-wise cumulative cases of COVID-19 affected population and death tolls were acquired from multiple government databases (Table 13.1). The Landsat 8 satellite data with Operational Land Imager (OLI) sensor's data for March to April 2020 was obtained from USGS. The spatial resolution of OLI data was 30 m with 16 days of temporal resolution and utilized to derive urban extents. Temperature and relative humidity data were obtained from power NASA for the period January 2020 to May 2020 for select cities (Table 13.1). Sentinel-5P from Copernicus hub was used for mapping air pollutants like CO and $NO_2$. In this study, pollutant data for April to May 2019 and 2020 period were obtained from Copernicus mission, and these pollutant data were processed using the API code developed in Google Earth Engine (GEE) [14].

## 13.3 Methodology

### *13.3.1 COVID-19 Infection Rates and Population Density*

The total number of infections of COVID-19 and total population was used to calculate the percentage of the infected population for select cities. The death tolls are also tabulated. The infection rate and population density were computed using the following equations:

**Table 13.1** Data used for this study, including sensor characteristics

| Data used | Resolutions | Purpose | Source/websites |
|---|---|---|---|
| *Landsat 8 (OLI)* | Spatial: 30 meter<br>Spectral: 9 bands<br>Temporal: 16 days<br>Acquisition dates: March to April 2020 | Urban density mapping | https://earthexplorer.usgs.gov |
| *Sentinel-5P/ TROPOMI* (CO, $NO_2$ conc.) | Spatial: 1 km<br>Temporal: daily<br>Duration: 2019–2020 (April to May) | Pollution variation | Copernicus mission: https://cds.climate.copernicus.eu |
| *Weather data*<br>Temperature and humidity | Daily<br>*Duration:* January to May 2020 | Variation of temperature and humidity with infection spread | https://power.larc.nasa.gov |
| *COVID-19 statistics*<br>Infection<br>Death tolls | March to August 2020 | Infection rate | https://www.worldometers.info https://www.covid19india.org https://coronavirus.jhu |

$$\% \text{ infected population} = \frac{\text{Total no.of infection}}{\text{Total population}} * 100 \quad (13.1)$$

$$\% \text{ infection rate} = \frac{\text{Number of infection}}{\text{Number of days}} \quad (13.2)$$

$$\% \text{ populaton density} = \frac{\text{Total population of the city}}{\text{Area of the city}} \quad (13.3)$$

To relate the infection rate with the actual population, population density has been calculated. Urban density map was prepared using the Landsat 8 satellite data with Operational Land Imager (OLI) sensor's data, wherein actual urban areas across select cities are extracted. Fine-scale false color composite (FCC) was used to classify urban areas more accurately by using the three bands such as green, red, and NIR. Training samples were collected based on tones of FCC characteristics. Urban areas show cyan tone in FCC image in which urban training samples were acquired. For extracting urban areas, a decision tree-based algorithm and random forest classification were used in Google Earth engine (GEE) platform, which eventually takes training data as inputs and produces high-quality urban classifications. The significance of RF classifier is nonparametric in nature and runs the iteration using the training samples until it reached the optimum accuracy level. After converting urban raster pixels into vector points, point density function was used in ArcMap environment for creating high- and low-density areas of urban. Then a morphological filter was applied with window size 3 × 3 for smoothing the urban density. Accuracy of urban map varied between 90 and 95% for all the five metropolises.

Data of the number of infections for selected five cities across various countries from January to June was recorded. The maximum and minimum temperature together with humidity was used for comparative analysis of the spread of infection with environmental variables and urban population density in five cities.

### *13.3.2 SVM-Based Predictive Modelling for the Number of Infections*

There are several models available for predicting the number of cases: clustering model, forecast model, outlier model, and time series model. In this study, statistical data-based predictive modelling was performed from 11 August to mid-November 2020 in Python-3 platform. The advanced machine learning algorithm, the support vector machine (SVM) model, was employed to analyze and predict the effect of the spread of COVID-19 pandemic. The SVM was applied by importing required libraries. Input parameters used daily are the total number of confirmed cases from 1

February to 10 August 2020 and another is the number of days of prediction. In the case of tuning parameters, it needs test and training data for running the model. Test data should be sized according to the number of total cases (in this case 25%), and training data can be either remaining data after test data or any other linked data to the same input including the number of recoveries daily. SVM kernel functions, such as polynomial, sigmoid, and radial basis functions, were applied for training the model. By deciding the best parameters to be fitted, it forecasts the number of cases based on the selected test and training datasets. Pre-calibration estimation was carried out by selecting a proper test size which showed the low difference between the mean square and mean absolute error. Post-calibration in machine learning is the comparison between actual and predicted values which has been carried out in the form of bias estimation. Possible retreat in the number of cases was calculated using the percentage increase or decrease of new cases per day.

## 13.4 Results

### 13.4.1 *COVID-19 Infections Cases and Mortality Across Five Cities*

Figure 13.1 represents the cumulative growth of the percentage of the infected population across five cities due to coronavirus COVID-19 as of May 2020. The study revealed only 0.12% of the total population in Delhi are infected, whereas 0.88%, 1%, 2%, and 1.8% of the total population are infected in cities of Madrid, Lombardy, New York, and New Jersey, respectively. Cities of the United States showed maximum numbers of COVID-19 cases followed by European cities. New York City has demonstrated the highest death tolls as the percentage of infection rate was also

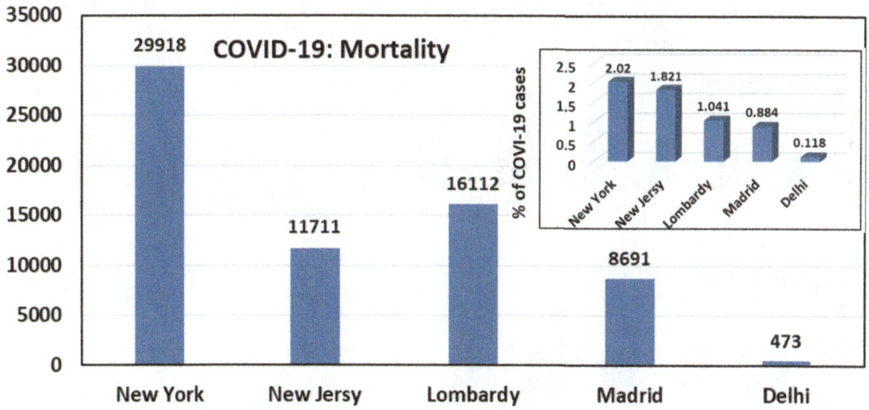


**Fig. 13.1** Total mortality due to COVID-19 and % infected population of select cities (inset plot) to the total population as of 31 May 2020

high. Delhi showed little infection despite having a larger population due to earlier deployment of lockdown in India as compared to other countries. Due to delay in lockdown, infection rose abruptly, and more death tolls occurred in Madrid, New Jersey, and Lombardy. About 29,918 deaths occurred in New York which is highest among selected cities, while 16,112 deaths occurred in Lombardy which is second highest, 11,711 deaths occurred in New Jersey, 8691 deaths occurred in Madrid, and 473 deaths occurred in Delhi till May 2020.

### *13.4.2 Association of Climatic Variables and Population Density with the Spread of Cases*

Adjacent cities New Jersey and New York revealed almost similar temperature range as well as humidity (Fig. 13.2a, b). In New Jersey, the number of cases in March was 18,696, whereas in April the case rose by 99,957 and reached up to 118,652 at the end of April (Table 13.2). This increase in the number of cases in New Jersey in April is due to a decrease in humidity (Fig. 13.2a), whereas in May, the cases increased by 43,160 and reached up to 161,812 at the end of May, which is less than the observation of April because temperature increased by 3 °C and lockdown was also imposed. In New York, the number of cases in March was 76,946 and rose by 233,443 and reached up to 310,389 in April (Table 13.2) due to decrease in humidity, and temperature was also suitable to stabilize the virus in the environment (Fig. 13.2b), whereas in May, the cases reduced sharply by 45,627 and

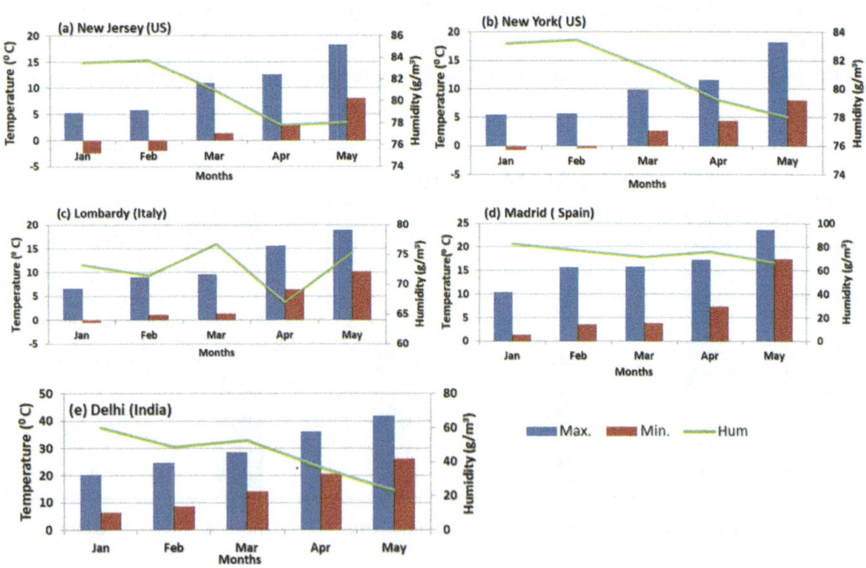


**Fig. 13.2** Variation of temperature and humidity across select cities from January to May 2020

**Table 13.2** The number of COVID-19 infection cases and death for five select cities from March to June 2020 (cumulative numbers). The lockdown timeframe indicates mostly referring to the restriction to industrial and transport activities

| | March | | April | | May | | June | | |
|---|---|---|---|---|---|---|---|---|---|
| Cities/provinces | Cases | Death | Cases | Death | Cases | Death | Cases | Death | Lockdown timeframe |
| New Jersey | 18,696 | 267 | 118,652 | 7228 | 161,812 | 11,711 | 173,122 | 15,090 | 16 March–15 June |
| New York | 76,946 | 2677 | 310,389 | 23,780 | 380,253 | 29,918 | 409,822 | 32,129 | 21 March–15 June |
| Madrid | 30,997 | 3865 | 61,799 | 8176 | 68,920 | 8944 | 70,299 | NA | 14 March–9 May |
| Lombardy | 43,208 | 7199 | 75,732 | 13,860 | 88,985 | 16,112 | 93,980 | 16,644 | 10 March–10 April |
| Delhi | 120 | 2 | 3515 | 59 | 19,819 | 473 | 90,089 | 2742 | 23 March–18 May |

reached up to 380,253 (Fig. 13.2b and Table 13.2) because temperature started to increase with decreasing humidity and the lockdown as well as prevention parameters has been adopted by the people.

In Lombardy (Northern Italy), COVID-19 virus has spread rapidly in the starting phase (February) because humidity and temperature both supported the condition of virus spread. The humidity was always less than 75 g/m$^3$ as compared to other cities (Fig. 13.2c). In February, Lombardy witnessed only 984 cases, but due to less temperature up to 5.5 °C in the next month (March), the number of cases rose to 43,208 (Table 13.2). Cases started to decline from April to May because temperatures started to increase, and also lockdown prevention measures were undertaken. Similarly, Madrid's temperature was only a critical factor in the increased number of cases in that region in February and March when humidity was 71–82 g/m$^3$ (Fig. 13.2d). The temperature crossed the threshold of 10 °C only in April and May when humidity was between 67 and 76 g/m$^3$.

In Delhi (India), the COVID-19 cases were detected in mid-March 2020, and by the end of the month, the number of cases was 120 (Table 13.2). The numbers increased to 3515 by the end of April 2020. The maximum temperature was 32.4 °C in March to April, with a humidity level of 37–53 g/m$^3$ (Fig. 13.2e). The number of cases further increased to 19,819 by May, while the average temperature was 42 °C in May with humidity level 23 g/m$^3$. Humidity is observed as a critical factor in increased cases in Delhi as it remained lower in April to May.

### *13.4.3 Association of COVID-19 Infection Rate and Population Density*

Considerable urban density and compactness were observed in New York and Delhi having almost similar populations (Fig. 13.3). The urban density was relatively lower in New Jersey as compared to New York, USA. The urban density was also higher across Milan, Lombardy, and Madrid, Spain. These results indicated that with high urban density and compactness, the infection rate and mortality were higher in all four cities except Delhi in India.

Infection rates are calculated for the number of days, and it has been compared with population density across five cities (Fig. 13.4). The results showed that infection rate and population density are directly correlated in New York, New Jersey, and Madrid. Conversely, infection rate and population density are not directly connected in Delhi and Lombardy, which can be attributed to early confinement following the lockdown in Delhi and delayed lockdown in Lombardy. Despite having high urban density and more compactness (Figs. 13.3 and 13.4), Delhi has witnessed less number of infection rate as well as death tolls till May 2020 owing to timely lockdowns. By contrast, Lombardy, Italy, had less urban density, but it witnessed devastating conditions due to delayed lockdown decisions. COVID-19 pandemic started in mid-February, and it imposed a lockdown on 10 March, and so concerning pandemic starting date, the lockdown was delayed. Madrid, Spain, had a significant urban density and a compact built-up pattern, and it displayed more number of

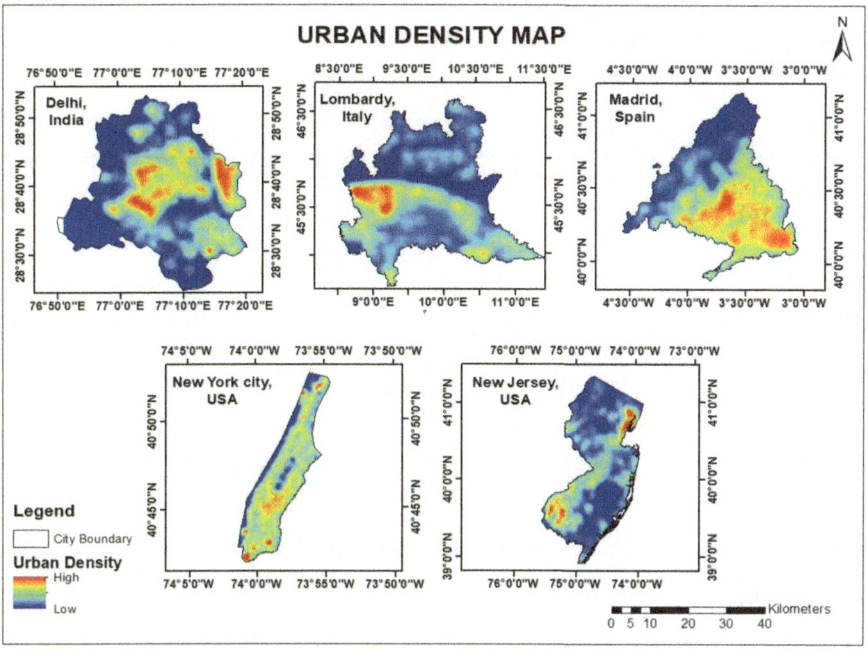


Fig. 13.3 Satellite-derived urban density of five cities using Landsat 8 satellite data

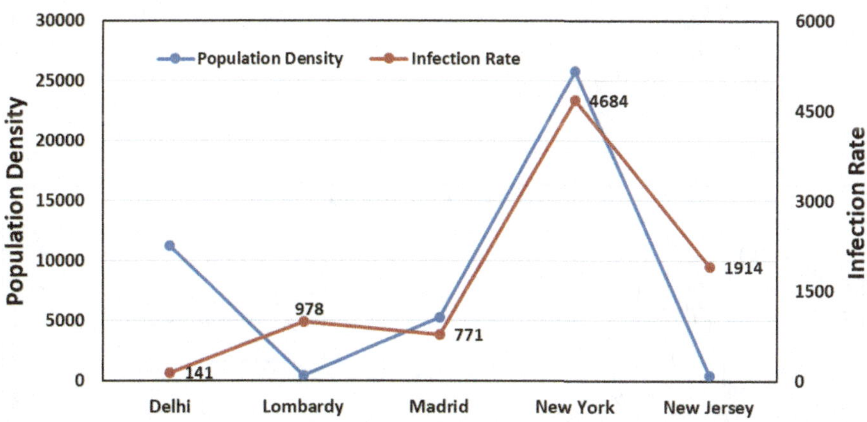


Fig. 13.4 COVID-19 infection rate up to May 2020 in relation to the population density of five cities

infections till date. New York and New Jersey in the USA had a very high population density (Fig. 13.4), but the delayed deployment of lockdown witnessed the worst condition.

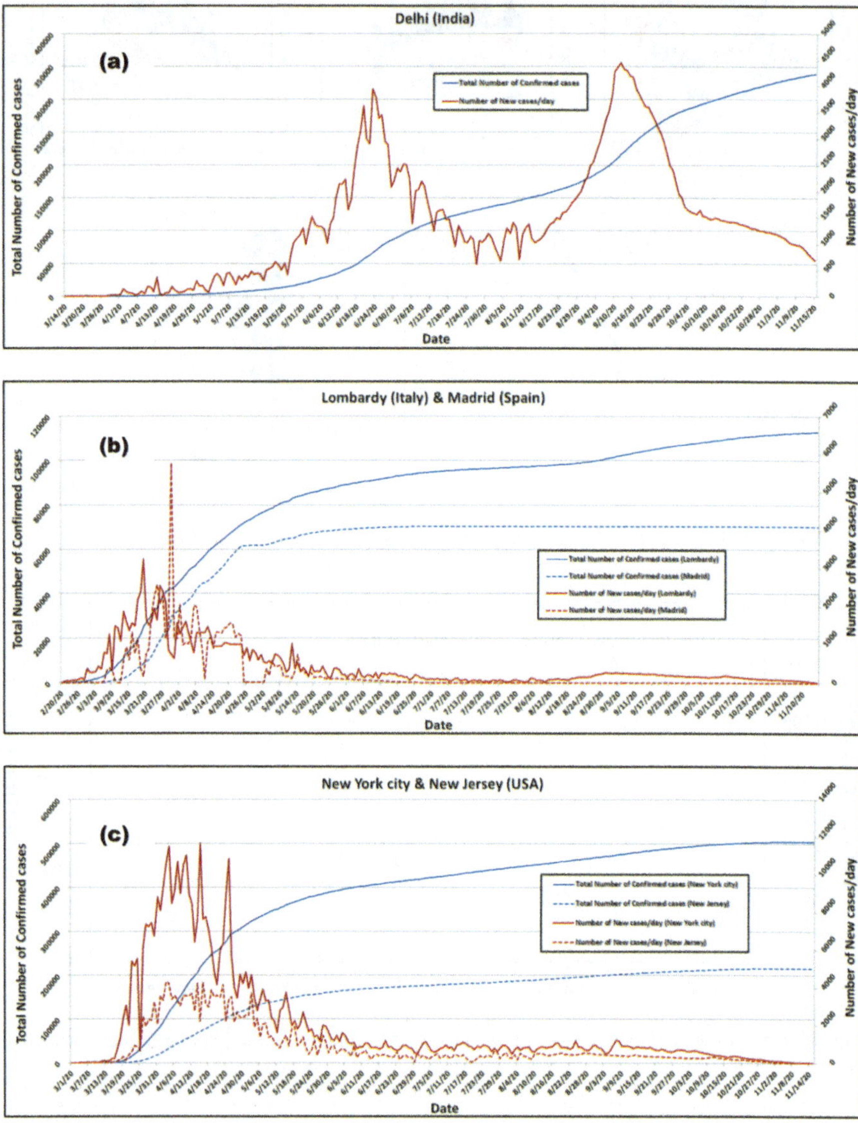


**Fig. 13.5** Predictive modelling for COVID-19 cases during August to November 2020 over five cities across the globe

### 13.4.4 Predictive Modelling for the Number of Infections

Predictive analysis using SVM machine learning based on the statistical dataset for the select cities is presented in Fig. 13.5. The changes in the number of infections are based on many factors, such as the number of tests carried out, violation of social distancing, etc. Delhi reported 19,819 cases till 31 May 2020, and the cases abruptly increased to 90,089 by 30 June and may increase to 339,042 till mid-November 2020 (Table 13.3). It observed a sharp peak nearly 4000 new cases per day during the third week of June and predicted a second peak almost 4447 new cases per day during the second week of September due to de-escalation of lock-down. Thereafter, it may retreat gradually from November 2020 in Delhi, and the normalcy may prevail by the end of the year 2020 (Fig. 13.5a).

Lombardy, Italy, is getting control over this pandemic as the number of new cases per day gradually decreased from June (Fig. 13.5b). So far Lombardy has reported 88,985 cases as of 31 May 2020 due to late deployment of lockdown. The infections predicted to increase to 100,695 till August and 112,900 till mid-September 2020 (Table 13.3). A flattening of the curve of new cases per day was observed in July to August but again rises in September. The pandemic may be retreated by the end of the year 2020, and thereafter, the normalcy may prevail. Madrid, Spain, has reported 68,920 cases till 31 May 2020, and it started flattening its curve from July (Fig. 13.5b). Its cases reached up to 70,299 till 30 June followed (Table 13.3) by a continuous decreasing pattern of new cases per day. Based on a decrease of new cases per day, Madrid may notice normalcy with no new cases from July 2020.

New York City was adversely affected due to COVID-19 pandemic by following a late lockdown strategy in the USA. It reported 380,253 cases till 31 May 2020 and showed some spiked peak cases on 15 and 25 April 2020 when the number of new cases per day was 11,661 and 10,868, respectively (Fig. 13.5c). It was recorded that from May, New York also exhibited flattening of its curve with 1000 to 4000 new cases per day and ended with 1282 cases on 31 May 2020. It was observed that total cases raised to 409,822 by the end of June, and it was predicted that the case might rise to 468,837 by the end of August 2020 and 492,072 by the end of September 2020 (Table 13.3). Predictive modelling revealed that there will be no COVID-19 cases from the end of the year 2020. New Jersey, USA, reported 161,812 COVID-19

**Table 13.3** Predicted COVID-19 cases for August to November 2020 using the SVM model

| Cities | 31 Aug 2020 | 30 Sept 2020 | 31 Oct 2020 | 15 Nov 2020 | Remarks |
|---|---|---|---|---|---|
| New Jersey | 198,818 | 209,663 | 215,932 | 216,047 | Marginally increasing over Aug to Nov |
| New York | 468,837 | 492,072 | 503,917 | 504,641 | Increasing over Aug to Nov |
| Madrid | 70,299 | 70,299 | 70,299 | 70,299 | No change since 1 July |
| Lombardy | 100,695 | 107,494 | 111,930 | 112,900 | Increasing over Aug to Nov |
| Delhi | 177,163 | 278,798 | 324,127 | 339,042 | Increasing over Aug to Nov |

cases till 31 May 2020, with the highest spike of 4300 new cases on 3 April. In April, there are multiple peaks of single-day highest cases up to 4000 (Fig. 13.5c). Since the first week of June, the number of cases was decreasing possibly due to implementation of various governmental measures. It recorded 848 new cases on 31 May 2020 with a total number of cases nearly 161,812. It was observed that total cases increased to 173,122 by the end of June (Table 13.3). Predictive modelling indicated that there would be less or no new cases from mid-November 2020. The bias on the number of new cases during 11–25 August 2020 for each city was presented in Table 13.4. The results displayed that the estimated bias was between 5 (Lombardy) and 11.5% (New Jersey).

### *13.4.5 Effect of Lockdowns on Air Pollutants Across Select Cities*

Impact of the pandemic on the atmospheric pollutants has been studied using spatiotemporal satellite-based products related to $NO_2$ and CO across five select cities (Figs. 13.6 and 13.7). In Delhi, the tropospheric $NO_2$ column number density ranges between 0.00003 and 0.00007 mol/m$^2$. The higher concentration of $NO_2$ was observed in April to May 2019 in almost all the five cities (Fig. 13.6). There has been a reduction of more than 40% in concentration in 2020 (during lockdown) in Delhi as against the same time period in 2019 (pre-lockdown). A similar condition can be observed in the other four cities (Fig. 13.6). Significant reduction in eastern parts of Delhi in the levels of $NO_2$ was observed between years 2019 and 2020. In the city of Madrid in Spain, the considerable reduction can be seen in the central part of Madrid in 2020 as compared to 2019 (Fig. 13.6). The reduction of $NO_2$ was also quite significant in the central part of the city of Lombardy in Italy in 2020. New Jersey and New York in the USA show very substantial changes from 2019 to 2020 in the $NO_2$ concentration.

The mean CO column number density based on daily observation of Sentinel-5P TROPOMI exhibits a concentration range between 0.01 and 0.06 mol/m$^2$. Delhi, New Jersey, New York, and Madrid observed a significant reduction in CO concentration in 2020 when compared to 2019 (Fig. 13.7). However, Lombardy experiences almost negligible change in concentration, which might be due to delayed lockdown in the city. The CO concentration in the city of Delhi in India showed a considerable variation from the years 2019 to 2020. The reduction of CO over the

**Table 13.4** The bias in the predicted model on new COVID-19 cases from 11 to 25 August 2020

| Predicted cases | Actual | Predicted | Bias (%) |
|---|---|---|---|
| New Jersey | 6059 | 6759 | +11.5% |
| New York | 12,093 | 13,039 | +7.8 |
| Lombardy | 1687 | 1768 | +4.8 |
| Delhi | 18,237 | 19,576 | +7.3 |

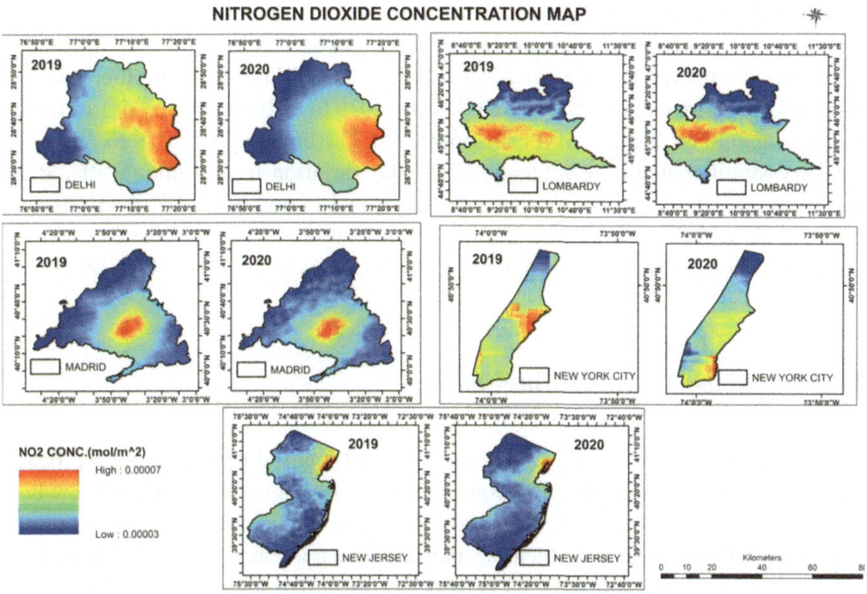


**Fig. 13.6** Satellite-derived mean $NO_2$ variation from April to May in 2019 and 2020 across select cities

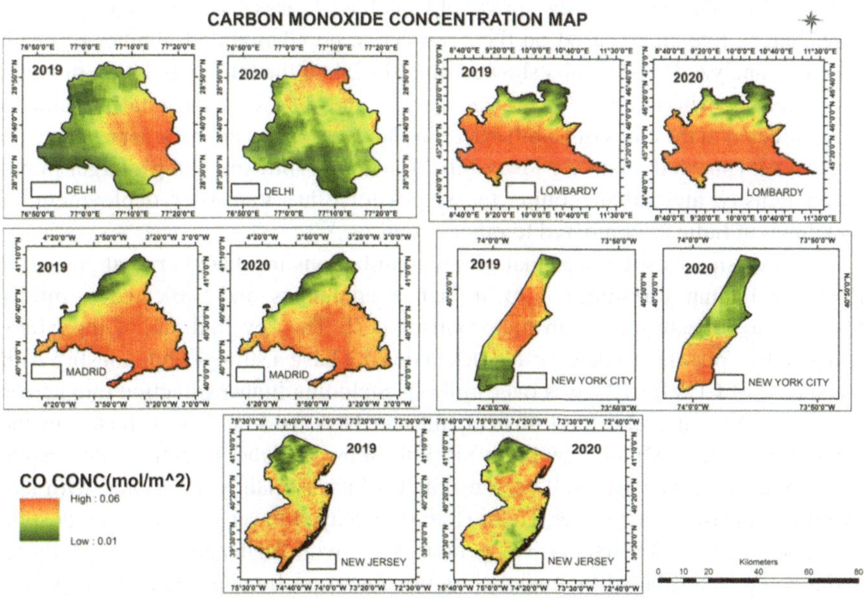


**Fig. 13.7** Satellite-derived mean CO variation from April to May in 2019 and 2020 across select cities

eastern side of Delhi was seen due to decline in the amount of anthropogenic $CO_2$ emissions attributed to total slowdown of transport as well as industrial production in 2020 as compared to the year 2019 (Fig. 13.7). In Madrid, Spain, there was an insignificant change in the amount of CO from 2019 to 2020. In the city of Lombardy in Italy, again the variation of the air pollutant CO from the year 2019 to 2020 was not very significant. In New Jersey, USA, the variation in the amount of carbon monoxide was noticed. There was a decrease in CO concentration from 2019 to 2020. In New York City, USA, a significant amount of reduction in the CO concentration was noticed in 2020 as against the pre-lockdown year 2019 (Fig. 13.7).

## 13.5 Discussion and Conclusions

The novel coronavirus SARS-CoV-2 (COVID-19) caused panic and public health emergencies across more than 188 countries since the beginning of 2020. The whole world is eager to know its end, and simultaneously, the research community started analyzing various controlling factors, such as social and environmental. The present study investigated the spread of COVID-19 cases in five selected cities concerning social factors as population density, urban factor as urban density, and climatic factor as temperature and humidity. Besides these factors, other preventive measures, such as social distance, imposed lockdowns by governments, and restriction on citizen mobility, also influence the spread of COVID-19 cases. The temporal spread of cases across five cities based on their respective population and number of death tolls was analyzed. The results showed only 0.12% of the total population in Delhi was infected, whereas 1.04%, 0.88%, 2.02%, and 1.82% of the total population were infected in the cities of Lombardy, Madrid, New York, and New Jersey, respectively. Delhi showed relatively lower infection rate in spite of having a larger population density and urban compactness, possibly due to earlier deployment of lockdown in India as compared to other countries.

Previous studies suggested that urban conurbations incubated critical chains of human-to-human transmission of influenza epidemics and indicated a milder response to climate factors in metropolises [15]. The key findings of this study revealed that population density and urban density have a stronger relationship with the spread of COVID-19 cases over millions including higher infection rate across the three cities, namely, Madrid in Spain and New York and New Jersey in the USA. By contrast, Milan (Lombardy) in Italy showed higher infection rate despite lower population density (420 persons/km$^2$), which is mainly associated with late lockdown measures. However, Delhi (India) displayed lower infection rate despite higher population density (11,312 persons/km$^2$) with higher urban compactness, and it could be attributed to timely restriction measures by imposed lockdowns and social distancing. These contrasting results of COVID-19 spread in Delhi and Milan (Lombardy) to the social factor of population density and urban factor represented by urban density suggested that other co-variants, such as climatic factors (temperature and humidity), may be playing a crucial role in spreading COVID-19.

The investigation on climatic factors (temperature and humidity) showed that especially in Milan (Lombardy, Italy) there was the highest spread of COVID-19 cases in March to April 2020 when both temperature (10–15 °C) and humidity (67–77 g/m$^3$) were lower. In Madrid, Spain, there was the highest spread of COVID-19 cases in March to April 2020, which can be associated with lower temperature (15–17 °C), albeit humidity level was 71–76 g/m$^3$. However, the delayed imposition of lockdown is another major factor which caused an abrupt spread of COVID-19 cases. In New York and New Jersey in the USA, the highest spread of COVID-19 cases occurred in March to April 2020, and it is possible that lower temperature (10–12 °C) may have increased the spread of the virus, albeit the humidity level was higher (78–81 g/m$^3$). In Delhi (India), the highest spread was April to May 2020 which can be linked to lower humidity level (23–37 g/m$^3$), but higher temperature (36–42 °C) during April to May has offset the spread of the virus. Therefore, infection rates are meagre as compared to the other four cities across the globe. Earlier studies have suggested that the climatic factors (humidity and temperature) played crucial roles in spreading infectious diseases for SARS-COV-1, 2003 [16, 17]. The spread of SARS-COV-1 was much higher in low temperature than the higher temperature [18]. When the relative humidity was below thresholds of ~11–12 g/kg, it caused an influenza epidemic in the USA and Vietnam [15, 19]. By contrast, these climatic factors might not have a significant association with disease transmission in the tropical region.

Variability in atmospheric pollutants ($NO_2$, $SO_2$, CO, $PM_{2.5}$) due to total lockdown in cities has also concern on the number of deaths due to spread of COVID-19. Notably, imposed lockdowns have reduced concentration of gaseous pollutants due to marginal vehicle movements and minimal industrial activities. The key findings indicate that the satellite-derived mean $NO_2$ and CO pollutants concentration were lower in 2020 as compared to the pre-lockdown period of 2019 across five select cities. The lower level of pollutants could have abetted in lowering the number of deaths but not the spread of the virus. The reduced concentration of gaseous pollutants was also reported by many recent studies across the world [4, 5, 20].

The present study suggested that urban density and population density catalyze the spread of infection across various cities of the world regarding their built-up pattern and population. The climatic variables, viz., temperature and humidity, played an important role for disease spread especially over cities (European cities, New York and New Jersey in the USA) located in temperate regions where the temperature is less than 10 °C. In Delhi, higher temperature with 42 °C in May might offset the spread, but lower humidity level 23 g/m$^3$ abetted the spread of the virus. We concluded that social factors (human-to-human transmission, social distancing, mass gathering, migrant laborers, illegal migrants, among others) and urban factors (urban compactness and population density) had catalyzed the abrupt spread of infection across various cities of the world.

The climatic factors (temperature and humidity) have also abetted the spread of the virus, especially in temperate regions with temperature $<10$ °C with a humidity level between 60 and 77 g/m$^3$. Predictive analysis of COVID-19-affected cases showed good correlation with statistical data that revealed European countries might notice normalcy of no new cases from July 2020. However, in Lombardy, the normalcy may prevail by the end of the year 2020. It portrays possible substantial reduction of COVID-19 cases or no new cases by December 2020 for the USA and India, although real-time changes in data may affect the future predictions. It was predicted that the spread of COVID-19 cases would be marginal from July in Madrid and Milan (Lombardy, Italy). Some of the limitations of SVM predictive model was difficulty in selecting the test size for calibration as wrong test size results in a large difference between mean square and mean absolute errors and the kernel functions and their individual impacts. Nevertheless, these findings would assist policymakers in making appropriate decisions for preventing the spread of COVID-19 novel virus.

**Acknowledgments** Authors thank various government sources for providing daily COVID-19 statistics. Authors also thank the USGS for providing access to Landsat 8 data and GEE portal for TROPOMI satellite data.

## References

1. Wu, J. T., Leung, K., & Leung, G. M. (2020). Nowcasting and forecasting the potential domestic and international spread of the 2019-nCoV outbreak originating in Wuhan, China: A modelling study. *The Lancet, 395*, 689.
2. WHO. (2020). *World Health Organization (WHO) Characterizes COVID-19 as a Pandemic.* Available online: https://www.Who.Int
3. JHU. (2020). *New cases of COVID-19 in world countries. COVID-19 Dashboard by the Center for Systems Science and Engineering (CSSE) at Johns Hopkins University (JHU).* Available online: https://Coronavirus.Jhu.Edu/Data/New-Cases. Accessed on 5 Oct 2020.
4. Tobías, A., Carnerero, C., Reche, C., Massagué, J., Via, M., Minguillón, M. C., Alastuey, A., & Querol, X. (2020). Changes in air quality during the lockdown in Barcelona (Spain) one month into the SARS-CoV-2 epidemic. *Science of the Total Environment, 726*, 138540.
5. Kanniah, K. D., Kamarul Zaman, N. A. F., Kaskaoutis, D. G., & Latif, M. T. (2020). COVID-19's impact on the atmospheric environment in the Southeast Asia region. *Science of the Total Environment, 736*, 139658.
6. Otmani, A., Benchrif, A., Tahri, M., Bounakhla, M., Chakir, E. M., El Bouch, M., & Krombi, M. (2020). Impact of Covid-19 lockdown on $PM_{10}$, $SO_2$ and $NO_2$ concentrations in Salé City (Morocco). *Science of the Total Environment, 735*, 139541.
7. Kraemer, M. U. G., Yang, C.-H., Gutierrez, B., Wu, C.-H., Klein, B., Pigott, D. M., Open COVID-19 Data Working Group, du Plessis, L., Faria, N. R., Li, R., Hanage, W. P., Brownstein, J. S., Layan, M., Vespignani, A., Tian, H., Dye, C., Pybus, O. G., & Scarpino, S. V. (2020). The effect of human mobility and control measures on the COVID-19 epidemic in China. *Science, 368*, 493.
8. Ferguson, N., Laydon, D., Nedjati Gilani, G., Imai, N., Ainslie, K., Baguelin, M., et al. (2020). *Report 9: Impact of Non-Pharmaceutical Interventions (NPIs) to reduce COVID19 mortality and healthcare demand.* London: Imperial College.
9. Stoecklin, S. B., Rolland, P., Silue, Y., Mailles, A., Campese, C., Simondon, A., Mechain, M., Meurice, L., Nguyen, M., Bassi, C., Yamani, E., Behillil, S., Ismael, S., Nguyen, D., Malvy, D., Lescure, F. X., Georges, S., Lazarus, C., Tabaï, A., Stempfelet, M., Enouf, V., Coignard, B., Levy-Bruhl, D., & Investigation team. (2020). First cases of coronavirus disease 2019 (COVID-19) in France: Surveillance, investigations and control measures. *Eurosurveillance, 25*, 2000094.

10. Casanova, L. M., Jeon, S., Rutala, W. A., Weber, D. J., & Sobsey, M. D. (2010). Effects of air temperature and relative humidity on coronavirus survival on surfaces. *AEM, 76*, 2712.
11. Bu, J., Peng, D.-D., Xiao, H., Yue, Q., Han, Y., Lin, Y., Hu, G., & Chen, J. (2020). Analysis of meteorological conditions and prediction of epidemic trend of 2019-NCoV infection in 2020. Infectious Diseases (except HIV/AIDS).
12. Chan, J. F., Yuan, S., Kok, K., To, K., Chu, H., Yang, J., et al. (2020). A familial cluster of pneumonia associated with the 2019 novel coronavirus indicating person-to-person transmission: A study of a family cluster. *The Lancet, 395*, 514.
13. Zhou, Z. X., & Jiang, C. Q. (2004). Effect of environment and occupational hygiene factors of hospital infection on SARS outbreak. *Chinese Journal of Industrial Hygiene and Occupational Diseases, 22*, 261.
14. Gorelick, N., Hancher, M., Dixon, M., Ilyushchenko, S., Thau, D., & Moore, R. (2017). Google Earth Engine: Planetary-scale geospatial analysis for everyone. *Remote Sensing of Environment, 202*, 18.
15. Dalziel, B. D., Kissler, S., Gog, J. R., Viboud, C., Bjørnstad, O. N., Metcalf, C. J. E., & Grenfell, B. T. (2018). Urbanization and humidity shape the intensity of influenza epidemics in U.S. cities. *Science, 362*, 75.
16. Chan, K. H., Peiris, J. S. M., Lam, S. Y., Poon, L. L. M., Yuen, K. Y., & Seto, W. H. (2011). The effects of temperature and relative humidity on the viability of the SARS coronavirus. *Advances in Virology, 2011*, 1.
17. Monaghan, A. J., Moore, S. M., Sampson, K. M., Beard, C. B., & Eisen, R. J. (2015). Climate change influences on the annual onset of Lyme disease in the United States. *Ticks and Tick-Borne Diseases, 6*, 615.
18. Yuan, J., Yun, H., Lan, W., Wang, W., Sullivan, S. G., Jia, S., & Bittles, A. H. (2006). A climatologic investigation of the SARS-CoV outbreak in Beijing, China. *American Journal of Infection Control, 34*, 234.
19. Tamerius, J. D., Shaman, J., Alonso, W. J., Bloom-Feshbach, K., Uejio, C. K., Comrie, A., & Viboud, C. (2013). Environmental predictors of seasonal influenza epidemics across temperate and tropical climates. *PLoS Pathogens, 9*, e1003194.
20. Collivignarelli, M. C., Abbà, A., Bertanza, G., Pedrazzani, R., Ricciardi, P., & Carnevale Miino, M. (2020). Lockdown for CoViD-2019 in Milan: What are the effects on air quality? *Science of the Total Environment, 732*, 139280.

10. Casanova, L. M., Jeon, S., Rutala, W. A., Weber, D. J., & Sobsey, M. D. (2010). Effects of air temperature and relative humidity on coronavirus survival on surfaces. *AEM, 76*, 2712 [illegible]
11. [illegible] Liang, L. D., Xiao, H., [illegible] (2020). Analysis of meteorological conditions and prediction of epidemic trend of 2019-nCoV infection in [illegible]
12. Chen, [illegible]
[illegible]

# Chapter 14
# Chatbots for Coronavirus: Detecting COVID-19 Symptoms with Virtual Assessment Tool

**Aasma Chouhan, Supriya Pathak, and Reshma Tendulkar**

## 14.1 Introduction

> When we emerge from this crisis, Chatbots are likely to become digital portals for interactive healthcare. –Venkataraman Sundareswaran, Kay Firth-Butterfield [1]

December 2019 accounted for the worst case of sudden onset of pneumonia among masses in the south Chinese seafood market in Wuhan, Hubei Province, China. When the professionals from the National Health Commission investigated further, a novel coronavirus (eventually COVID-19 for coronavirus disease 19) was identified by the Laboratory of Virology, Chinese Center for Disease Control and Prevention on 7 January 2020. By then the number of pneumonia cases had increased significantly in the Chinese province as well as internationally [2].

As stated by the World Health Organization (WHO), coronavirus disease (COVID-19) is an infectious disease caused by a newly discovered coronavirus, and the best way to prevent transmission is be well informed about the COVID-19, the disease it causes, and how it spreads. Organizations like the Centers for Disease Control and Prevention (CDC) and the WHO have initiated the use of Chatbots to share details and facts related to the pandemic, propose behavior, and provide emotional reassurance [3].The CDC has titled theirs "Clara" [4]. Since the advancement of Internet and mobile phone applications, Chatbots are the latest development. It is established that these apps are the software programs, developed for automatic communication utilizing artificial intelligence (AI) between the users and computers [5]. These agents are further expanding in the fields of education, agriculture, healthcare, banking, etc. The first company to use a Chatbot for

A. Chouhan (✉) · S. Pathak · R. Tendulkar
H K College of Pharmacy, Mumbai, India



S. Kautish et al. (eds.), *Computational Intelligence Techniques for Combating COVID-19*, EAI/Springer Innovations in Communication and Computing,
https://doi.org/10.1007/978-3-030-68936-0_14

detection of coronavirus was Buoy Health; they are working for state of Massachusetts since then. Chatbots proffer strong prospective for curated information. The information can be personalized to the requirements and symptoms of the individual. Numerous companies and organizations are preeminently taking the charge in employing Chatbots to furnish COVID-19 information. The two most accredited voices of the pandemic, WHO and CDC, have also incorporated Chatbots in their websites to provide contemporary particulars to billions on the spread of the disease and its symptoms. Chatbots can be used or produced in a range of capabilities, which means it is highly scalable. Whether an individual needs some help or the whole community does, Chatbots can reach out every one of them provided there's an Internet connection. People can benefit from it in the comforts of their own homes. Chatbots are a just a click away for the people in need of information and help.

"AI increasingly integrates our daily lives with the creation and analysis of intelligent software and hardware, called intelligent agents. Intelligent agents can do a variety of tasks ranging from labor work to sophisticated operations. A Chatbot is a typical example of an AI system and one of the most elementary and widespread examples of intelligent human-computer interaction (HCI)." "It is a computer program, which responds like a smart entity when conversed with through text or voice and understands one or more human languages by Natural Language Processing (NLP)" [6]. In the lexicon, a Chatbot is defined as "a computer program designed to simulate conversation with human users, especially over the Internet" [7]. Chatbots are also known as SmartBots interactive agents, digital assistants, or artificial conversation entities.

## 14.2 Fundamentals of Chatbots

### *14.2.1 What Is a Chatbot?*

AI led to various developments in conversational interfaces, one of which is the Chatbot. Mauldin coined the term "Chatbot." A Chatbot is considered to be software program, which runs various actions via interaction with the individuals. These interactions might be about a precise theme or a certain zone that is carried out in a typical, colloquial manner utilizing text and voice. Chatbots have been implemented in the market for various purposes such as education, marketing, customer service, and healthcare. Conversations with technology are possible due to contemporary developments in this field, either by text or voice-speech; that is why users gradually prefer digital interaction.

## *14.2.2 Evolution of Chatbots*

### 14.2.2.1 1950s: The Turing Test

Alan Turing, in 1950, wrote a paper initially starting with the "Can machines think?" question. Turing thereby proposed an experimental game called, "The Imitation Game." In the very first procedure of the experiment, there were three rooms or compartments with computers out of which one room consisted of a male, another one consisted of a female, and the last room consisted of a judge. The judge had to recognize which room consist the male and which room consisted the female. Judge asking or communicating with the participants utilizing the computer did this, whereas the participants would send hints or deceits to complete the tasks.

A modification to this experiment was done by Turing which now contains three rooms or compartments with one occupied by the judge; another by a human, either a male or a female; and the last room or compartment which was initially occupied by another human will be replaced with a machine conversing like a human. The judge on the basis of identification of compartments or room containing human now analyzes this experiment. The possibility of machine being able to imitate the human conversation more than 50% of the time will decide the intelligence factor of the machine. The test is known commonly as Turing test [8].

### 14.2.2.2 1964: ELIZA

ELIZA was the first ever computer program to pass the Turing test and made publicly available. ELIZA utilized the (NLP). "NLP is the branch of AI," a technology that translates human conversations to the computer programs by breaking the words, sentences, and statements.

Professor Joseph Weizenbaum implemented computer "scripts," which enabled ELIZA to examine user input, elucidate the inputs entered, and further supply the user with a suitable response [9].

The widely implemented script was the one named as DOCTOR, which directed to imitate the Rogerian psychotherapist.

### 14.2.2.3 1980s: Jabberwacky

Jabberwacky.com
A British programmer, Rollo Carpenter, designed Jabberwacky. The main objective of this program is to create interesting and humorous interactions making it to be a conversational bot. The program is entirely based on context and feedback and is not controlled by any rules and relies. The Jabberwacky program has the capability to continually learn from the conversations and interactions [10].

#### 14.2.2.4 1990s: A.L.I.C.E

Dr. Richard Wallace designed Artificial Linguistic Internet Computer Entity free Chatbot program in 1995. Inspired by ELIZA, the program managed to bag the Loebner Prize in the year 2000. Dr. Wallace also implemented the Artificial Intelligence Markup Language (AIML), thereby upgrading the A.L.I.C.E. as Program A, Program B, Program C, and Program D [11].

#### 14.2.2.5 2000s: SmarterChild Arrives

Facts-based Chatbots were commercially introduced in the form of SmarterChild in the year 2001. Questions such as "What is the population of Indonesia?" or "What movies are playing near me tonight?" can be easily answered using this Chatbot. The program has the capability to fairly converse and continue an interaction [12].

#### 14.2.2.6 2010s: Chatbots and Personal Assistants

Contemporary developments have led to upgrade of conversational interfaces such that Chatbots are now not just a novelty but slowly making its way into daily needs. Chatbots have its applications spread in various fields such as education, healthcare, customer service, trading, etc.

Some of the most popular assistants occupying the markets are Amazon's Alexa, Apple's Siri, Google Assistant, and Microsoft's Cortana.

## 14.3 Types of Chatbots

There are different types of Chatbots each having their own capability to interact with the users and make their lives easier. The broad classification of Chatbots can be done as follows.

### *14.3.1 Entertainment Chatbots*

Chatbots, which are used by the customers to have conversations for a longer duration of time, come under this classification. Assessment can be done through Turing test; other ways include finding out the extent of conversation, time invested by the users with the bots, and other quantitative measures [13].

### *14.3.2 Enterprise Chatbots*

These Chatbots are more business oriented: the length of conversation is usually short and informative. They are more focused on providing the needs and requirements of their customers.

### *14.3.3 Classification of Chatbots*

Using different parameters such as knowledge domain, service provided, goals, input distilling, and the construction, Chatbots are classified as follows.

#### 14.3.3.1 Knowledge Domain

The knowledge domain classification contemplates the assessment of Chatbot on the basis of the knowledge or data it is upskilled with. It is further classified as open-domain Chatbots and closed-domain Chatbots [14, 15].

#### 14.3.3.2 Service Provided

The service provided classification deals with the integral accessibility with the user. The details of conversation describe the Chatbots as interpersonal Chatbots, intrapersonal Chatbots, and inter-agent Chatbots. Examples of each of the above category are as follows: for interpersonal Chatbots, restaurant booking, flight booking, and FAQ bots; for intrapersonal Chatbots, Messenger, Slack, and WhatsApp; and for inter-agent Chatbots, Alexa and Cortana.

#### 14.3.3.3 Goals Achieved

The goals achieved by a Chatbot can be classified into chat-based/conversational Chatbots, informative Chatbots, and task-based Chatbots. Conversational Chatbots aim to achieve the primary goal of having successful continuous conversation with the user and implementing interactions as per user's need. Informative Chatbots provide the user with the information needed or asked by the individual such as FAQ Chatbots. Task-based Chatbots comply with the user request and achieve the given task such as hotel bookings, ticket bookings, etc.

#### 14.3.3.4 Input Distilling

Chatbots are also classified on the basis of input distilling. Depending on the responses produced, the three models used for input distilling are rule-based model, retrieval-based model, and generative model. Initially, Chatbots were built on rule-based model, where the program generated response over a predefined memory instilled within it and the program stored no new information. However, the retrieval-based model retrieves some data from the ongoing conversation with the user and interacts with suitable responses. The generative model thereby satisfies the user with better answers as compared to the other two. However the built-up and design of such models are made with various complications and difficulties, thereby making it difficult in training [16].

#### 14.3.3.5 Construction

The construction of Chatbots simplifies the task given and works according to the implementation of platforms. The construction of Chatbots can be classified as open-source platforms and closed-source platforms.

## 14.4 Architecture and Design of Chatbots

### *14.4.1 Architecture*

The Chatbot is designed based on the requirement of the developer. The Chatbot can generate responses through two mechanisms: by creating a response from square one, consistent with machine learning models, or it can use some probing to elect a suitable response from a collection of preformed responses.

#### 14.4.1.1 Generative Models

The smart bots which require special skills are designed through this model. Since very complex algorithms are required for this model, it is not used very often (Fig. 14.1).

Generative models are very intricate; thus they are complicated to assemble. For training this model, billions of examples are needed which is extremely time-consuming. Due to this the deep learning model is able to hold a conversation. But even after this, we are not sure what will be the exact response generated by the model [18].

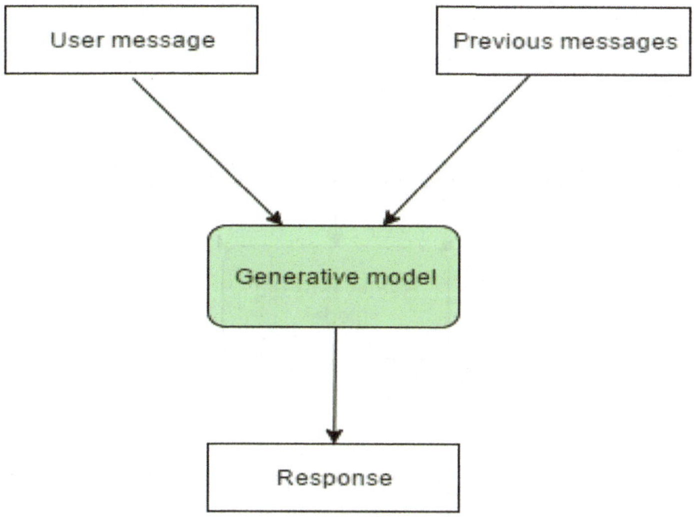


**Fig. 14.1** The workflow of generative model [17]

#### 14.4.1.2 Retrieval-Based Models

Retrieval-based model is much more straightforward and can be assembled conveniently. But for this type of Chatbot, we need to pre-assign appropriate responses in order to avoid imprecise and impertinent responses during the conversation (Fig. 14.2).

These models are used far more frequently as compared to the generative models because of its simple algorithm. In this type of Chatbot, the responses are pre-feeded, thus generating text-related responses during the conversation [18].

#### 14.4.1.3 Mechanism for Response Generation

There are two different ways for the Chatbot to figure out the context of the conversation or to understand their intent.

Pattern-Based Heuristics

Response generation can be done either by machine learning or by using if-else conditional system. Following a set of rules and preframed responses, a pattern can be generated through which the correct responses will be given. The most commonly used programing language for Chatbot development is AIML.

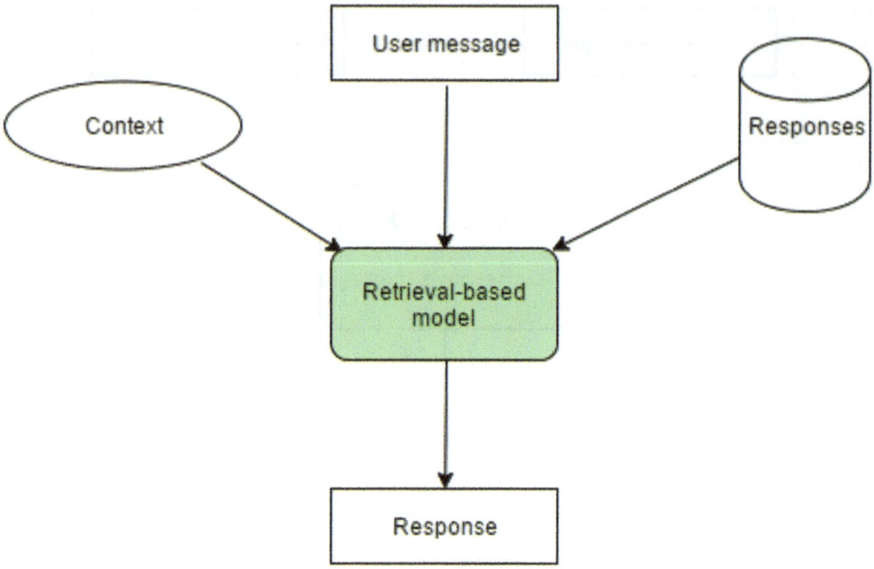


**Fig. 14.2** The workflow of retrieval-based model [18]

```
<category>
<pattern>What is your name</pattern>
<template>My name is Bob Cooper</template>
</category>
```

AIML is used for constructing SmartBots; because of its flexibility and user friendliness it is a very popular choice. It helps to create human interfaces while being easy to program, easily accessible, and understandable. Synonyms, figure of speech, and other grammatical functions can be carried out through these Chatbots. Nonetheless these bots are required to be specially programmed to use other APIs and machine learning algorithms [18].

Intent Classification Using Machine Learning

The pattern-based heuristics has to have all the programs to be programmed by developers manually. This work is very tiresome since millions of responses are to be added and the Chatbot should be able to differentiate the intent of the users in diverse situations.

Hence intent classification is required. It is dependent upon machine learning technology which is used for the training of the Chatbots. From this training, which encompasses hundreds of example responses, the bot forms a pattern through which it learns [18].

#### 14.4.1.4 Generation of Response

After figuring out the intent of the user, the bot needs to generate a response. There can be two ways to do it: the Chatbot can simply generate a static response or it can have template responses which were programmed beforehand. Based on the purpose of the Chatbots, the response mechanism is computed by the manufacturers.

The response to every user varies. The Chatbot examines the user's previous conversation and forms a pattern of responses to use and hence personalizing each and every response. The given schematic representation shows the mechanism for response generation (Fig. 14.3).

Creating a Chatbot is a very intricate procedure, so professional help should be sought. The Chatbot development agencies help build the bot in such a way that it gives out customized responses to each and every user in a hassle-free manner [18].

## *14.4.2 Chatbots and Its Functionality*

The medical organizations are firmly linked with human interaction, and it appears unreasonable that virtual conversational tools such as Chatbots are recognized and accepted. Health managements are occupying their time in appointment organizing and replying frequent questions asked by the patients. Jobs such as repeating the same actions or words can be carried out easily by Chatbots. It is evident that assembling user data to maintain patient records can also do patient feedback evaluation. During the global pandemic chaos like COVID-19, healthcare bots seem to be an addition to clinicians and emergency medications (Battineni 2020) [19] (Fig. 14.4).

The Chatbot is designed to operate user inquiry and recognize messaging styles with the help of an AIML.

The Chatbot functionality is defined either by request analysis or return response. Initially, Chatbot assesses the gravity of the virus using series of responses received from a predetermined set of questions. Therefore, if the individual is unable to confess correct answers, the Chatbot will further fail to issue the correct response. In the response return of the Chatbot, after the assessment of a patient's condition, it conveys an apparent response through either common text or text recovered from the knowledge base response. Following is the Chatbot design.

#### 14.4.2.1 AIML Fundamental Design

The AIML operates according to impetus-response methodology and issues easy, straightforward conversation description. As referred, it is based on markup language with a tag basis. These tags are modifiers, which insert instructions and assemble code fragments in the Chatbots. With the implementation of AIML in the

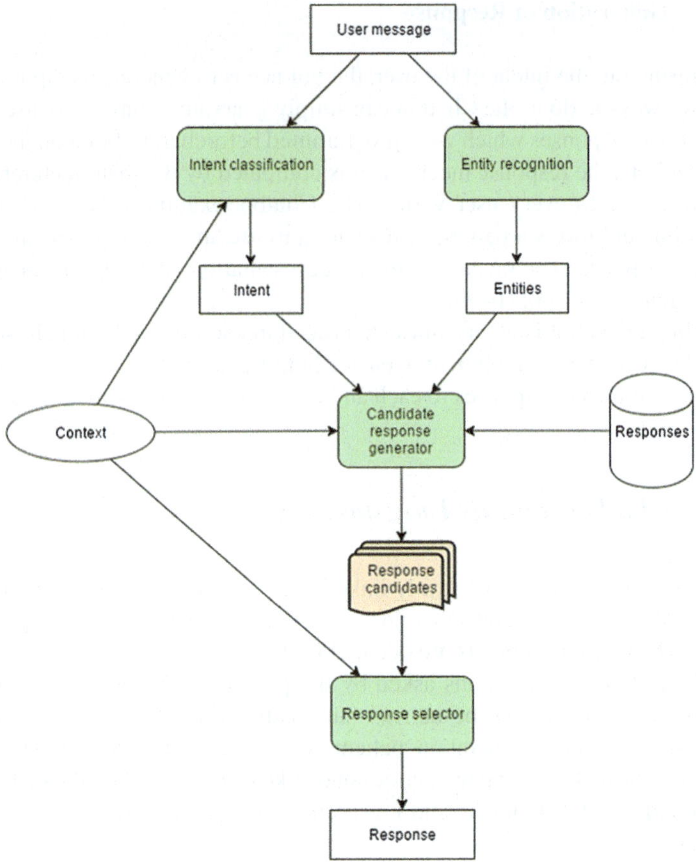


**Fig. 14.3** The workflow of response generation [17]

Chatbot, it is able to identify user messages pattern and displays clear and correct response. The Chatbot further identifies if the individual user ought to either examine the infection position or be aware of the primary estimates and characteristic conduct of the COVID-19 virus.

#### 14.4.2.2 Paradigm Identification Using Snippets

Particularly, a Chatbot should recognize the paradigms of user's appeals with predetermined tags of the AIML component. Within AIML, a predetermined tag paradigm ([paradigm]) assists Chatbot in identification of virus symptoms, which if matches, the specific set of questions shall be displayed [20]. For example, let's say the user doubts that they have been infected; the subsequent illustrative paradigms with snippets may proceed as follows:

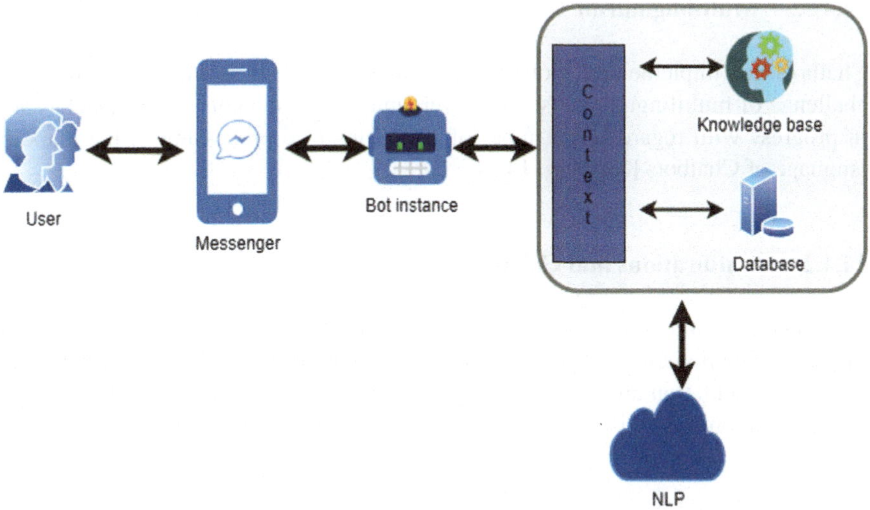


**Fig. 14.4** The workflow of a Chatbot [19]

> [paradigm] I am having fever since three days [paradigm] I am experiencing dry cough as well [paradigm] I lived with infected patient [paradigm] I had travel history of migration in the last two weeks [paradigm].

In the abovementioned paradigm, the Chatbot examines for attainable occurrences of being infected, or if it crosses the portal value instantly, it will subjoin to the healthcare specialists.

#### 14.4.2.3 Portal Value Assessment

The Chatbot should be as natural as possible when responding to user's queries, thereby consisting of precise data collection and feasible backend sagacity for outcome generation [19].

#### 14.4.2.4 Instrumentation

The Chatbot engine applies principal backend logic using WEB API method, which is a validated input. The tool follows two routines, that is, communication with a healthcare professional and instant investigation of basic preventative measures, once the evaluation of infection is obtained [19].

All of the symptoms attribute to a numeral, which evaluates gravity score of infection. After the aggregation symptomatic statistics is obtained, the Chatbot activates a healthcare expert consultation.

#### 14.4.2.5 Multilingualism

Chatbots are implemented globally in various sectors of services, although the challenge of multilingualism is yet to overcome. Developments and researches are in progress with regard to the input of multi-language processing in the markup language of Chatbots [21] (Fig. 14.5).

#### 14.4.2.6 Calibrations and Collation

The AI conversational tool building organizations often consider various aspects to assess the functionality and performance of the Chatbot. This is done to evaluate the visual representation and its implementation and also to caliber the understanding of conversation capabilities and interaction skills of the Chatbot [19].

## 14.5 Applications of Chatbots

### *14.5.1 Chatbots in Education*

Chatbots are widely in use for educational services since it is easily accessible to everyone anytime of the day.

#### 14.5.1.1 Language Study

With the help of Chatbots, students are ensured to have a learning environment where they can have access to the languages 24/7. It allows students to have a conversation as many times as they want with the Chatbot, thus providing a mistake-free friendly environment. Due to this the stress and anxiety of students regarding face to face communication is reduced significantly. This has helped in encouraging them to learn foreign languages such as ALGOL 68, CLOJURE, Hayashi, etc. However, in the recent years, the use of Chatbots as language learning facility has reduced significantly. This is due to increased utilization of human assistants such as Alexa and Siri (Fryer and Gibson 2017b) [9, 22].

#### 14.5.1.2 Performance Reviewer

Chatbots can be developed to issue feedback about the performance of students throughout the year. Performance review has been shown to encourage students to function better. The Chatbot is much more approachable since it is nearly impossible to have an individual formative feedback during the ongoing semester. This formative feedback helps in motivating the students and hence improving

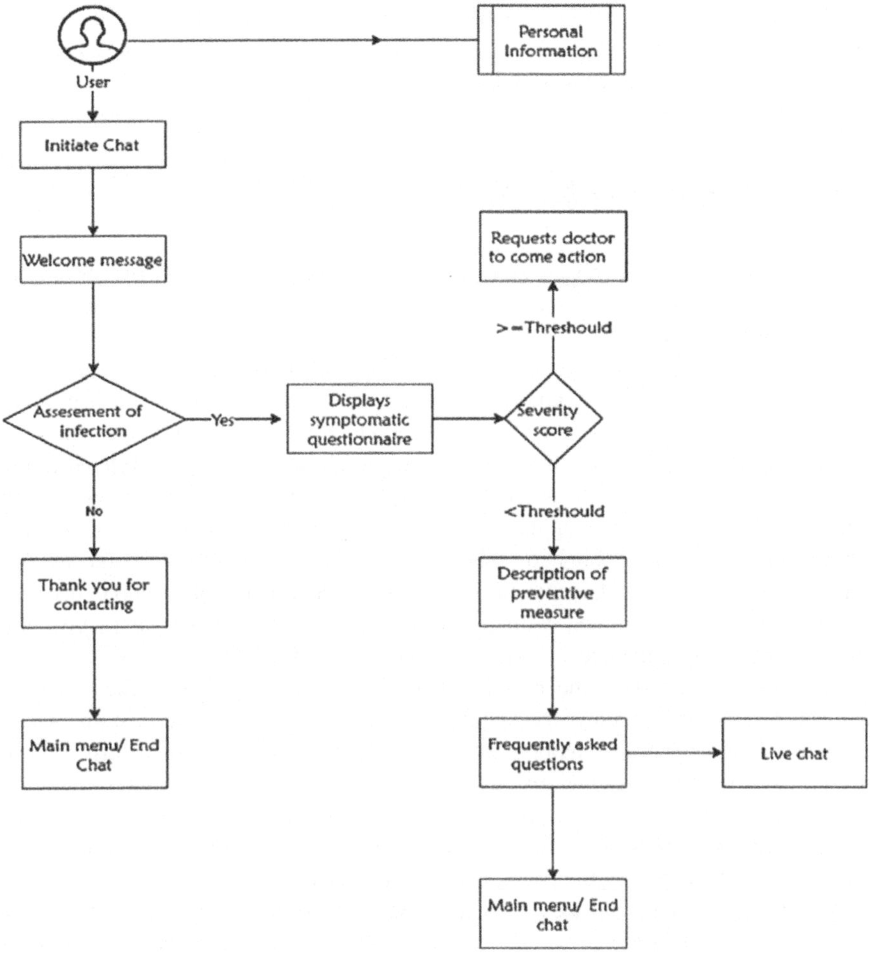


**Fig. 14.5** The working of a Chatbot [19]

performance. Chatbots as performance reviewer has an added advantage as it can be used by the students to have a conversation with the bot and ask questions related to their review. The bots can also be used to enhance the metacognitive thinking of the students [23, 24].

#### 14.5.1.3 Motivation Builder

Chatbots can be utilized to boost the confidence of the students and also motivate them to learn more. This can be done by making the students in charge of their learning experience, thus building up their self-belief. Chatbots enhance self-efficacy by making students curious and challenging them to test their skills. Motivation and self-efficacy are one of the most important factors of learning success [23–25].

All things considered, Chatbots have a range of function in the education field. They help in the learning process, performance reviewing, and a variety of things. Chatbot is a boon in the education industry.

### *14.5.2 Chatbots in Client Service*

Customer service or client service is the support which is offered to the customers before, after, and during the purchase. This field has a variety of purposes which are fulfilled by the Chatbots.

Customer service is a real-time business, Chatbots in this field is very beneficial since it can be used 24/7, and mistakes can be avoided. The bots are becoming popular day by day in the e-commerce market [26]. The customer can have an individual assistant anytime of the day whom they can ask questions related to the product, have assistance to solve technical issues, etc. In recent times human interacting agents are often replaced by AI bots like Chatbots which are programmed to chat with the customers in natural language [27]. Nonetheless, some users are not satisfied by the Chatbots because of the lack of human touch. For example, because the Chatbot is programmed with a set of responses, it is not able to give the satisfactory reply to the user which further creates complications.

To solve these issues, the new age Chatbots are equipped with the feedback collector in order to record the suggestions and feedback by the customers and improve from it. These Chatbots are programmed to respond in a turn-by-turn fashion to avoid mistakes and give a human touch. Some Chatbots are programmed anthropomorphically to give a touch of social presence and have conversations which seem more personal. The Chatbots today also give verbal anthropomorphic design cues like thanking the users, excusing themselves, etc. [28].

Chatbots nowadays are designed to be more flexible and empathetic in their response rather than the previous versions of crude responses. These are built to increase user friendliness and have an adapting nature [26, 29].

## 14.6 Chatbots for COVID-19 [30]

Novel coronavirus COVID-19 causes infection primarily via the respiratory tract by spread of either droplets or respiratory secretions and at times through one to one contact and thus has emerged as an acute respiratory infectious disease. Among the various possibilities of multiple routes of transmission, it had been reported that severe acute respiratory syndrome coronavirus 2 (SARS-CoV-2) was isolated from fecal swabs and blood of a severe pneumonia patient [31, 32].

However, some health experts have commented on concerns related to the transmissions of SARS-CoV-2 through tears and conjunctiva secretions of the patients infected with COVID-19 SARS-CoV and SARS-CoV-2 have been reported to be genetically similar with similarity of greater than 80% [33].

It is evident through research and data that the presence of SARS-CoV in the tears of the infected patient was studied during the SARS outbreak in 2004.

Likewise, the reports consisting details of the infected ophthalmologists are found to be in large numbers due to the ongoing pandemic. Evaluation of the infectivity of COVID-19 due to tears of patients has been found in some of the recent studies.

### 14.6.1 Detecting COVID-19 Symptoms

With various ongoing researches and studies on confirmed cases of COVID-19, the authoritative sources have come to the conclusion that the most common clinical symptoms of COVID-19 include fever, cough, fatigue, sputum production, shortness of breath, sore throat, and headache. Some additional symptoms included gastrointestinal symptoms with diarrhea and vomiting. Among all the symptoms, fever and cough have been the superior ones. The geriatric and those affected with disorders such as diabetes, cardiovascular disease, and hypertension take up the respiratory distress rapidly at times even leading to death.

Frequently applied technique used for the identification of SARS-CoV-2 is reverse transcriptase polymerase chain reaction (RT-PCR) real-time reverse transcription polymerase chain reaction. This technique involves reverse transcription of the SARS-CoV-2 RNA to form cDNA followed by amplification of the specific gene fragments from cDNA utilizing target specific primers. However, various contrasting studies suggest that CT should be considered as a primary tool for the detection of COVID-19. This is due to the results obtained with CT that are far more accurate when compared with RT-PCR technique.

The drawback of using CT technique is that it possesses the risk of exposing the patients undergoing the test to the infection. Hence, CT can be considered as an additional symptom-detecting tool primarily for individuals who show symptoms.

The use of Chatbots in healthcare system has been increasing rapidly. They not only assist with appointment and medicine management, but they can also identify symptoms and guide on possible diagnoses. The global threat of COVID-19 pandemic has led to the urgent need of Chatbots in healthcare, rather than it being a luxury or novelty. Then how exactly can Chatbots lend a helping hand to the healthcare professionals amid the pandemic chaos?

### 14.6.2 Information Device

The healthcare system can use Chatbots as information-distributing source for patients as well as the healthy individuals. Chatbot users can directly ask questions related to their health and the status of pandemic worldwide and get immediate answers from an authoritative source. The need for online healthcare device is set to grow due to a combination of factors such as self-isolation, heightened demand for remote healthcare information, instant panic-induced symptom searching, and many more. To add on the chaos of global pandemic, circulation of misinformation about the COVID-19 disease is rampant leading to infodemic. The plethora of information is making it hard for people to distinguish fact from fiction.

### *14.6.3 Interactions and Guidance*

Apart from users asking Chatbots questions, Chatbots can cross-examine users for information too. With this, Chatbots in healthcare can assist people get a preluding diagnosis. Hereby, they can ask about symptoms and then offer possible diagnosis and advice on what to do next.

In a pandemic, people who worried that they might have the coronavirus often face a feeling of disquiet. Unless the need to visit the intensive care unit arises, there are no appointments for them. Meanwhile, the doctors are extremely busy. And, with a limited number of appointments in a day, patients have to come to blows to access the help they need.

Owing to COVID-19, Chatbots in healthcare come up with ways for people to ascertain about their own health and well-being.

Chatbots do so by dispensing coronavirus help which is assisting concerned individuals whether or not he/she may be infected with the novel coronavirus and if so the need to put in quarantine from their family. Asking the individual users a few questions related to the symptoms characteristic of the coronavirus does the mentioned procedure. From the answers obtained, they can prompt a suggestion of whether the person is symptomatic of infection. Thereby, Chatbots can offer specific advice on what to do next which might be either providing a number to call or how to self-isolate and might as well offer advice about what to do and how to manage the symptoms.

### *14.6.4 Examples*

Some of the well-known Chatbots that were recognized on a World Health Organization lists of systems supporting the fight against pandemic are "Clara, MyGov Corona Helpdesk, Rapid Response Virtual Agent program, Microsoft Azure, and many more" [34]. The framework of the Chatbot is rooted on official WHO guidelines that are further verified by team of doctors. The Chatbot provides individuals with guidelines and advice, depending on the scanning of their answers (Fig. 14.6).

The tool validates users to examine whether they are in the threat group without the requirement to contact a health professional personally, thereby helping shrink the outspread of COVID-19.

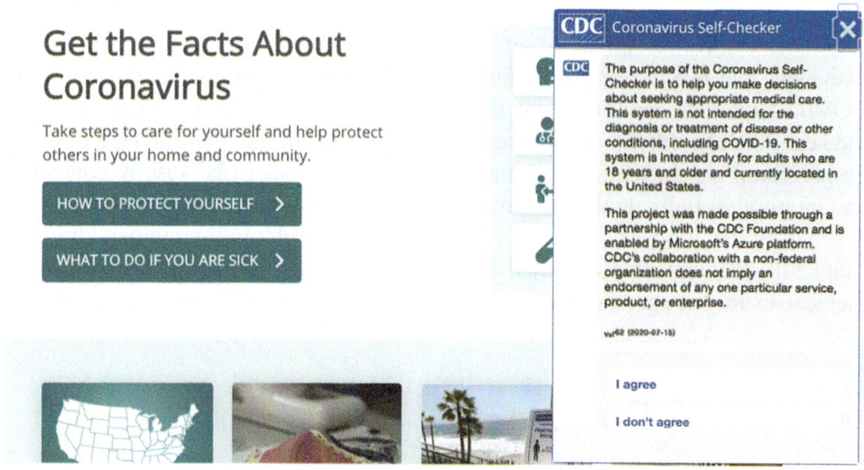


**Fig. 14.6** Screenshot of publically displayed Coronavirus Self-Checker Chatbot "Clara" by CDC on its official website [35]

In the course of a pandemic, both individuals and organizations want to perceive how and where contamination is spreading. Individuals want to steer clear of getting infected, and organizations such as health center or provincial governments require data-informed strategy to escalate the capacity for ordering more testing kits and to plan social interventions such as operating businesses during pandemic. However, attempts to rapidly and accurately congregate population-level infection rates are hampered by individuals' panic that divulging symptoms may torment their professional and social lives.

Chatbots may be uniquely adapted for symptom screening in a pandemic since individuals with denounced conditions more so circumvent seeking healthcare and education. According to a research, individuals tend to share personal information regarding their health to a Chatbot instead of humans. This alludes that individuals may be more approaching with Chatbots than other humans, providing prompt and more specific personal triage and population-level infection rate evaluation.

Precaution and anticipation are very much important during the ongoing pandemic, as there is no authorized therapy or treatment for its infection. Factors such as vague characteristics of the disease, communal transmission from asymptomatic individual, as well as patients with clinical-recovery records and prolonged incubation period cause hindrance with the prevention from virus infection.

Patients with confirmed or suspected infection with some of the manifestation are advised to quarantine themselves at their house. In order to fight the virus and its infection, proper sanitation and hygiene are to be maintained. Every individual must follow various health practices such as coughing and sneezing hygiene or to use a cloth while doing so, practice to wear surgical masks, and follow hand hygiene every 20–30 min.

Protection and safety measures of healthcare professionals must be the top priority to control the spread of infection to others and to provide optimum care. It is evident that healthcare professionals and workers are exposed to the spread of COVID-19 disease more than any other individual. At the time of SARS spread in the year 2002, healthcare workers contributed to 21% of the total infected ratio. To ensure complete prevention, communal transmission has to be strictly controlled and monitored. Individuals must avoid nonessential trade and travel and should be asked to follow proper cough and sneeze hygiene, thereby following hand hygiene frequently. Patients infected with the same should practice mask wearing and isolate themselves for the specified period.

### 14.6.5 Antiviral Therapies

Primarily used drugs such as ganciclovir, acyclovir, zanamivir, etc. for treatment of influenza virus seem to have no effect on coronavirus and hence are invalid for the treatment of COVID-19 [33, 36–38].

When administered to the first COVID-19 patient in the USA, remdesivir has shown some effective pharmacological action. Remdesivir is a prodrug, which shows wide range of antiviral activity when administered to treat various RNA viruses [33, 39].

Another widely used drug amidst ongoing pandemic is chloroquine [40]. It has shown beneficial use for treating malaria since ages and further exhibits considerable prospective for the treatment of COVID-19. However, the mechanistic action of chloroquine is still not clear as it seems to have some effect on the viral infection and transmission [33, 41].

### 14.6.6 Ongoing Treatment

Since no great effect has been observed after the administration of antiviral treatment against the coronavirus disease, therapies are now pneumonia centered which is caused by COVID-19 [42]. The treatments are structured according to the manifestations and treatment of pneumonia. Among the most accepted and responded treatments, symptomatic and respiratory support along with oxygen therapy has proven to ease the respiratory distress [43]. The authoritative sources such as WHO has recommended extracorporeal membrane oxygenation (ECMO) and rescue treatment to critical patients respective to their condition.

## 14.6.7 *Bots Already in Use for COVID-19*

### 14.6.7.1 Orbita COVID-19 Screening Chatbot and Knowledge Base

Orbita was one of the first companies to come up with a Chatbot in this pandemic, "The COVID-19 Screening Chatbot" & Knowledge Base is serving two main purposes: As a screening virtual assistant: Since the rise of COVID19 cases, people are worried and turning up to the hospitals and clinics with very mild symptoms increasing the load on the already burdened healthcare system. This Chatbot can help lessen some of the workload by detecting the symptoms of the users and providing them with options. As an education provider for patients: False information is the major problem during this pandemic. Chatbot presents with credible, clinically-reviewed data directly from the Centers of Disease Control and Prevention (CDC). Presently the Orbita Chatbot is accessible in the US Healthcare market, in English language only [44].

### 14.6.7.2 NHS WhatsApp Bot

The government of UK had recently launched a Coronavirus Information Centre on WhatsApp; its aim was to provide accurate and up-to-date information on the coronavirus scenario.

As stated by the UK government officials on their website, "The GOV.UK Coronavirus Information Service is an automated Chatbot service which will allow the British public to get answers to the most common questions about coronavirus direct from government." This assures that misleading information would not be circulated among the masses. To connect with the Chatbot in the UK, users just need to send "hi" to +44 78600 64422 using WhatsApp. For the users outside of UK, WhatsApp in association with the World Health Organization (WHO) has generated another contact providing the same services. Individuals need to send "hi" to +41 22 501 76 55 on WhatsApp [46].

### 14.6.7.3 Corona Helpdesk Chatbot on Facebook

Reading the situation Facebook also came up with a Chatbot in order to provide credible information in this chaotic situation. The government of India with the help of Facebook's messenger app came up with a Chatbot, the Corona Helpdesk. This can be accessed through MyGovIndia's page. Users can reach out to gather reliable news, real-time updates, emergency contact numbers, etc. The Chatbot answers in both English and Hindi. Relying upon the question asked, individuals will receive authentic information in the form of text, videos, news articles, or infographics [44].

#### 14.6.7.4 Microsoft's Coronavirus Self-Checker Bot

The USCDC now has got a "coronavirus self-checker" bot on their website. This Chatbot was built by utilizing Microsoft's healthcare bot service. The Chatbot is not designed for diagnosis or treatment of COVID-19 but for the patients to upload their symptoms and get to know the appropriate measures to be taken for their condition. The bot gathers personal data such as the age of the user, if they are taking care of someone or they themselves are not well, their age, address, and the symptoms they are having and thus giving a detailed response on further steps to be taken. Currently you can converse with this Chatbot on CDC website [44].

## 14.7 Challenges

Chatbots may be uniquely functional in a pandemic; however, defiance in information dissemination, symptom tracking, and behavior change are noteworthy. Providing well-grounded evidence-based information is scathing in a pandemic, and issues such as varying advices between global and local authorities and inaccuracy of information have material impact [30].

Chatbots designers must determine whose opinion to magnify and should provide authentic information from authoritative sources like the WHO while also systematizing with regional authorities. If employed for symptom screening, which is happening at present for COVID-19, sharing health-related statistics between companies and governments tests constitutional and regulatory boundaries.

These challenges, if only addressed immediately during an emergency, may bring out imprecise results from a lack of testing. In addition to a billion voice searches per month, any health-related misinterpretation, such as mystifying key symptoms, would be increased with immense harmful consequences. Furthermore, medical and public health specialists must notify what Chatbots say and how they say it. Interpreting medical information into advice for the users needs expertise and evaluation to prevent unforeseen circumstances. Chatbots might create confusion instead of helping the users if it is not designed properly.

The following are some of the most common challenges.

### *14.7.1 Communiqué Elucidate*

Among the most common challenges with using Chatbots in customer support is identifying the individual's purpose and interpreting correct information. With humans known to different ways of expression, they say things in a variety of ways in contrast to machines that do it in one and only possible way. One of the several solutions to this is cautioning the user to be expressive using general terminologies, which will in turn simplify the processing of the request [45, 46].

### 14.7.2 Gadget-to-Human Leap

In certain cases, there must be swift shifting from Chatbots to humans from authoritative sources. Solution to this is based on severe analysis of the nature of responses with prearranged sequences to contemplate whether the human advice is needed. In certain cases, there must be swift shifting from a Chatbots to humans from authoritative sources. Solution to this is based on severe analysis of the nature of responses with prearranged sequences to contemplate whether the human advice is needed [45].

### 14.7.3 Personalization

Once the bot is user friendly, the next immediate step could be personalization. The best way to achieve this is by maintaining the individual records intact [45].

### 14.7.4 Chatbot Style

Additionally, what needs to be scrutinized is the style of Chatbot. The user would prefer an affecting interaction rather than dealing with answering machine which Chatbot basically is. It simply attributes to Chatbots having some style or attitude; one of the possibilities is selecting the gender of a bot. However, the most widely deployed practice is choosing several ways of interaction such as informal, more formal, or conservative [45].

### 14.7.5 AI Uncertainty

The opacity of the Chatbots develops hesitancy and uncertainty among the users due to which they are hesitant to utilize virtual device as healthcare assessment tool. The caliber, dependability, and precision of medical information are also doubted due to the mechanical complication of the Chatbots. The fear of misidentifying the manifestations and the incorrect interpretations of data contributes to one of the many obstacles in using Chatbots [46].

## 14.8 The Virtual Assessment Tool and Its Possibilities

Chatbots acted as a guardian angel for the entire customer service and healthcare organizations, which used to have thousands of panicked calls from the people due to this pandemic.

Some companies like Microsoft came up with a Chatbot, which will assist the recovered COVID-19 patients to donate plasma in order to facilitate treatment and further researches [47].

It is named CoVIg-19 Plasma Bot and is a part of CoVIg-19 Plasma Alliance, which is a collaboration of pharmaceutical companies, healthcare providers, and scientists that work together in order to receive donations for plasma research.

The CoVIg-19 Plasma Bot screens the individuals before they donate plasma by asking questions about their health status post COVID-19, last checkup, age, blood donation frequency, and records on STDs. The bot can also give information about the nearest plasma donation center by utilizing the data provided by the user.

This is a boon for the researching facilities, since the research on application of plasma to treat COVID-19 has been initiated. They use the recovered patient's plasma to give it to the diseased patients' transfusions and secondly to develop a possible treatment known as polyclonal hyperimmune globulin (H-Ig).

As stated by Hadas Bitran, group manager of Microsoft Healthcare Israel; Jean Gabarra, general manager of Health AI; and Dr. Greg Moore, corporate vice president of Microsoft Health on a post, "Through the product manufacturing process, multiple plasma donations are pooled together and the antibodies are concentrated to consistent and reliable levels, meaning the medicine can be delivered in lower volumes and therefore would likely take less time to administer to patients than plasma itself." Microsoft and the CoVIg-19 Plasma Alliance are focused on development of H-Ig treatment.

**Why Do We Need This?**

As per the latest World Health Organization statement, the global COVID-19 cases have exceeded 36.5 million. Researches are carried out worldwide in order to find out potential treatments. Plasma therapy is one of the promising treatments, and hence the CDC emboldened the COVID-19 survivors to donate plasma to facilitate research. The UK's NHS is also encouraging their recovered patients to help with the clinical trials. To overcome this pandemic, new treatment are required.

### *14.8.1 Product Service Bots on Webpage*

For instance, organizations, be it business, health institutions, or government that are overburdened with queries for coronavirus assessment and guidance, inquiries regarding stock availability, or simple questions about reduced operating time of essential services, can be assisted with these virtual assessment tool known as Chatbots.

### 14.8.2 Communication via SMS Chatbots

SMS bots will not only notify the individual of immediate information but also respond to the recipients solitarily. Various institutions and organizations are deploying voice-enabled devices to gain information hands-free. These tools are essential in health institutions and organizations, where individuals are more comfortable with speaking their request than to type it somewhere, more so to diminish the spread of infection and maintain sanitation. In a hospital, a voice-enabled bot can deliver an urgent message to healthcare professionals, request additional supplies, or keep track of quarantine records completely hands-free.

### 14.8.3 Teams Bots for Internal Maintenance

If the organization is deploying Microsoft Teams, a Chatbot can easily function via keeping everyone updated with information, whether it's a small school, which needs to maintain student's record, or an institution itself that needs to ensure standard and simple communications are encompassing all its employees.

### 14.8.4 Wearable Devices

Wearable tools are the devices which are worn by the users, and it has got an alert system to update them about the possible infections of COVID-19 before they are too ill, by the utilization of an early detection algorithm (EDA). Wearables with the help of EDA can detect the symptoms in their initial stages, thus providing users' time to seek help, quarantine themselves, and reduce the transferal of the infection. The users at the comfort of their houses, thus mitigating the transmission of the infection to the medical professionals and preserving hospital resources, can also use these devices [48].

With the help of remote patient monitoring, there can be development of more efficient ways to treat patients and reduce cost of treatment, and the balance between nurses and patients can be maintained.

Development of this technology has led to detection of the physiological symptoms much more precisely, which is very helpful in following the pandemic progression. This device has a broad spectrum of functions including identifying of patients under self-isolation who need critical care or a neighborhood where there's outbreak of the pandemic and need of an early interference. The major hindrance in utilizing the wearables faced by patients is the controversy of data confidentiality, underreporting, and information distribution. The companies making the wearables should ensure the users that they will maintain data privacy and use it for coronavirus research only. Countries like Germany have shown immense development in securing the patients' data. There may be requirement of privacy agreements and consent for information sharing to give superior care and reduce health discrepancies. Presently these devices are used in the COVID-19 crisis for molecular testing, gathering information from the users and providing data, but in the future it can be used for other outbreaks too. The devices can be improved by further development of the EDA to detect the fluctuations in the health of the population. The device can be accurately designed with the proficiency of scientists, engineers, doctors, and nurses if there's another outbreak of this pandemic.

## 14.9 Future Possibilities

When we see the success of Chatbots, we are convinced that we have finally found the bots which can have a conversation just like humans, but still they prove to be a disappointment sometimes since they don't know what the customer is expecting. This is because the uses of Chatbots are often exaggerated. We expect the bots to do everything without thinking if it is possible or not. Even a human assistant will get confused in those circumstances. But as long as the Chatbots do the work they are programmed to do, there are no worries. Without using artificial intelligence, the bots will become more like telephonic services that text and say "Press 1 for English, press 2 for French." This is helpful since it would consume less time and be accessible anytime. Following are the challenges the Chatbots face in today's world and what can be done to enhance the quality of the bots. These will make the Chatbots much more personalized.

### *14.9.1 Situation Awareness*

Nowadays the Chatbots are not aware of the context of the conversation. For example, when the individual says "Text mom to book the concert tickets from the website at 10 am," the Chatbot should be able to check the user's calendar and make sure it's free and be able to anticipate what the user is trying to say. Or if the user says, "Schedule the meet at noon" and then says "cancel it," the bot should be able to conclude what the user is talking about and hence identify the factor [14].

### *14.9.2 Types of Responses*

The Chatbots as of today are not able to differentiate between the responses to be given, i.e., if it should respond with the one set reply or choose between the series of responses. The future bots should be programmed in such a way that they can assess the circumstances and respond appropriately. They could be trained to have a pattern-based response [14].

### *14.9.3 Objective-Based Responses*

If the responses were generated on the basis of intention or the objective of the conversation, it would give rise to a variety of responses. But the Chatbots today have a fixed set of replies they give. When the information matches its data, it gives out the predefined response. So there is always a possibility of imprecise or inexact responses [14].

### *14.9.4 Identity*

In the future we would want our Chatbots to have a personality of their own. As we move forward, we need to add a human touch to the bots by instilling them with personality traits. For this the bots will have to be trained by adding a set of patterns and responses in particular situations according to the personality of the bot. This will be a very tiresome job to do. But this will ensure the humanizations of the Chatbots [49].

### *14.9.5 Customer Awareness*

For user friendliness the Chatbot should be aware of the individuals utilizing it. The bot should be able to recognize the user and know their predilection. This can be done by having access to the user's social media accounts, but it would be rather difficult to know the preference of the individuals who are not on such handles. For this research it is to be done on the user by the bot to collect all the significant data. This will make sure that the bot is personalized as per the needs of the customers [14].

### *14.9.6 Continuity*

For the Chatbot to behave as a personal assistant, it should be able to continue the conversations that were deserted halfway. If the user was previously talking about a location and mentioned any item and then asks "Do you recall the station where I left my luggage?" then the bot should be able to remember where the user is referring to and respond accordingly [14].

### *14.9.7 Narrative*

The Chatbot should always be able to narrate the sequence of events it was part of. For example, if the user has set up a calendar with events to be followed throughout the week, the bot should be able to recall them and narrate it to the users. And it should also add in its own reaction to the process. This has to be done in order of the sequence. As the bots are personalized, they should be able to remember the conversations they had with other family members and narrate them to the users [14].

## 14.10 Conclusion

Contemporary developments in Chatbots over various fields have made the implementation and utilization of these conversational agents in every walk of life. The worldwide authoritative sources such as WHO had recently asked for innovative pandemic responses [50]. For this purpose, Chatbots were utilized to battle against COVID-19. Chatbots have a crucial role in curbing the disease and all the consternation and confusion regarding its information. They can help in symptom detection, induce infection-reducing practice, and minimize the psychiatric health burden. In the near future, applications of Chatbots in healthcare will keep on flourishing. Now the Chatbots are not just a novelty to healthcare, they are an immediate addition to the medical management and preventive medicine. They are providing a bridge between the patients and healthcare [75, 76].

## References


1. Sudareswaran, V., & Firth-Butterfield, K. https://www.weforum.org/agenda/2020/04/chatbots-covid-19-governance-improved-here-s-how/
2. WHO. (2020). Novel Corona virus, emergencies preparedness, response. *Disease Outbreak News*. https://www.who.int/csr/don/12-january-2020-novel-coronavirus-china/en/
3. WHO. (2020). WHO Health alert brings COVID-19 facts to billions via WhatsApp. *WHO*. https://web.archive.org/web/20200323042822/https://www.who.int/news-room/feature-stories/detail/who-health-alert-brings-covid-19-facts-to-billions-via-whatsapp
4. CDC. (2020). Coronavirus disease 2019 (COVID-19)—symptoms. *Centers for Disease Control and Prevention*. https://www.cdc.gov/coronavirus/2019-ncov/symptomstesting/symptoms.html; https://www.cdc.gov/coronavirus/2019-ncov/community/general-business-faq.html
5. He, J., Baxter, S. L., Xu, J., et al. (2019). The practical implementation of artificial intelligence technologies in medicine. *Nature Medicine, 25*, 30–36. https://doi.org/10.1038/s41591-018-0307-0.
6. Vosoughi, S., Roy, D., & Aral, S. (2018). The spread of true and false news online. *Science, 359*, 1146–1151.
7. Vaidyam, A. N., Wisniewski, H., Halamka, J. D., Kashavan, M. S., & Torous, J. B. (2019). Chatbots and conversational agents in mental health: A review of the psychiatric landscape. *Canadian Journal of Psychiatry, 64*, 456–464.

8. Mauldin, M. L. (1994). ChatterBots, TinyMuds, and the Turing test: Entering the Loebner Prize competition. In *Proceedings of the 12th national conference on artificial intelligence*.
9. Ayedoun, E., Hayashi, Y., & Seta, K. (2015). A conversational agent to encourage willingness to communicate in the context of English as a foreign language. *Procedia Computer Science, 60*(1), 1433–1442. https://www.sciencedirect.com/science/article/pii/S1877050915023467.
10. Raine, R. (2009). Making a clever intelligent agent: The theory behind the implementation. In *2009 IEEE international conference on intelligent computing and intelligent systems. Deep Learning for Chatbots* (p. 53).
11. alicebot.org. *Alicebot technology history*. [Online]. Available: http://www.alicebot.org/history/technology.html
12. Chatbots.org. *Smarterchild.* [Online]. Available: https://www.chatbots.org/chatterbot/smarterchild/; https://chatbotslife.com/chatbots-past-present-future-13a5cb026b18
13. Priyadarshini, A. (2019). *A complete guide to Chatbots*. https://blog.kore.ai/a-complete-guide-to-chatbots
14. Nimavat, K., & Champaneria, T. (2017). Chatbots: An overview types, architecture, tools and future possibilities. *International Journal of Scientific Research and Development, 5*, 1019–1024. https://www.researchgate.net/publication/320307269_Chatbots_An_overview_Types_Architecture_Tools_and_Future_Possibilities.
15. Hien, H. T., Cuong, P.-N., Nam, L. N. H., Nhung, H. L. T. K., & Thang, L. D. (2018). Intelligent assistants in higher-education environments: The FIT-EBot, a chatbot for administrative and learning support. In *Proceedings of the ninth international symposium on information and communication technology* (pp. 69–76). New York: ACM. https://dl.acm.org/doi/abs/10.1145/3287921.3287937.
16. Wu, Y., Wu, W., Xing, C., Zhou, M., & Li, Z. (2016). *Sequential matching network: A new architecture for multi-turn response selection in retrieval-based Chatbots*. https://arxiv.org/abs/1612.01627
17. Surmenok, P. (2016). *Chatbot architecture*. http://pavel.surmenok.com/2016/09/11/chatbot-architecture/
18. Smith, A. (2020). *Understanding architecture models of Chatbot and response generation mechanisms*. https://dzone.com/articles/understanding-architecture-models-of-chatbot-and-r
19. Battineni, G., Chintalapudi, N., & Amenta, F. (2020). AI Chatbot design during an epidemic like the novel coronavirus. *Healthcare, 8*, 154. https://www.mdpi.com/2227-9032/8/2/154.
20. Li, Q., & Chen, Y. P. (2010). Personalized text snippet extraction using statistical language models. *Pattern Recognition, 43*, 378–386.
21. Lommel, A., & Cirillo, C. (2017). *Chatbots from Czech to Chinese (and everywhere in between) chief marketer*. https://www.chiefmarketer.com/chatbots-czech-chinese-everywhere/
22. Lundqvist, K. O., Pursey, G., & Williams, S. (Eds.). (2013). *Design and implementation of conversational agents for harvesting feedback in eLearning systems*. Springer. https://link.springer.com/chapter/10.1007/978-3-642-40814-4_79.
23. Oudeyer, P.-Y., Gottlieb, J., & Lopes, M. (2016). Chapter 11 – Intrinsic motivation, curiosity, and learning: Theory and applications in educational technologies. In B. S. A. S. Knecht (Ed.), *39 Progress in brain research: Motivation theory, neurobiology and applications* (Vol. 229, pp. 257–284). Elsevier. https://www.sciencedirect.com/science/article/pii/S0079612316300589.
24. van der Meij, H., van der Meij, J., & Harmsen, R. (2015). Animated pedagogical agents effects on enhancing student motivation and learning in a science inquiry learning environment. *Educational Technology Research and Development, 63*(3), 381–403. https://link.springer.com/article/10.1007%252Fs11423-015-9378-5.
25. Schunk, D. H. (1991). Self-efficacy and academic motivation. *Educational Psychologist, 26*(3–4), 207–223. https://www.tandfonline.com/doi/abs/10.1080/00461520.1991.9653133.
26. Mero, J. (2018). The effects of two-way communication and chat service usage on consumer attitudes in the e-commerce retailing sector. *Electronic Markets, 28*(2), 205–217. https://link.springer.com/article/10.1007/s12525-017-0281-2.

27. Weizenbaum, J. (1966). ELIZA—A computer program for the study of natural language communication between man and machine. *Communications of the ACM, 9*(1), 36–45. https://dl.acm.org/doi/abs/10.1145/365153.365168.
28. Adam, M., Toutaoui, J., Pfeuffer, N., & Hinz, O. (2019). Investment decisions with robo-advisors: The role of anthropomorphism and personalized anchors in recommendations. In *Proceedings of the 27th European conference on information systems (ECIS)*. Sweden: Stockholm & Uppsala. https://aisel.aisnet.org/ecis2019_rp/33/.
29. Adam, M., Wessel, M., & Benlian, A. (2020). AI-based chatbots in customer service and their effects on user compliance. *Electron Markets*. https://doi.org/10.1007/s12525-020-00414-7.
30. Miner, A. S., Laranjo, L., & Kocaballi, A. B. (2020). Chatbots in the fight against the COVID-19 pandemic. *NPJ Digital Medicine, 3*, 65. https://doi.org/10.1038/s41746-020-0280-0.
31. Zheng, J. (2020). SARS-CoV-2: An emerging coronavirus that causes a global threat. *International Journal of Biological Sciences, 16*(10), 1678–1685. https://www.ncbi.nlm.nih.gov/pmc/articles/PMC7098030/.
32. Zhang, W., Du, R. H., Li, B., Zheng, X. S., Yang, X. L., Hu, B., et al. (2020). Molecular and serological investigation of 2019-nCoV infected patients: Implication of multiple shedding routes. *Emerging Microbes & Infections, 9*(1), 386–389. https://www.tandfonline.com/doi/full/10.1080/22221751.2020.1729071.
33. Guo, Y., Cao, Q., Hong, Z., et al. (2020). The origin, transmission and clinical therapies on coronavirus disease 2019 (COVID-19) outbreak – An update on the status. *Military Medical Research, 7*, 11. https://doi.org/10.1186/s40779-020-00240-0.
34. WHO. https://www.who.int/news-room/feature-stories/detail/who-and-rakuten-viber-fight-covid-19-misinformation-with-interactive-Chatbot
35. CDC. Coronavirus disease 2019 (COVID-19)—symptoms. *Centers for Disease Control and Prevention*. https://www.cdc.gov/coronavirus/2019-ncov/symptoms-testing/testing.html
36. Zumla, A., Chan, J. F., Azhar, E. I., Hui, D. S., & Yuen, K. Y. (2016). Coronaviruses - drug discovery and therapeutic options. *Nature Reviews. Drug Discovery, 15*(5), 327–347. https://www.nature.com/articles/nrd.2015.37.
37. Li, H., Wang, Y. M., Xu, J. Y., & Cao, B. (2020). Potential antiviral therapeutics for 2019 Novel Coronavirus. *Chinese Journal of Tuberculosis and Respiratory Diseases, 43*(0), E002.
38. Wang, D., Hu, B., Hu, C., Zhu, F., Liu, X., Zhang, J., et al. (2020). Clinical characteristics of 138 hospitalized patients with 2019 novel coronavirus-infected pneumonia in Wuhan, China. *Journal of the American Medical Association*. https://doi.org/10.1001/jama.2020.1585.
39. Agostini, M. L., Andres, E. L., Sims, A. C., Graham, R. L., Sheahan, T. P., Lu, X., et al. (2018). Coronavirus susceptibility to the antiviral remdesivir (GS-5734) is mediated by the viral polymerase and the proofreading exoribonuclease. *MBio, 9*(2), e00221-18. https://mbio.asm.org/content/9/2/e00221-18.short.
40. Vincent, M. J., Bergeron, E., Benjannet, S., Erickson, B. R., Rollin, P. E., Ksiazek, T. G., et al. (2005). Chloroquine is a potent inhibitor of SARS coronavirus infection and spread. *Virology Journal, 2*, 69.
41. Golden, E. B., Cho, H. Y., Hofman, F. M., Louie, S. G., Schonthal, A. H., & Chen, T. C. (2015). Quinoline-based antimalarial drugs: A novel class of autophagy inhibitors. *Neurosurgical Focus, 38*(3), E12.
42. National Health Commission of the People's Republic of China. (2020). *Diagnosis and treatment of pneumonia caused by 2019-nCoV (version 6)*. http://www.gov.cn/zhengce/zhengceku/2020-02/19/content_5480948.htm
43. WHO. *Clinical management of severe acute respiratory infection when novel coronavirus (nCoV) infection is suspected*. https://www.who.int/publications-detail/clinical-management-of-severe-acute-respiratory-infection-when-novel-coronavirus-(ncov)-infection-is-suspected
44. Medeiros, J. (2020). 4 helpful Chatbots guiding people through the pandemic. *Voice*. https://www.voicesummit.ai/blog/4-helpful-chatbots-that-are-guiding-people-through-the-pandemic
45. Wade, M. (2019). Useful Chatbot Solution ideas to help during COVID-19. How to quickly scale up customer service ops with Chatbots. *Blog on AtBot*. https://blog.getbizzy.io/useful-chatbot-solution-ideas-to-help-during-covid-19-4421f1a06c8e

46. Nadarzynski, T., Miles, O., Cowie, A., & Ridge, D. (2020). Acceptability of artificial intelligence (AI)-led Chatbot services in healthcare: A mixed-methods study research article digital health-2019 National Health Commission of the People's Republic of China. *Diagnosis and treatment of pneumonia caused by 2019-nCoV (version 6)*. https://journals.sagepub.com/doi/full/10.1177/2055207619871808
47. Lovett, L. https://www.google.com/amp/s/www.dailymail.co.uk/sciencetech/article-8241623/amp/Microsoft-set-launch-plasmabot-help-recovered-coronavirus-patients-donate-plasma.html
48. Sohrabi, C., Alsafi, Z., O'Neill, N., Khan, M., Kerwan, A., Al-Jabir, A., Iosifidis, C., & Agha, R. (2020). World Health Organization declares global emergency: A review of the 2019 novel coronavirus (COVID-19). *International Journal of Surgery, 76*, 71–76. https://www.sciencedirect.com/science/article/pii/S1743919120301977.
49. Jokinen, K., & Wilcock, G. (2003). Adaptivity and response generation in a spoken dialogue system. In J. van Kuppevelt & R. W. Smith (Eds.), *Current and new directions in discourse and dialogue. Text, speech and language technology* (Vol. 22). Dordrecht: Springer. https://doi.org/10.1007/978-94-010-0019-2_10.
50. WHO. (2020). Director-general's opening remarks at the media briefing on COVID-19. *WHO*. https://www.who.int/dg/speeches/detail/who-director-general-s-opening-remarks-at-the-media-briefing-on-covid-19
51. Byers, D. (2020). The US wants smartphone location data to fight coronavirus. Privacy advocates are worried. *NBC News*. https://www.nbcnews.com/tech/tech-news/u-s-wants-smartphone-location-data-fight-coronavirus-privacy-advocates-n1162821
52. Larson, H. J. (2018). The biggest pandemic risk? Viral misinformation. *Nature, 562*, 309.
53. Brooks, S. K., et al. (2020). The psychological impact of quarantine and how to reduce it: Rapid review of the evidence. *Lancet, 395*, 912–920.
54. Mak, I. W., Chu, C. M., Pan, P. C., Yiu, M. G., & Chan, V. L. (2009). Long-term psychiatric morbidities among SARS survivors. *General Hospital Psychiatry, 31*, 318–326.
55. The Behavioral Insights Team. Covid-19: How do we encourage the right behaviours during an epidemic? *The Behavioral Insights Team*. https://www.bi.team/blogs/covid-19-how-do-we-encourage-the-right-behaviours-during-an-epidemic/
56. Sharma, M., Yadav, K., Yadav, N., & Ferdinand, K. C. (2017). Zika virus pandemic-analysis of Facebook as a social media health information platform. *American Journal of Infection Control, 45*, 301–302.
57. Intermountain Healthcare. *Covid19 Symptom Checker*. https://intermountainhealthcare.org/covid19-coronavirus/covid19-symptom-checker/
58. Michie, S., West, R., & Amlot, R. Behavioural strategies for reducing covid-19 transmission in the general population. *BMJ*. https://www.nature.com/articles/s41562-020-0887-9
59. Bickmore, T. M., Pfeifer, L. M., & Jack, B. W. (2009). Taking the time to care: Empowering low health literacy hospital patients with virtual nurse agents. In *Proceedings of the SIGCHI conference on human factors in computing systems* (pp. 1265–1274). New York: Association for Computing Machinery.
60. Ho, A., Hancock, J., & Miner, A. S. (2018). Psychological, relational, and emotional effects of self-disclosure after conversations with a Chatbot. *The Journal of Communication, 68*, 712–733.
61. Huremović, D. in Psychiatry of pandemics: A mental health response to infection outbreak (Huremović, D) 95–118 (Springer Nature Switzerland AG, Basel, 2019).
62. Mak, W. W., et al. (2009). A comparative study of the stigma associated with infectious diseases (SARS. AIDS, TB). *Hong Kong Medical Journal, 15*, s34–s37.
63. Berger, M., Wagner, T. H., & Baker, L. C. (2005). Internet use and stigmatized illness. *Social Science & Medicine, 61*, 1821–1827.
64. Lucas, G. M., Gratch, J., King, A., & Morency, L. P. (2014). It's only a computer: Virtual humans increase willingness to disclose. *Computers in Human Behavior, 37*, 94–100.

65. Steinhubl, S. R., & Topol, E. J. (2018). Now we're talking: Bringing a voice to digital medicine. *Lancet, 392*, 627.
66. Jadhav, K. P., & Thorat, S. A. (2020). Towards designing conversational agent systems. In *Advances in intelligent systems and computing*. Berlin: Springer.
67. Yan, R. "Chitty-chitty-chat bot": Deep learning for conversational AI. In *Proceedings of the twenty-seventh international joint conference on artificial intelligence (IJCAI-18)*. Stockholm, Sweden, 13–19 July 2018.
68. Aguiar, A. C. C., Murce, E., Cortopassi, W. A., Pimentel, A. S., Almeida, M., Barros, D. C. S., et al. (2018). Chloroquineanalogs as antimalarial candidates with potent in vitro and in vivo activity. *International Journal for Parasitology: Drugs and Drug Resistance, 8*(3), 459–464.
69. Savarino, A., Boelaert, J. R., Cassone, A., Majori, G., & Cauda, R. (2003). Effects of chloroquine on viral infections: An old drug against today's diseases? *The Lancet Infectious Diseases, 3*(11), 722–727.
70. Lee, P. I., & Hsueh, P. R. (2020). Emerging threats from zoonotic coronaviruses-from SARS and MERS to 2019-nCoV. *Journal of Microbiology, Immunology, and Infection*. https://www.sciencedirect.com/science/article/pii/S1684118220300943.
71. Hamming, I., Timens, W., Bulthuis, M. L., Lely, A. T., Navis, G., & van Goor, H. (2004). Tissue distribution of ACE2 protein, the functional receptor for SARS coronavirus. A first step in understanding SARS pathogenesis. *The Journal of Pathology, 203*(2), 631–637.
72. Jin, Y. H., Cai, L., Cheng, Z. S., Cheng, H., Deng, T., Fan, Y. P., et al. (2020). A rapid advice guideline for the diagnosis and treatment of 2019 novel coronavirus (2019-nCoV) infected pneumonia (standard version). *Military Medical Research, 7*(1), 4.
73. Poutanen, S. M., Low, D. E., Henry, B., Finkelstein, S., Rose, D., Green, K., et al. (2003). Identification of severe acute respiratory syndrome in Canada. *The New England Journal of Medicine, 348*(20), 1995–2005.
74. Huang, C., Wang, Y., Li, X., Ren, L., Zhao, J., Hu, Y., et al. (2020). Clinical features of patients infected with 2019 novel coronavirus in Wuhan, China. *Lancet, 395*(10223), 497–506.
75. Rani, S., & Kautish, S. (2018). Association clustering and time series based data mining in continuous data for diabetes prediction. In *2018 second international conference on intelligent computing and control systems (ICICCS)* (pp. 1209–1214). IEEE. https://ieeexplore.ieee.org/document/8662909.
76. Sampathkumar, A., Rastogi, R., Arukonda, S., Shankar, A., Kautish, S., & Sivaram, M. (2020). An efficient hybrid methodology for detection of cancer- causing gene using CSC for micro array data. *Journal of Ambient Intelligence and Humanized Computing*, 1–9.


**Aasma Chouhan** is a fourth year B. pharmacy student at H.K College of Pharmacy, Mumbai India. She has received numerous accolades in her field. Her major thrust areas for research include pharmaceutical chemistry, biochemistry, and drug analysis.

**Supriya Pathak** is studying in final year B. pharmacy at H.K college of Pharmacy, Mumbai India. She has been part of various curricular and co-curricular activities. Her main area of interests includes drug discovery and development, formulation designing, and biotechnology.

**Reshma Tendulkar** is working as an assistant professor, HOD of Pharmaceutical Chemistry department in H.K. College of Pharmacy, Jogeshwari, Mumbai. She is having 12 years of experience in teaching. She has completed her PhD from C.U. Shah College of Pharmacy, S.N.D.T University. Main areas of research are drug synthesis and computer-aided drug designing.

# Chapter 15
# Enabled IoT Applications for Covid-19

**A. Gasmi**

## 15.1 Introduction

Coronavirus is an acute respiratory-contagious pneumonia, linked to the SARS-CoV-2 family, deadly attack on human organs via 1-beta hemoglobin chain synthesis 1–5% of multiple linear regressions analyzed to have evolved from Puglia, sardine, and Sicilia. The beta thalassemia heterozygote affects the human immune system, causing temperature increase above 380°, dry cough, fatigue, breathing difficulty, dyspnea, and diarrhea. Some patients may report thrombotic complication known as acute pulmonary infection [44].

The global surge in demand for personal protective equipment and overwhelming demand placed on medical care facilities made it critical to seek for an alternative invention of screening tools, infection tracking, and vaccine development. Research presently going on will explore emerging technologies for achieving innovative concepts during quarantine, social distancing, use of Internet of Things (IoT) to detect errors, change requirements, and process future treatments [73].

Ravi et al. [28] introduced "Internet of Medical Things" (IOMT), to confront Covid-19 pandemic issues, just as it was previously used to diagnose orthopedic patients. Orthopedic IOMT was successfully used for data sharing, report monitoring, patient tracking, information gathering, hygiene optimization. as well as providing medical care for sick patients [45]. The same can be said about the recent introduction of industry 4.0 technologies that aid proper isolation, reduce the spread of Covid-19, and are used for telemedicine and manufacturing of personal protective equipment. IOMT testing methods involve PCR assay called "RRT-PCR,"

A. Gasmi (✉)
Interuniversity Laboratory of Motor Biology, University of Claude Bernard, Lyon, France

Société Francophone de Nutrithérapie et de Nutrigénétique Appliquée, Villeurbanne, France



S. Kautish et al. (eds.), *Computational Intelligence Techniques for Combating COVID-19*, EAI/Springer Innovations in Communication and Computing,
https://doi.org/10.1007/978-3-030-68936-0_15

a molecular assay that will not only control the pandemic but also act as a lateral flow immunoassay tool that detects human transmission via serum [65].

Internet of Medical Things device called the "POC LFIA" device can detect IgG and RGM antibody level during screening to show asymptotic carriers of Covid-19 within 20 minutes. Other lateral flow immunoassay tools (LFIA) are used as home-testing kits that show positive test results via specimens, referred to as "Nucleo-Capsid" (N) or "Spike" proteins from nasal swabs [63].

Another unique IoT tool called nano-biosensing system acts as an intelligent healthcare device used to investigate Covid-19 early development since it shows low-level detection by demonstrating disease biomark Pm level [60].

However, Cognitive Internet of Medical Things (CIOMT) was developed to tackle Covid-19 issues using CR-based dynamic spectrum technique that offers rapid diagnosis by referring to previous reports. It also clusters, screens, and surveys medical workload for preventing control of the infection [27].

Elijah et al. [85] disclose dozens of IoT applications implored online for medical care and health services for checking vital signs, detecting viral infections, and handling medic-data analytics. IoT platform through fog and cloud network can control potential spread of Covid-19 and estimate quarantine timing, contact tracing, and social distancing. Below image demonstrates the IoT platform implemented using fog/cloud network to forecast Covid-19 outbreak (Fig. 15.1).

According to the image, there are five sections: implement, prevention/control, diagnosis and monitoring, contact tracing, and social distancing. IoT can be used to prevent the spread of Covid-19, especially its wearable sensors. It's necessary for gathering information, notification of signs/symptoms, and sensing data transmitted on Wi-Fi/4G and 5G that monitors human activities. The fog network consists of nodes deployed with network connections (like physical LAN connected processor). It can also compute data generated from IoT sensors [86]. Fog layer implements time sensitivity for monitoring quarantine, predicting contact tracing, and social distancing.

Enabled IoT for predicting Covid-19 involves data streaming in a centralized cloud server capable of tracing outbreak and controlling CoV-2 mutation. Vishwakarma and Agrawal [102] discussed the use of perception layer to sense the environment and acquire real-time data for medical investigations. Perception layer

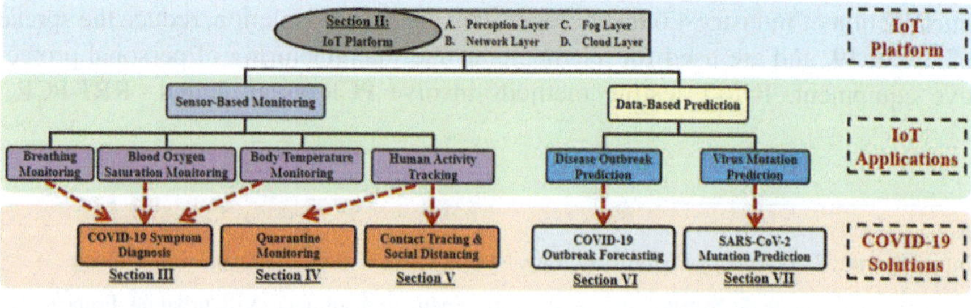


**Fig. 15.1** IoT platform implemented on fog/cloud network, predicting/forecasting covid-19 outbreak [85]

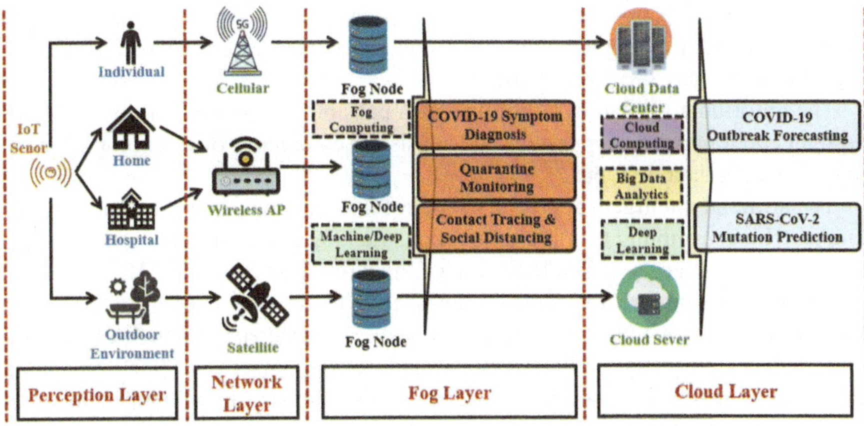


**Fig 15.2** IoT platform for controlling, preventing and managing covid-19 [103]

devices include a camera, inertial sensor, magnetometer, microphones, commodity Wi-Fi, MW-wave radar, and RFID [87, 92]. The diagram below shows the interrelationship between perception layer, network, and fog layers (Fig. 15.2).

According to the above diagram, the perception layer devices in the form of camera and other IoT sensors generate data from the hospital, individuals, and homes. The generated datasets are linked to either wireless app, satellites, and cellular data connection using 3G and 4G networks. The authenticated data linked to networks are placed on fog layers and interconnected to fog nodes to predict Covid-19 symptoms and monitor quarantine and contact tracing. The cloud layer stores generated data in the data center/cloud server after the forecast [88–91].

### *15.1.1 Context and Background*

Coronavirus outbreak commences 2019 December in Wuhan, China, and has excessively spread around the globe. The World Health Organization advises governments to enforce lockdown and travel restrictive measures to combat the spread of this virus. China launched the IoT application health status code tool that shows green, red, or yellow code that can be used to know if the applicant is fit to travel and can move around and have social contact with people. According to Chinese Government Classification, if the test results show red or yellow codes, it signifies that the applicant is unfit to travel and may need further medical tests to verify if they need 7–14 days of quarantine [11].

Despite the effort exercised by WHO and Public Health Emergency of International Concern (PHEIC) and global regulatory rules of government and the struggle of the healthcare system, inferred behavioral statistics shows that people infected are mostly diabetic patients, elderly, and health compromised people.

Patient's recovery patterns show records of different methods of recuperation; people get infected via droplets and direct contact with infected person. Incubation period ranges from 2 to 14 days [61].

The unfortunate situation of not finding a possible vaccine or cure of Covid-19 brought about preventive measures and consistent emergence of technologies in the best of AI, big data, IoT, etc.

The artificial intelligent approach to control the pandemic follows clinical symptom matching, sampling to confirm infection, tracking and treating, monitoring, and recovering phase analysis and later conducting a retest on patients [22].

Furthermore, Internet of Medical Things (IOMT) means connecting nodes to the Internet and in turn analyzes patient complexes and evaluates its high error rates, time and cost, privacy and limitations, and security, necessary for eradicating Covid-19 ailments. The process involves numerous computational models to structure protein to protein interactive network (PPIN), in turn, to predict amino acid of basic and advanced biological features of the patient. The network IOMT interaction passes through discrete wavelength and entropic sequence. The network IOMT process is monitored using partial tree and non-nested generalized exemplar (NNGE) that identifies human protein complexes, experiments, and provides useful outcomes. The results can further be integrated with mining algorithms such as Bayesian probability network (BN) and random forest to determine its accuracy and efficiency and provide the needed privacy [66].

The connection of computing nodes to medical equipment allows to discover aliment, preventive and protective equipment and measures, and cures regarded as IOMT.

During the lockdown, some patients with other medical conditions find it impossible to access routine treatments and regular follow-ups. For instance, patients with orthopedic issues face the challenges of medical inaccessibility to resolve fractures and obtain surgery, joint replacement, and arthroscopic and spinal repair. IOMT approach has been researched to enable integrated healthcare appliance for treatment, data collection, report monitoring, and handling of the patient database reviewing x-ray images, analyzing, and connecting medic workflow [67]. IOMT can enable proactive supervision, diagnosis, and treatment, whereas the cost of medicare will be reduced and emergency handled and monitoring made easier.

Some experts referred to IoT as an application that supports biometric test like blood pressure and vital signs. The essence of IoT is to reduce the chances of mistakes made while handling Covid-19 issues, lessen the cost of implementation, and to have better treatment and effective and efficient control while providing an enhanced diagnosis. It can also minimize workloads for healthcare practitioners; monitor remote area access, virtual management, and communication; analyze received data; and follow up on reports [64]. The Indian Government on the Covid-19 crisis launched Aarogya Setu application and China introduced the close contact application to demonstrate how users get infected by being closer to others. Taiwan militarizes its regulation to suppress Covid-19 increase and provide database and uses big data analytics to subdue travel while scanning and separating infected from non-infected. They also used QR barcode screening to report identities and travel history [67].

## 15.2 IoT and Its Interrelated Discoveries for Alleviating Covid-19 Problems

Covid-19 gave rise to new habits and innovative space discovery of 5G network, necessarily significant in telemedicine consulting and advancement of artificial intelligence (AI) in contextual medical diagnosis like tomography scan for pandemic diagnosis [77]. The demand for personal health applications and remote medical surveillance system known as M-health is quite increasing in Pakistan. M-health can be used to capture and store health statistics via integrating sensors and biomedical acquired systems [38].

The M-health IoT offers full care to patients using flexible systems to determine health conditions while providing necessary diagnoses. Shun et al. [37] designed M-health coordinating device called Dim/COAP that shows HTTP performance, packet loss rates, and syntax using JSON and XML. The COAP can transmit packets to HTTP and XML without consuming more resources than JSON.

Huang et al. [49] believed that MNS (medical nursing system) can support IoT, when implemented with 2G–3G, WSN, RFID, sensor, Zigbee, Wi-Fi, and Bluetooth. The essence is to aid Covid-19 vaccine research by enabling its drug accuracy. Fan et al. [76] conducted SOA research ontology for resource allocation and rehabilitation to aid patients recovering from Covid-19 [76].

Some experts furthered M-health research by analyzing open gateway that will work with 5G networks, while Dr. Salah's medical sensing device helped to minimize queues, monitor patient's physical conditions, and implement social distancing [34]. Further research shows coronavirus impact on body organs led to CAD algorithms that show abnormalities in the kidney ultrasonic image of the FPGA files, using two models known as LUT and Sum, supported by vector and Kintex machines [26].

Chavan et al.'s [39] objective assumptions on the pneumonia effect of Covid-19 on the heart can easily be detected using the ECG monitoring wave device. The ECG monitoring process at this Covid-19 era aids design of IoT for tracking the patient's heart rate value, represented as a band or smart health band.

Li et al. [10] used his OSA (obstructive sleep apnea) device to demonstrate sleep problems in aging adults and monitor aging patient's respiratory unrest and other related health issues. Chinese IoT experts [74] study cardiac signal of patients with Covid-19 focusing only on entropy heart rates using some mathematical models to monitor the process. Kaushik et al. [56] emphasize that IMUs (inertia measurement units) can be utilized to boost IOMT accuracy, improve sensing algorithms, and enable IoT flexible devices.

Deep learning cardiac image processing can manage and monitor data collected via IOMT using wearable devices. IoT has been promoted as an intelligence small sensor electronics interacting with Internet access and other features such as biological sensor nodes that use wireless transmitters to check abnormalities in patients' vital signs; physiological signals like temperature, heartbeats, and blood pressure; and cardiac images [46].

It consists of wearable sensors that transmit and sense data to a wireless channel, comes in small size, and is lightweight and power-constrained. There are recognizable techniques for energy optimization, which enhances battery life, maximize access control (MAC), physical layer, network topology, and power control transmission in IOMT. Such technique includes self-adaptive power control base that enhances energy-aware approach (EEA), conventional TPC, DL-IOMT framework, PLR, RSSI indicators, and full-battery model [39].

The Cloud Plus Terminal, known as "nCapp", is an intelligent assisted diagnosis and treatment tool that will help to alleviate the spread of Covid-19. nCapp has IoT functionality that executes management, command, and diagnosis in one click; it possesses eight functions which are register, consult, diagnose, treat, list specialist on duty, identify the location using maps, offer protection, and information [74].

When nCapp is compared with P4 traditional medicine of predicting, preventing, personalizing, and participatory form of medical service, NCAPP ensures to beat the procedure since it conducts online monitoring, location tracking, etc. To perfect diagnosis, nCapp offers intelligent assisted diagnoses by confirming suspected patients' status whether it is mild, moderate, severe, or critical while suggesting antiviral or antibacterial treatment and scheduling an online appointment or physical visit to the hospital [9].

nCapp according to Shanghai respiratory clinical quality control center will ensure proper respiratory support in case of HFNO/NIV respiratory distress to relieve patients using oxygen therapy. Some patients suffer respiratory distress within 2 hours that requires an invasive mechanical ventilator to decrease the tidal volume of 4–8 ml/Kg and plateau pressure (30cmH2O), with other sedative strategies that can salvage patients with severe acute respiratory distress [47]. nCapp circulates fluid resuscitation and administers vasoactive drugs to improve microcirculation and hemodynamic status. nCapp is intelligent enough to use CT images and activate an inflammatory response to recommend dosages of glucocorticoid drugs equivalent to 1–2 mg/kg of methylprednisolone daily. For Covid-19 issues, it can suppress immune-compromised with immunosuppressive effects while administering regulators to maintain intestinal balance and prevention of repetitive infection [48].

nCapp works as an assisting IoT tool to perfect self-prevention and management via handling isolation and protection and reserving qualified and sufficient protective materials while disinfecting mask, protective equipment, isolation gowns, etc. It can also be used to strengthen measures for preventing viral transmission through droplets and airborne transmission [66].

nCapp can be used for staffing to identify and recommend experts, online consultation, QC consensus, science education, and expert forums [68].

**How Enabled IoT Applications Help Patients to Recover from Covid-19**

Hernandez et al. [93] affirm that breathing rates and patterns can reveal physical condition of patients. IoT wearables improve breath monitoring whereas IoT inertia sensors, mm-wave & radar are used to monitor breath rates. Hernandez et al. [93]

mentioned biowatch accelerometer and gyroscope mounted wrist device for analyzing breath rates. Biowatch helps to monitor Covid-19 patients recovering from the infection by showing their band-pass digit filtered frequency from 0.13 to 0.66hz.

Murpthy et al. [94] enhance data accuracy extracted from breathing and posture patterns from inertia sensor data to predict changes in breathing, specifically to determine whether a patient is gradually recovering. Murpthy et al. [94] measure SPO2 breath rate using thermal cameras to capture exhaled air flows, as illustrated below.

Petkie et al. [95] monitored breath motion using RF sensing technique on radar WIF to reveal continuous wave Doppler radars while measuring chest displacement. IoT applications monitor blood oxygen saturation (SPO2) of patients with Covid-19 since infected patients experience low blood SPO2. Low blood spo2 is an early symptom that can be treated with supplemented oxygen to boost blood spo2 level. It can monitor changes of blood spo2 which predicts Covid-19 virus. Chan et al. [96] suggest the use of IoT pulse oximeter and noninvasive device that measures patient's spo2. High temperature is another known symptom of Covid-19. Sixty-six advise hospitals to set up infrared IoT temp-sensors that check patient's body temperature on entry points. The diagram below demonstrates hybrid sensory IoT networks for monitoring healthcare against Covid-19 (Fig. 15.3).

Chan et al. [96] explored the use of IoT infrared thermography (IRT) camera to screen out patients with fever. IRT can be placed in public places (airports) to trace infected patients and to isolate immediately.

The objective behind the use of IoT applications relies on tracing, predicting, and isolating infected patients. IoT tools according to Baker et al. [97] help to maintain quarantine monitoring by ensuring that infected individuals are separated from non-infected individuals.

IoT conventional quarantine procedure consists of checking patients' vital signs and monitoring their activities during isolation. Catarinnurcci et al. [98] discussed the integration of RFID with WSN architecture to lower costs of screening patients and power consumption during patients' monitoring. The procedure evaluates patients' physiological data like heartbeat and pulse to monitor recovery during quarantines.

The diagram below illustrates IoT magnetometers based on contact tracing and social distancing (Fig. 15.4).

IoT application offers tremendous support to hospitals seeking to achieve contact tracing and social distancing. Some IoT devices have GPS, microphones, and magnetometer for proximity detection [99].

Recent researchers adopted microphone and IoT ambient sound and calculated the acoustic power spectrum by estimating the distance from one person to another [100].

Liu et al. [101] combined RF-based signs (e.g., Bluetooth and Wi-Fi) to explore proximity. The Table 15.1 below demonstrates IoT applications that offer solutions to Covid-19 virus.

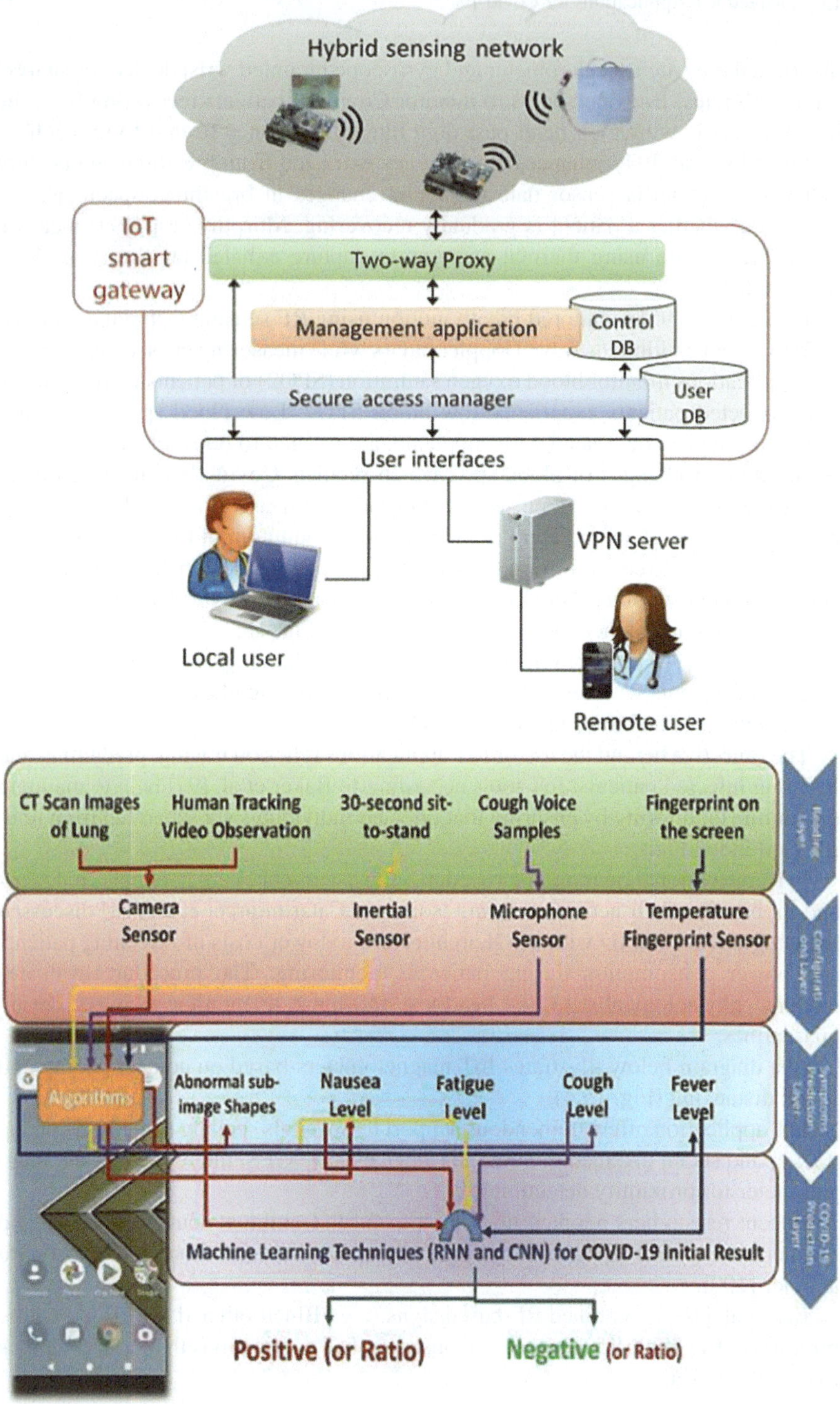


**Fig 15.3** Sensory IoT network for monitoring healthcare against covid-19 [104]

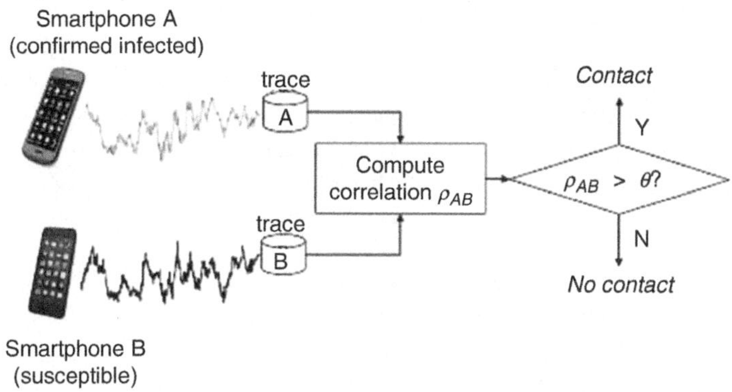


**Fig 15.4** Smart IoT magnetometers showing computable contact tracing and social distance matrix [98]

## 15.3 IoT Significance to Covid-19 Pandemic

IoT may help researchers to obtain a convenient and cheap outcome that can improve patient's recovery and minimize person to person transmission and managing of disease. For upgraded IoT technologies to experience countless enhancements and meet clinical requirements, lots of testing, experiments, and implementation are needed whereby polymerase chain reaction (PCR) will be utilized to diagnose diseases due to its level of accuracy. The serologic and antigen testing technique helps to demonstrate immune and antibody situations using 15–30-minute quick test [44].

To predict and classify infections using surveillance systems, BlueDot was invented to scan viruses via imploring algorithms in pneumonia cases. Such prediction needs metabiota natural language processing to alert people of the result using different languages [48].

Due to predictable errors in big data transmission that can lead to inaccurate diagnosis, IoT in healthcare gives an immediate data analysis and real-time decision without delays from mobile end user to cloud server. Fog layer aids cloud server implementation using IoT-based sensor to generate data processing, store, and provide results. Fog computing is quite essential in IoT-based health service due to its effective utilization for resource management, quality assurance, accessibility of medical information, and operating of medical emergencies. Fog layer provides middle layer IoT sensor and cloud computing operations that can identify Covid-19 infected users and show visible results to end users [49].

Allam and Jones [52] analyzed urban health and its interlinked technological tools and laboratory's ability to share data, devise tools for the cure of diseases, and guarantee public safety. Allam and Jones [52] proposed a smart city array technology plan to assist early detection of outbreak through thermal cameras, IoT sensors, and supportive open IoT protocols.

Buckley et al. [51] discussed urban data collection, especially via airport screening and monitoring via installing it in airports, bus terminals, market places,

**Table 15.1** IoT solutions for controlling/preventing covid-19 [99]

| COVID-19 solutions | IoT applications | Perception layer | Network layer | Fog layer | Cloud layer |
|---|---|---|---|---|---|
| COVID-19 symptom diagnosis | Breathing monitoring | Inertial sensor | Cellular | ✓ | – |
| | | Depth camera | – | – | ✓ |
| | | Microphone | – | ✓ | ✓ |
| | | mmWave radar | – | – | – |
| | | WiFi | WiFi | ✓ | – |
| | Blood oxygen saturation monitoring | Oximeter | – | – | – |
| | | PPG sensor | – | – | – |
| | | RGB camera | – | – | – |
| | Body temperature monitoring | Infrared temperature sensor | – | – | – |
| | | IRT camera | Cellular | – | ✓ |
| | | RFID | – | – | – |
| Quarantine monitoring | Human activity tracking | RFID | – | | ✓ |
| | | Smart devices | WiFi, Cellular | ✓ | ✓ |
| | | Ear sensor, motion sesnor | Cellular | – | ✓ |
| | | Smartphone | WiFi, Cellular | ✓ | ✓ |
| | | Drone, GPS | Radio | ✓ | – |
| Contact tracing social distancing | | WiFi, Bluetooth | WiFi, Bluetooth | – | ✓ |
| | | RFID | Cellular | ✓ | – |
| | | Cellular trace | Cellular | – | – |
| COVID-19 outbreak Forecasting | Disease outbreak Prediction | Wearable device | – | ✓ | ✓ |
| | | Mobile phones and body sensor | Wireless Mode | ✓ | ✓ |
| | | GPS | Cellular | ✓ | ✓ |
| SARS-CoV-2 mutation prediction | Virus mutation prediction | – | – | – | – |

subways, and health facilities. For smart city to be possible with the IoT sensor, it is important to install and allow the reception of distributed data in a real-time digital network. Buckley et al. [51] believed that urban health wearable sensors can help the tracking of viruses and reveal blood pressure and body temperature rise and other vital signs needed to confirm case earlier than normal.

Hence, Abdel-Basset et al. [20] highlight the process of using spatiotemporal mapping, cloud computing, and remote monitoring to observe symptoms, identify causes, and enforce the quarantine. To avoid data and privacy breach, security requirements may be updated with blockchain and quantum cryptography to render a wealth of data collection in medicine, smart city operations, and better information management.

Bai et al. [24] mentioned the functional significance of using IoT for Covid-19 cases, which includes online monitoring, location tracking, alarm linkage, command and control, plan management, security and privacy, remote maintenance, online upgrading, command management, and statistical decision. Among the above-stated functions, devices like mobile phone/tablet, PC, Arduino, data center, and cloud platform are needed to implement an adequate E-health system. IoT as a fifth-generation (5G) technology has unique network requirements that aid network liquidity, efficiency, high load and capacity, and three linkages to IoT clouds [50].

Prior to the 3G and 4G network, 5G has 20Gbps for downlink and 10Gpbs for uplink with reduced latency and improved overall network efficiency that is superior to other previous networks.

**Importance of Fog and Cloud Layer Integration with IoT Applications**
Wireless sensor network generates and controls large amount of data and helps to remove irrelevant data connected to IoT sensors to monitor patients at risk of Covid-19. Fog and cloud layers handle task analysis, data aggregation, and storage passing through IoT sensors. Thus, fog and cloud layers act as an infrastructure linking cloud server to IoT device. Chiang et al. [8] defined fog layer as a computing architecture for storage, control, and network distribution from patients to cloud servers which integrate IoT continuum fog architecture that works in both mobile and wireless scenarios and traverses across software and hardware using network edge control. Sinisha et al. described the fog layer is an extension of computing due to its heterogeneous and centralized pattern. Fog layer aids cloud computing, reduces processing burden, and automates data using an automated controller. Fog network supports the prediction of patients' data when integrated to work with IoT sensors; it can collect datasets, implement using fog nodes, and offer the required prediction.

## 15.4 Enabled Applications for Covid-19

Applications necessary for possible diagnoses are wearable IoT sensor, fog, and cloud layers. The wearable and non-wearable IoT shows collected data from different healthcare, specifically their sensor data, location, drugs, environmental description, and meteorology. The data collected from wearable IoT sensors are transferred to the fog layer, in turn, to perform real-time processing and diagnosis of infected patients [53].

Toward the conclusion of the diagnosis, the fog layer generates alert messages, which are sent to users' mobile devices as a precaution message and further transferred to the cloud layer for calculations of spread probability and warning sent to non-infected people [40].

Advanced technology development of IoT in 5G will aid telecommunication networks, AI, machine learning algorithms, decision trees, NB, extreme and reinforcement learning, CNN, deep learning, big data, cloud computing, 4.0 industrial revolution, blockchain, etc. [30].

Above-enabled technologies have been claimed to improve viral diagnosis, treatment, and prevention of diseases due to its ability to handle real-time data, remote area IoT processing, forecasting, decision making, interpreting, and backing up of data for security purpose. For quality assurance, Internet of Things and quality of service (QoS), cognitive radio, and other wireless devices are mentioned to provide dynamic spectrum allocation techniques that accommodate a massive number of other devices and data. It can accommodate device for body temperature checks, EEG and ECG, oxygen level, and speech expression [19].

Generally, IoT deals with physical objects interconnected and utilized as sensors, smart meters, home and office appliances, autonomous vehicles, and healthcare monitoring tools. Hence, IoT data traffics are expected to reach about 4394 EB in the future. Due to the rapid increase in bandwidth requirements, CLOMT technique used during spectrum insufficiencies are allocated to radio channels in exchange for data needed to combat covid-19 issues.

The discovery of cloud, fog, and edge computing application has brought new perspectives in health paradigms via aiding sensor data processing, storage of multiple nodes, and locating of users using edge node with smartphones, smart watches, and other portable devices. Some come as a single-board microcontroller device. Fog layer node works with local server and gateways that have physical distance from sensors and actuators. The essence of fog and edge computing depends on its limited computable capacity especially in reducing high data transmission costs evident in the mobile cloud computing model (MCC) and mobile edge computing model (MEC) [7].

An accelerometer is a good IOMT architecture that elevates heart rate, and filters expected situations using microcontrollers to gather patients data used in E-health platforms. Orha and Onia [8] analyzed physiological data of the human body using an Arduino microcontroller that can transfer data from PC to E-health sensors. Yakut et al. [43] measured ECG signals using an E-health sensor linked to the Raspberry Pi. Magana et al. [13] handle professional detecting and alerting of patients' health analysis with an event-based monitor that reports tachycardia and bradycardia heart rates via sensors or triple-axis accelerometer using LCP2148 ARM7 microcontroller (a sensor encrypted to report abnormal event reporting).

Azimi et al.'s [19] approach to virus classification using Linux-based PC or GPU hardware will enable remote healthcare to monitor temperature and heart rate with sensors that partitioned ECG sensors using linear SVM. Muhammad et al. [18] used a voice-enabled pathological detecting tool connected to smartphones to capture date via IoT which are sent to Bluetooth devices to monitor body temperature and ambient humidity.

Dubey et al. [17] developed speech monitoring watches with microphone dynamics for time warping using mining patterns and time series to detect diseases. Ravi et al.'s [53] Covid-19 prescreening device configured with Raspberry Pi Camera V2, FLIR Lepton 3.5 Radiometry long-wave infrared camera, and Google Coral USB accelerator can segment, detect, and access temperature using lip images in a visible spectrum. Greco et al. [15] enabled anomaly to contain accelerometer, gyroscope, and magnetometer that work on Raspberry Pi 3, for edge layer streaming and computing to detect HTM algorithms and physiological well-being of patients.

Yeh et al. [14] presented a secured IoT-based communicator architecture that is a local processing unit that works perfectly with mobile device and fog server to show crypto primitive transmission, confidentiality, and entity authentication of objects and data.

When WESN (Wi-Fi-Bluetooth-GPS) is connected using smartphones, watches, or compact embedded systems, it can be linked to fog and clouds via Wi-Fi or Bluetooth to achieve field sensor networking on a local server that will further achieve a high-performance data storage in clouds [55].

Abdel-Basset et al. [29] introduced different wearable sensor activities and LSTM recurrent neural network activities that can run on a local fog server with GPU accelerator. It can also employ other sensors to move tracking and investigation to a new level using a support vector machine (SVM) and random forest classifier (RF) [70].

To further classify Covid-19 abnormalities, Azimi et al. [19] used Hierarchical Fog-Assisted Computing Architecture for Healthcare (HICH) to create variant MAPE-K model that can distribute data in three-layer forms. The three-layer forms are instituted as edge, fog, and cloud with four main computable elements First is a "monitor" element that handles the implementation between sensors and edge. The second element provides preprocessing aggregation and data storage that analyzes the element of cloud machines utilized computing complex tasks. The third element is "plan" that allocates edge location, handles periodic updates, runs the trained model, and offers local decisions. The fourth element will test with the linear machine partition and deployable deep learning (nonlinear algorithm) [33].

For patients with Covid-19 to recover effectively, a postoperative situation with the IOMT solution will aid the detecting of infection and complications arising during rehabilitation. Mathura et al. [71] predicted health status residual monitoring edge devices that can capture and send fog station data while performing ML-based prediction. Villeneuve et al. [72] added a measuring tool with low-power accelerometers placed on the forearms to simplify the kinematic health process.

## 15.5 Arising Issues and Solutions of the Study

Covid-19 has affected everything globally, and its contained treatment is still far to be grasped, even with consistent research from diverse laboratories to develop vaccines; yet the accuracy still contains errors. TJM2 vaccine by I-Mab Biopharma and several drug options like hydroxychloroquine and azithromycin are still suspected to offer anecdotes to the virus. Some claimed HIV retroviral drugs have a promising remedy. Thus, WHO maintains that the use of surgical masks and protective gear, sanitizing, ventilators, and proper hygiene are better ways to subside the spread of the virus. Some countries with high medical standards used testing kits to isolate infected people from non-infected, while social distancing is maintained in a crowded environment. With the high economic, environmental, and psychiatric impact of Covid-19, there are sustainable benefits experienced in environmental productivity in medicine and business sectors, advancement felt in ICT, and the growth of fifth-generation and industrial 4.0 [1].

Some possible solution to control Covid-19 can be found in AI tool since AI apps have computer vision and natural language process that models big data for recognizing patterns, which can be used to predict outbreak and readdress wrong information relevant in clinical trial of vaccines, CT scanning, detecting of pneumonia virus, and manufacturing of equipment [2].

Unlike AI, IoTs are available in the form of wearable sensory devices, drones for surveillance, and other epic devices that aid epidemiologist to search, remedy, and monitor in-house patients [4]. Big data and virtual reality can be found reliable during the forecast of data, VR improvement of data efficiency and upgrading of communication tool [5]. Microscopy et al. [3] maintained that laser-based electron holograph with 3D photography can offer to webcast for live events/conferencing and prevent people from gathering together causing unnecessary crowds. Cloud computing as part of IoT may influence everyday life by introducing digital live styles in the form of Zoom video, Slack and Netflix, Amazon Web Services, Microsoft Azure, Google Cloud, etc.

Different countries adopted autonomous robots this pandemic season to ensure social distancing is maintained. They also used the robot to conduct police patrol and enhance vehicle and medical ambulance movement. 3D scanning with non-contact techniques can be useful for detecting and quantifying the virus, because it conducts VR, motion capturing, robotic mapping, industrial design, etc. [69]. Also, 3D printing has supported the manufacturing of N95 respirators and masks, aiding the development of NanoHack 3D printed recyclable mask. A biosensor is a possible solution that is capable of providing cost saving, has high accuracy, and is used in glucose monitor and wireless biosensor patch 1AX that conducts temperature check, ECG trace, and respiratory track recordings [6].

## 15.6 Methods, Hypothesis, and Literature Review

Low-level disease detections might be the alternative to eliminate viral infections since some virus-like Covid-19 has asymptotic cases of people with the virus without acknowledging their role in spreading the infectious disease. Under therapeutic procedures, bioinformatic collection of data and correlated biomarking of the level of pathogen diseases is realized through nanotechnology enabled unit's fabric device that will integrate, interface, package, sense, and record point of care performance before rendering diagnostic procedure to manage the diseases. The process is known as Geno-sensor, which is a molecular immune-assay sensor process supported by IoT/AI and data analytics that show contact tracing, targeted sensing, quarantine monitoring, and homestay prediction [12].

Methodologically, IoT interface uses wearable POC system and fog/edge/cloud layers for data sharing, raid assessment, and post-pandemic assessment. Biosensor has been discovered as an emergent nanotechnology that enables to translate data analytic prototypes to diagnostic tools for clinical applications [21]. In the USA, biosensor tool referred to as smart ultrathin graphene layer is fabricated with Au substrate integration which works perfectly with spectrophotometric genetics. The Raman spectrophotometer (RNA) is extracted from stem cell and performs material detection, especially when optimizing with artificial cell to combine nano-transmitter, bio-cyber interface, and electronic tattoo to be monitored using threat-based chemical and physical sensors [32].

Allam et al. [54] introduced surface-enhanced Raman scattering (SERS) phenomena as a selective base for sensitive genetic sensing using DNA neuro-biomarker to detect active dye-label probe to DNA oligonucleotide. For DNA and Covid-19 human immunity research, Internet of Bio-Nano Things (IOBNT) was proposed by Akyildiz et al. [23] to handle intra-bodily sensing, environmental control of toxic, and polluting of substance.

Research believes that some immune systems are resistant to Covid-19, whereas electronic artificial tattoo process designed for the bio-cyber interface may help to translate biochemical information to the cyber domain for proper communicating of the result. This transmission of data is referred to as artificial cell nanotechnological application for genetic therapeutic process and artificial blood cell production. According to Yang et al. [58], such emergent technology will support thread acting 3D microfluidic channels to sense and monitor health electronically.

The microfluidic network works with chemical and physical sensors connected to hydrophilic traits to control and deliver body fluids to sensing platforms. This process is performed by nanomaterial conductive traits measured with electrodes that examine pH level, temperature, glucose, and stress level. It also exhibits the result via a wireless communicator or signal processing unit of a smartphone or PC. Recent expansion to IoT wearable and non-wearable is channeled to further develop electrochemical, optical, thermal, and piezoelectrical transduction, remarkably important for testing blood glucose, cholesterol, triglycerides, PT, infections, drug and vaccine discovery, blood gas, etc. [59].

In spite of the updated sensing technologies, it is significant to adopt the picomolar (PM) level to achieve low-level detection and targeting of bio-market using the femtomolar (FM) process. Femtomolar promotes sensitive and selective infectious disease management via reporting with biosensing material that will show bioactive enzymes. The method of achieving the process is to use a biosensing prototype chip that can integrate the miniature-potentiostat (M-P) utilized as micro-nano-electronics to perform POC diagnosis. For a smartphone to perform M-P diagnosis, there are needs to manage and store data and review data accuracy, its high performance, and reliability [16, 42].

The nano-enabled smart sensing substrate system can perform biopolymer, metal oxide, gold, and carbon nanotube test. It can also handle graphene, quantum dots, and composite and hybrid tests. An explored electro-active functional surface for nanostructures has been effectively fabricated to form interdigitalized microelectrodes (IDμE), utilized in developing biosensing PM and FM low-level detector that monitors progress during quarantine and therapy.

A successful approach has been adopted during Ebola and Zika virus using polymerase chain reaction (PCR) and enzyme-linked immunosorbent assay (ELISA). However, nano-enabled IDμE was believed to outperform PCR and ELISA, due to its efficiency level in tackling cancer and stress issues. IDμE biosensing chips work with m-p applications, as well as micro-nano-enabled electronics, designed to reduce the basis for POC diagnostic application [59].

Shanghai et al. [75] examined a real-time MEMS/BIOMEMS approach for biosensing using pressure sensors, accelerometer, microfluidics, ultrasonic, and microphone sensors.

Although the medical sensing methodologies involve devices for capacitive/piezoelectric ultrasonic applications that show detection on mobile-based devices, specifically on healthcare smartphones, offering an easy operational solution for data recording, implementation of IOMT, and performance of E-health. The known E-health process uses smartphone-assisted personal electronic sensing for quick bioinformatic collection and recordings. It can also offer Do-It-Yourself (DIY) approach for self-aware diagnostics, given to stay-at-home patients [25].

Another established sensing prototype compatible with IoT application is the electrochemical biosensor that uses IDE-modified self-assembler that is appropriate for self-assembling of monolayer (SAM) and detects cortisol psychological stress via biomark (10-PM) tool, which shows result within 40 minutes of the test. The SAM biosensor test can be conducted with plasma or saliva samples and validated using ELISA [27].

However, the IDE-based cortisol immune-sensor can be integrated to form miniaturized microfluid for an automatic sampling of 10ul and customized M-P portable cortisol biosensing fabrication. The essence of IDE sensors is to offer user-friendly clinician performance via analytics and sharing of data [31].

## 15.7 Data Analysis

Sun et al. [78] used similar epidemiological mapping IoT visualization tools to create surveillance on the spread of Covid-19 and test the rate of infections.

Figure 15.5 illustrates the concept of IoT infection surveillance, targeting vital signs such as heart and respiration rates, the temperature of the body, and data generated on ambient temperature, GPS, and humidity.

The image above illustrates IP and GPS server information that records values obtained from vital signals and thermal images.

Liu et al. [79] extended data entries of Covid-19 screening and performed a bibliometric analysis to evaluate its median interquartile range (IQR) proportions, ranking, and descriptive statistics. He used Hirsch index (H-index) to put together quantity and quality to research the possible output and compiled datasets in Python

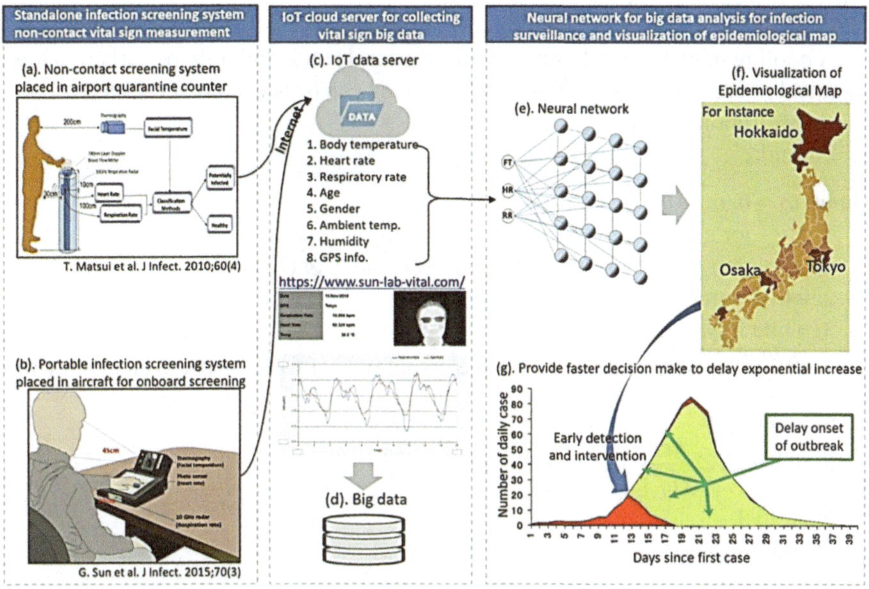


**Fig. 15.5** IoT infection surveillance and targeting of vital signs [78]

version 38.0 while showing data aggregates of the European Centre for Disease Prevention and Control [80].

However, the data followed some classifications such as types, topics, and medical specialties, whereby types outlined include observation, interventional, and protocol types. The protocol shows basic, mathematical study, analyzing epidemiological risk factors, characteristics, features, and diagnosis. The clinical features mentioned include patients' signal/symptoms, radiology results, and pathogenesis.

The pathogenesis result shows viral mechanisms, disease progress, counter-immune responses, and treatment. This Covid-19 test was conducted with IoT tools with simulation results showing test numbers, the number of Covid-19 cases, and ratios of asymptomatic/presymptomatic carriers. The IoT tool works as a PCR-based molecular testing tool for tracing and enabling group testing. The group test possesses feasible approaches that focus on the prevalent population regime by scanning samples and the number of tests and detecting defective elements. The group test algorithms will be formulated with an eq. $T = 0$ (K Log N), where O stands for the measurement of orders in the magnitude of the positive tests generated.

If the pooling rows and columns of PCR test go with 10X efficiency (which is 1.0–5%) in the calculation, the sample pooling number (for instance, 48 infected patients out of 384 tests conducted) will indicate 8X efficiency and 1% test prevalence.

The algorithm will be placed on a random pooling matric as demonstrated below:

**Algorithm 15.1** Random pooling

A pooling matrix is randomly initialized (step 1) and randomly perturbed to limit identical pooled samples (3–8), and new pooling can be accepted or rejected according to Metropolis sampling (steps 9–14).

Formula:

Input: $\varnothing = 0$, $\alpha = 0$, $n$, $m$, $k$, $p$

1: $\varnothing \leftarrow$ *for* each sample ($i$) pick ($k$) random pols out of m, for setting a distribution column while corresponding the set of rows $\varnothing$ (I,f) to 1

2: while iteration_no< Max_Iteration do

3: while i $\leq$*n do*

4: $\varnothing \frac{new}{i,f} \leftarrow$ swap each non − zero element of $\varnothing(i,f)$ with a zero element with a probability p

5: if $\exists j < i, \varnothing \frac{new}{(i,f)} = \varnothing\ (\frac{new}{i,f})$ then

6: go to 4

7: end if

8: end while

9: $\alpha\ new = k - \max\left\{\varnothing \frac{new}{i,f)} \mathrm{T}\varnothing new(i,f)\ \forall \mathrm{i,j} < \mathrm{n,i} \neq \mathrm{j}\right]$

10: if $\frac{\alpha\ new}{\alpha} > u \sim \frac{-}{u}(0,1)\ then$

11: $\alpha \leftarrow \alpha\ new,\ \ \varnothing \leftarrow \varnothing\ new$

12: end if

13: end while

Output: pooling matrix $\varnothing$ with m pools;each sample is added to exactly $k$ pools.

According to Metropolis algorithm [83], the sampling scheme set of 12 samples will be gathered in six pools and equated as $N = 12$, $M = 6$, and $k = 2$. Sinnott-Armstrong et al. [80] and Eberhardt et al. [81] proposed a data pooling sampling method represented in the bipartite graph below with the pooling scheme calculated with $k = 2$ and $k = 1$, respectively.

The pooling scheme illustrated in Fig. 15.6 sampled 6–12 pool samples in the bipartite graph and represent matrixes with the binary $\varnothing$. $\varnothing$sign represents the adjacent matrix used in organizing samples in column and row vertices, while calling-out samples use (I, J) denotations.

The result shows group tests using Bernoulli sampling simulation that drops within the range of 0.0005 and 0.2. By adopting Sinnott-Armstrong et al. [80] to evaluate row-column (grouping) and set up multistage testing with Eberhardt et al. [81] multi-staged (P16S3-P32S2). The final result according to Phatarfod and Sudbury's [82] adaptive row-column version of the simulation demonstrates mean of 1000 with an independent value and an underperforming denser area rate of 0.2–1%. The simulation result below demonstrates the efficiency gained while engaging the multi-pass test group scheme. Sinnott-Armstrong et al. [80] (row-column simulation) simulate 96–384 to 1536 set test plates (Fig. 15.7).

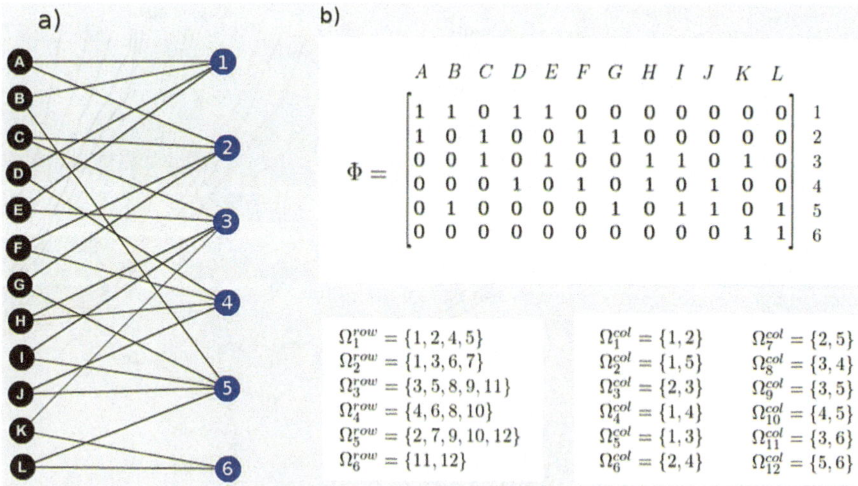


**Fig. 15.6** Pooling scheme with 6-12 pool samples [84]

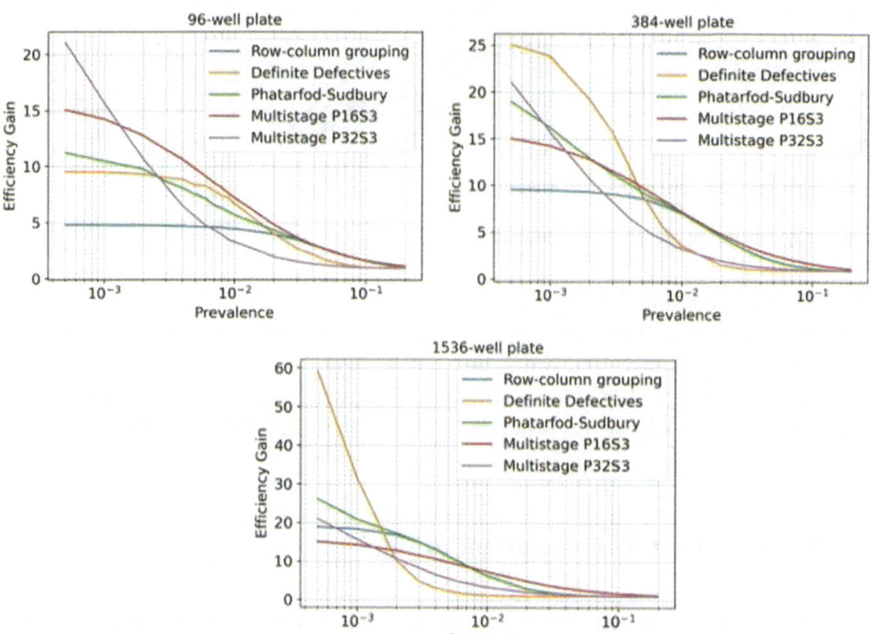


**Fig. 15.7** Phatarfod and Sudbury simulation 1 [82]

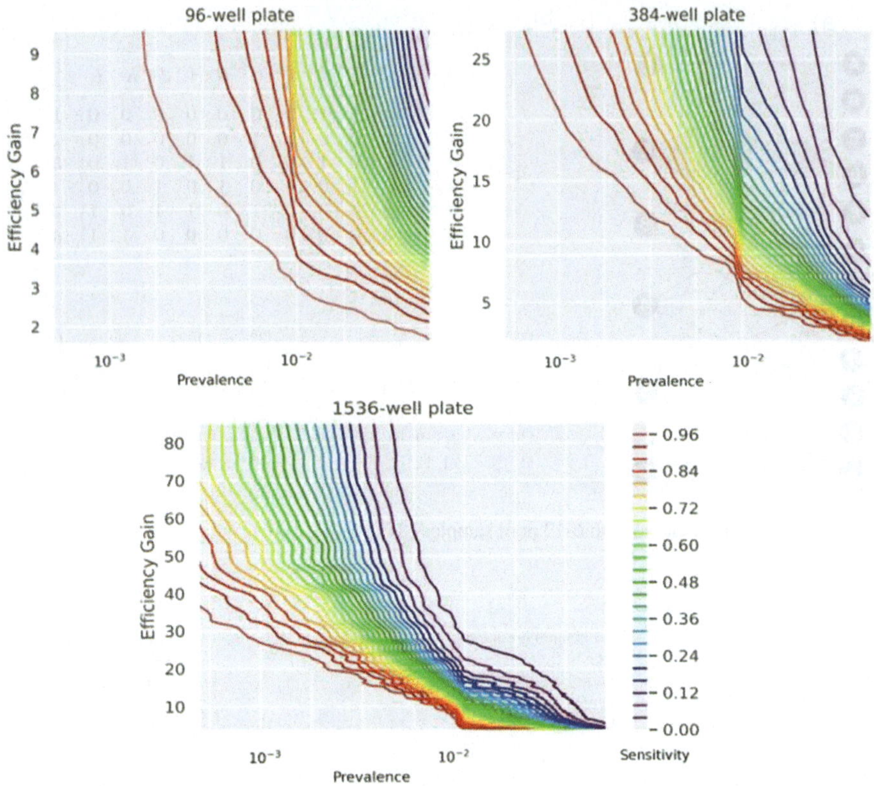


**Fig. 15.8** Phatarfod and Sudbury simulation 2 [82]

**Result Accuracy and Performance Metrics**

The performance metrics reflect the level of sensitivity in the operational success of mapping the group test. The simulation below shows the equal-sensitivity contour exhibits with greater slopes illustrating how the test prevalence gets smaller, as the efficiency increases while boosting the low-sensitivity level (Fig. 15.8).

## 15.8 Results and Recommendations

The US Federal Food and Drug Administration developed systematic approaches for approving scale-up research conducted for a clinical trial of the Covid-19 vaccine. Precisely, it follows a biosensing method that commences with a smart nanostructure to an enabled biosensing platform for sensing performance evaluation and validation [35]. The second phase includes the automation of operations using MEMS/BIOMEMS and IoT nano-electronic smart packaging, and an integrated sensing system is done on smartphone interface and data analysis using AI. Meanwhile, IOMT can be adopted to manage data, especially noninvasive biosensing applications that offer POC, home diagnostic analysis, bio-defense, environmental monitoring, and geological examination of food, beverages, and other wearable and non-wearable products [62].

IOMT serves as a medical device for connecting biosensing chip applications necessary for performing diagnostic analysis, bioinformatic data, handling of diagnostic processes, and developing protocols. IOMT devices enhance the processing of bioinformatic data relevant in drug development, disease profiling, treatment optimization, and personalized medicine. IOMT applications are utilized for accomplishing tasks in patient monitoring, disease management, and personalized health delivery [34].

The viewpoint remains that IOMT may constitute positively to intelligent healthcare and resolve minor and major health concerns. It can handle issues that do not require many clinic visits. IOMT may reduce the cause of serious illness if immediate diagnoses are visible with sensors, cyber-IoT systems, and cloud computing. Such devices can be multi-connected locally to network software, electronic sensors, or actuators to aid virus treatment, discovery, and radio-frequency energy emitted to read signal of asymptotic patients and minimize the spread of Covid-19 [57].

IoT may be viable when considering healthier, economic, and productive nations, whereas IoT wearable devices will function with an AI-based health monitoring system to deliver updates of patient health status using wireless sensing network (WSN). The IoT wearable, fog, IoT edge, and clouds are packages deployed with AI models to reduce complex computational task and collect data effectively via storing smart biosensing data accurately [5]. For AI models to be deployed, edge gateway must be predicted with anomaly data stream for proper action in generating healthcare wearable devices that are computed to send commands to IoT edge hub and further transmitted to machine learning to perform IoT edge function.

Covid-19 infection can be controlled by sensing supported AI and IoT detection and tracing, to manage Covid-19 spread. By using IDE-based SARS-CoV-2 biosensor and picking some anti-SARS-CoV-19 virus proteins from the antibody, the IDE-based biosensor can show sensitive positive or negative result within 30–40 minutes. The mentioned biosensor in healthcare can transform POC analytical devices to handle Covid-19 issues via generating bioinformatic understanding of disease progression. It can also offer error-free therapy to comprehend the relationship between CoV-19 level and bodily pathogens. MEMS are made to evaluate drugs which can be tested primarily on animals, while IoT biosensing wireless systems are plugged to detect disease. IOMT according to records may help to gain big data analytic breakthrough and Covid-19 vaccine development due to its relative features programmed to operate variably in the collection of associated data such as race, gender, and medical industry [36].

AI over the years was recommended to help the optimization of therapy and drugs/vaccines. It has supported direct testing, prediction, and social and physical distancing. Strategically, IoT has been accepted to minimize risk factors associated with tracking numbers of infected people, making decisions on lockdown, and assisting approaches of neuro-behavior alteration and safe work practice during the outbreak [41].

## 15.9 Conclusion

An IoT integration creates a functional operation between medical devices, connected to the Internet, especially how it sends messages and transits data to medical staffs on patients infected or not infected with Covid-19. This report analyzed the enabled application necessary for achieving remote location tele-device analysis and the ultimate strengthening and control of the virus. It has helpful tips on how to control Covid-19 spread. Alternatively, other applications useful for controlling the spread of Covid-19 include surveillance CCTV cameras, Trace-Together mobile applications, Bluetooth and GPS technology, remote working apps, and encrypted distance learning solutions like E-learning apps, drones, and robotic delivery technologies. IoT applications can improve quality of health and life at a low cost and effective diagnosing of illnesses. Primarily for Covid-19 diagnosis, it is essential to consider scanning computed tomography (CT) machine, x-rays, magnetic resonance imaging (MRI), AI, etc., which will help to interpret viruses.

IoT applications can support care coordination and system management for infected patients because it helps to capture images of pathological analysis. IoT might be a great resource for clinical decision support due to its enhanced AI guide features for extracting radiological images and making supportive decisions.

Conclusively, IoT will not be far-fetched when discussing modern technologies associated with social media, smart city development, chatbot, planning, and manufacturing. To achieve security and privacy, medical stakeholders are responsible for creating privacy regulations, have the right to protect data, identify data handling, and offer permission for the digital approach of medical data while creating encrypted electronic security for medical records using electronic health record (EHR) systems.

## References


1. Haleem, A. J., & Vaishya, M. (2020). Effects of COVID 19 pandemic in daily life. *Current Medicine Research and Practice*. https://doi.org/10.1016/j.cmrp.2020.03.011.
2. Naudé, W. (2020). *Discussion paper series artificial intelligence against COVID-19 an early: rev* (p. 13110). IZA Discussion Papers No.
3. Microscopy, E., Fields, M., Micro, E., Beams, E., & Boonendt, P. M.. (2001). *Techniques laser-based electron holography in phase space*: 1995.
4. Georgios, P. *Artificial intelligence in the fight against COVID-19* [internet]: Available from: https://www.bruegel.org/2020/03/artificial-intelligence-in-the-fight-against-covid-19/
5. Randy, B. *Big Data in the time of coronavirus (COVID-19) Co-network* [Internet]. Available from: https://www.forbes.com/sites/ciocentral/2020/03/30/big-data-in-the-time-of-coronavirus-covid-19/#161ff87558fc
6. Lawrence, C. (2020) *Is cloud computing the superhero of COVID-19? Dev hub* [Internet]. Available from https://www.codemotion.com/magazine/dev-hub/cloud-manager/cloud-computing-covid-19/google scholar
7. Hartmann, M., Hashmi, U. S., & Imran, A. (2019). Edge computing in smart health care systems: review, challenges, and research directions Trans. *Emergency Telecommunication. Technol.*, e3710.

8. Chiang, M., & Zhang, T. (2016). Fog and IoT: An Overview of Research Opportunities. *IEEE Internet of Things Journal, 3*, 1. https://doi.org/10.1109/JIOT.2016.2584538.
9. National health commission of the people's republic of china. *Diagnosis and treatment scheme for pneumonia of COVID-19* (interim version 6). http://www.nhc.gov.cn/yzygj/s7653p/202002/8334a8326dd94d329df351d7da8aefc2.shtml.
10. Li, D. (2019). 5g and intelligence medicine-how the next generation of wireless technology will reconstruct healthcare? *Precise Clinic Medicine, 2*(4), 205–208.
11. Montag, C., Becker, B., & Ganthe, C. (2018). Multipurpose application WeChat: A review on recent research. *Front Psychology, 9*(2247).
12. Yakut, O., & Solak, S. E. D. (2014). Bolt measuring ECG signal using e-health sensor platform. In *International conference on chemistry, biomedical and environmental engineering (Maccabee'14)* (pp. 65–69).
13. Magaña, P., Espinoza, R., Aquino-Santos, N., Cárdenas-Benitez, J., Aguilar-Velasco, C., Buenrostro-Segura, A., Edwards-block, et al. (2014). Wisph: a wireless sensor network-based home care monitoring system. *Sensors, 14*(4), 7096–7119.
14. Yeh, K. H. A secure IoT-based healthcare system with body sensor networks. *IEEE Access, 4*(2016), 10288–10299.
15. Greco, L., Ritrovato, P., & Xhafaan, F. (2019). Edge-stream computing infrastructure for real-time analysis of wearable sensors data. *Future Generation of Computer System, 93*, 515–528.
16. Hegde, C., Suresh, P. B., Zelko, J., Jiang, Z., Kamaleswaran, R., Reyna, M. A., & Clifford, G. D. (2020). Auto triage-an open-source edge computing raspberry pi-based clinical screening system. *medrxiv*. https://doi.org/10.1101/2020.04.09.20059840.
17. Dubey, H., Yang, J., Constant, N., Amiri, A. M., Yang, Q., & Makodiya, K. (2015). Fog data: enhancing tele-health big data through fog computing. In *Proceedings of the case big data & social informatics 2015* (p. 14). ACM.
18. Muhammad, G., Rahman, S. M. M., Allawi, A., & Alamri, A. (2017). Smart health solution integrating IoT and cloud: A case study of voice pathology monitoring. *IEEE Communications Magazine, 55*(1), 69–73.
19. Azimi, I., Takalo-Mattila, J., Anzanpour, A., Rahmani, A. M., Soininen, J. P., & Liljeberg, P. (2018). Empowering healthcare IoT systems with hierarchical edge-based deep learning 2018. In *IEEE/ACM international conference on connected health: applications, systems and engineering technologies (chase)* (pp. 63–68). IEEE.
20. Abdel-basset, M., Manogaran, G., Gamal, A., & Changa, V. (2019). Novel intelligent medical decision support model based on soft computing and IoT. *IEEE Internet of Things Journal*, 1–11.
21. SARS-CoV-2 IgM/IgG Antibody Rapid Test. Available online: https://www.surebiotech.com/rapid-test/coronavirus-covid-19-rapid-test/. Accessed on 14 Apr 2020.
22. Ting, S. K., Villano, R., & Dollery, B. (2018). Economies of Scale in Local Government Services: A Meta-Analysis. *International Journal of Service Management and Sustainability, 3*(1), 1–28. ISSN 2550-1569.
23. Akyildiz, I. F., Pierobon, M., Balasubramaniam, S., & Koucheryavy, Y. (2015). The internet of bio-Nano things. *IEEE Communications Magazine, 53*, 32–40.
24. Bai, L., Yang, D., Wang, X., Tong, L., Zhu, X., Bai, C., et al. (2020). Chinese experts' consensus on the Internet of Things-aided diagnosis and treatment of coronavirus disease 2019. *Clinical E-Health*.
25. Sohrabi, C., Alsafi, Z., O'Neill, N., Khan, M., Kerwan, A., Al-Jabir, A., Iosifidis, C., & Agha, R. (2020). World Health Organization declares global emergency: A review of the 2019 novel coronavirus (COVID-19). *International Journal of Surgery*.
26. Qureshi, F., & Krishnan, S. (2016). Wearable hardware design for the internet of medical things (IoMT). *Sensors, 18*(11), 3812.
27. Swati, S., & Chandana, M. (2020). Application of cognitive Internet of Medical Things for COVID-19 pandemic diabetes. *Metabolic Syndrome, 14*(5), 911–915. https://doi.org/10.1016/j.dsx.2020.06.014. Published online 2020 Jun 11. Internet of things (IoT) applications to fight against COVID-19 pandemic.

28. Ravi, P. S., Mohd, J., Haleem, A., & Rajiv, S. (2020). Diabetes. *Metabolic Syndrome, 14*(4), 521–524. https://doi.org/10.1016/j.dsx.2020.04.041. Published online 2020 May 5.
29. Abdel-Basset, M., Manogaran, G., Gamal, A., & Chang, V. (2019). A novel intelligent medical decision support model based on soft computing and IoT. *IEEE Internet of Things Journal*, 1–11.
30. Magaña, E. P., Aquino-Santos, R., Cárdenas-Benitez, N., Aguilar-Velasco, J., Buenrostro-Segura, C., & Edwards-Block, A. (2014). WiSPH: A wireless sensor network-based home care monitoring system. *Sensors, 14*(4), 7096–7119.
31. Mathur, N., Paul, G., Irvine, J., Abuhelala, M., Buis, A., & Glesk, I. (2016). A practical design and implementation of a low-cost platform for remote monitoring of the lower limb health of amputees in the developing world. *IEEE Access, 4*, 7440–7451.
32. Yeh, K. H. (2016). A secure IoT-based healthcare system with body sensor networks. *IEEE Access, 4*, 10288–10299.
33. IBM. (2020). *IBM Watson Assistant for Citizens*. Available at: https://www.ibm.com/au-en/watson/covid-response
34. Al-Majeed, S. S., Al-Mejibli, I. S., & Karam, J. (2015). Home Tele-health by the internet of things (IoT). In *Proceedings of the Canadian Conference on Electrical and Computer Engineering Halifax, Canada, May 3–6.*
35. Kumar, K. M. C. (2016). A new methodology for monitoring OSA patients based on IoT. *International Journal of Innovative Research & Development, 5*(2).
36. Chandel, V., Sinharay, A., & Ahmed, N. (2016). Exploiting IMU sensors for IoT enabled health monitoring. In *Proceedings of the First Workshop on IoT-enabled Healthcare and Wellness Technologies and Systems, June 30.*
37. Chun, S., Ge, S. M., Kim, H. S., & Park, J. T. (2016). Design and implementation of interoperable IoT healthcare system based on international standards. In *Proceedings of the 13th IEEE, Annual Consumer Communications & Networking Conference.*
38. De Mattos, W. D., & Gondim, P. R. L. (2016). *M- health solutions using 5G networks and M2M communications*. Published IEEE Computer Society.
39. Chavan, P., More, P., Thorat, N., Yewale, S., & Shade, P. (2016). ECG - Remote patient monitoring using cloud computing. *Imperial Journal of Interdisciplinary Research, 2*(2).
40. Sandeep, S. (2017). Wearable IoT sensor-based healthcare system for identifying and controlling chikungunya virus. *Computers in Industry, 91*, 33–44.
41. Vasyltsov, & Lee, S. (2015). Entropy extraction from bio-signals in healthcare IoT. In *Proceedings of the 1st ACM Workshop on IoT Privacy, Trust, and Security, April 14–17.*
42. Ni, Y., Bermudez, M., Kennebeck, S., Liddy-Hicks, S., Dexheimer, J.. (2019). A Real-Time Automated Patient Screening System for Clinical Trials Eligibility in an Emergency Department: Design and Evaluation. *JMIR Med Inform.* 7(3):e14185. https://doi.org/10.2196/14185.
43. Yakut, O., Solak, S., & Bolat, E. D. International Conference on Chemistry, Biomedical, and Environment Engineering (ICCBEE'14) 2014. In *Measuring ECG signal using e-health sensor platform* (pp. 65–69).
44. Verdict Medical devices screening for Covid-19. (2020). https://www.medicaldevice-network.com/features/types-of-covid-19-test-antibody-pcr-antigen/. Accessed 4 Apr 2020.
45. Vaishya, R., Javaid, M., Khan, I. H., & Haleem, A. (2020). Artificial intelligence (AI) applications for COVID-19 pandemic diabetes & metabolic syndrome. *Clinical Research & Reviews*. https://doi.org/10.1016/j.dsx.2020.04.012.
46. Özdemir, A., & Barshan, B. (2020). Detecting falls with wearable sensors using machine learning techniques. *Sensors, 14*, 10691–10708. https://doi.org/10.3390/s140610691.
47. Fan, Y. J., Yin, Y. H. L. D. X., Zeng, Y., & Wu, F. (2014). IoT-based smart rehabilitation system. *IEEE Transactions on Industrial Informatics, 10*, 1568–1577. https://doi.org/10.1109/tii.2014.2302583.

48. Diginomica. (2020). *Blue-Dot spotted coronavirus before anyone else had a clue*. https://diginomica.com/how-canadian-ai-start-bluedot-spotted-coronavirus-anyone-else-had-clue. Accessed 15th Mar 2020.
49. Huang, C., Wang, Y., Li, X., et al. (2020). Clinical features of patients infected with 2019 novel coronavirus in Wuhan, China. *The Lancet, 395*(10223), 497–506.
50. Pan, X. (2020). Application of personal-oriented digital technology in preventing transmission of COVID-19, China. *Irish Journal of Medical Science*. https://doi.org/10.1007/s11845-020-02215-5.
51. Buckley, C., & May, T. *Effects of coronavirus begin echoing far from Wuhan epicenter*. Available online: https://www.nytimes.com/2020/01/25/world/asia/china-wuhan-coronavirus.html. Accessed on 28 Jan 2020.
52. Allam, Z., & Joneson, D. S. (2020). The coronavirus (COVID-19) outbreak and the smart city network: Universal data sharing standards coupled with artificial intelligence (AI) to benefit urban health monitoring and management. *Healthcare (Basel), 8*(1).
53. Ravì, D., Wong, C., Deligianni, Berthelot, F., Andreu-Perez, M., Lo, J. B., & Yang, G. Z. (2016). Deep learning for health informatics. *IEEE Journal of Biomedical and Health Informatics, 21*, 4–21.
54. Yang, L., Lee, J. H., Rathnam, C., Hou, Y. J., Choi, W., & Lee, K. B. (2019). Dual-enhanced Raman scattering-based characterization of stem cell differentiation using graphene-plasmonic hybrid Nano-array. *Nano Letters, 19*, 8138–8148.
55. Mostafalu, P., Akbari, M., Alberti, K., Xu, A., Xu, Q., Khademhosseini, A., & Sonkusale, S. R. (2016). A toolkit of thread-based microfluidics, sensors, and electronics for 3D tissue embedding for medical diagnostics Microsyst. *Nano, 2*, 16039.
56. Kaushik, A., Yndart, A., Jayant, R. D., Sagar, V., Atluri, V., Bhansali, S., & Nair, M. (2005). Electrochemical sensing method for point-of-care cortisol detection in human immunodeficiency virus-infected patients. *International Journal of Nanomedicine, 10*, 677.
57. Krause, A., Smailagic, A., & Siewiorek, D. P. (2005). Context-aware mobile computing: Learning context-dependent personal preferences from a wearable sensor array. *IEEE Transactions on Mobile Computing, 5*, 113–127.
58. Yang, S., Zhou, P., Duan, K., Hossain, M. S., & Alhamidem, M. F. (2018). Health towards emotional health through depression prediction and intelligent health recommender system. *Mobile Networks and Applications, 23*, 216–226.
59. Dixit, C., & Kaushik, A. (2016). *Microfluidics for biologists*. Berlin, Germany: Springer.
60. Kaushik, A., Yndart, A., Kumar, S., Jayant, R. D., Vashist, A., Brown, A. N., Li, C. J., & Nair, M. (2018). A sensitive electrochemical immuno-sensor for label-free detection of Zika-virus protein. *Scientific Reports, 8*, 9700.
61. Kaushik, A., Tiwari, S., Jayant, R. D., Vashist, A., Nikkhah-Moshaie, R., El-Hage, N., & Nair, N. (2017). Electrochemical biosensors for early-stage Zika diagnostics. *Trends Biotechnol, 35*(2017), 308–317.
62. Yager, P., Domingo, G. J., & Gerdes, J. (2008). Point-of-care diagnostics for global health. *Annual Review of Biomedical Engineering, 10*, 107–144. [Google Scholar] [CrossRef] [PubMed].
63. Singh, R. P., Javaid, M., Haleem, A., & Suman, R. (2020). Internet of things (IoT) applications to fight against COVID-19 pandemic. *Diabetes and Metabolic Syndrome: Clinical Research and Reviews Impact Factor*.
64. Cecil, J., Gupta, A., Pirela-Cruz, & Ramanathan, M. P. A. (2018). IoMT based cyber training framework for orthopedic surgery using Next Generation Internet technologies. *Informatics in Medicine Unlocked, 12*, 128–137.
65. Joyia, G. J., Liaqat, R. M., Farooq, A., & Rehman, S. (2017). Internet of Medical Things (IOMT): applications, benefits and future challenges in healthcare domain. *Journal of Communication, 12*(4), 240–247.
66. Lin, B., & Wu, S. (2020). COVID-19 (Coronavirus Disease 2019): Opportunities and Challenges for Digital Health and the Internet of Medical Things in China. *OMICS, 24*(5), 231–232.

67. Iwendi, C., Khan, S., Anajemba, J. H., Bashir, A., & Noor, K. F. (2020). Realizing an efficient IoMT-assisted patient diet recommendation system through machine learning model. *IEEE Access, 8*, 28462–28474.
68. Montag, C., Becker, B., & Gan, C. (2018). The multipurpose application we-chat: A review on recent research. *Front Psychology, 9*(2247).
69. Li, D. (2019). 5G and intelligence medicine-how the next generation of wireless technology will reconstruct healthcare? *Precise Clinic Medicine, 2*(4), 205–208.
70. Ram, S., Padua, S., & Shiratori, R. N. (2019). *Machine learning framework for edge computing to improve prediction accuracy in mobile health monitoring in an international conference on computational science and its applications* (pp. 417–431). Cham: Springer: An architectural blueprint for autonomic computing, IBM white paper 31.2006(2006) 1–6.
71. Mathura, N., Paul, G., Irvine, J., Abuhelala, M., Buis, A., & Gleska, I. (2016). Practical design and implementation of a low-cost platform for remote monitoring of lower limb health of amputees in the developing world. *IEEE Access, 4*, 7440–7451.
72. Villeneuve, E. W., Harwin, W., Holderbaum, B., Janko, R. S., & Sherratt. (2016). Construction of angular kinematics from wrist-worn inertial sensor data for smart home healthcare. *IEEE Access*, 2351–2363.
73. Wang, Y., Hu, M., Li, Q., Zhang, X. P., Zhai, G., & Yao, N. (2020). Abnormal respiratory patterns classifier may contribute to the large-scale screening of people infected with COVID-19 accurately and unobtrusively. *Xiv preprint arXiv: 2002.05534*, 12.
74. Internet of things-aided diagnosis and treatment of COVID-19 Chinese experts group of clinical of E-health. (2020). Chinese experts consensus on the internet of things-aided diagnosis and treatment of COVID-19. *Fudan University Journal of Medical, 47*(2), 151–160.
75. Shanghai Respiratory Clinical Quality Control Center. (2020). Shanghai expert consensus for respiratory clinic quality control during epidemic 2019-NCOVtime Fudan university. *JMS, 47*(2), 143–150.
76. Fan, Y. J., Yin, Y. H., Xu, L. D., Zeng, Y., & Wu, F. (2014). IoT-based smart rehabilitation system. *IEEE Transactions on Industrial Informatics, 10*(2), 1568–1577.
77. Ozdemir, S. (2008). Secure Data Aggregation in Wireless Sensor Networks via Homomorphic Encryption. *Journal of the Faculty of Engineering and Architecture of Gasi University, 23*(2), 365–373.
78. Sun, G., Trung, N. V., Hoi, L. T., et al. (2020). Visualisation of epidemiological map using an internet of things infectious disease surveillance platform. *Critical Care, 24*, 400.
79. Liu, N., Chee, M. L., Niu, C., et al. (2020). Coronavirus disease 2019 (COVID-19): An evidence map of medical literature. *BMC Medical Research Methodology, 20*, 177.
80. Sinnott-Armstrong, N., Klein, D., & Hickey, B. (2020). Evaluation of group testing for SARS-CoV-2 RNA. *medRxiv*.
81. Eberhardt, J. N., Breuckmann, N. P., & Eberhardt, C. S. (2020). Multi-stage group testing improves efficiency of large-scale COVID-19 screening. *Journal of Clinical Virology, 128*, 104382.
82. Phatarfod, R., & Sudbury, A. (1994). The use of a square array scheme in blood testing. *Statistics in Medicine, 13*(22), 2337–2343.
83. Metropolis, N., Rosenbluth, A. W., Rosenbluth, M. N., Teller, A. H., & Teller, E. (1953). Equation of state calculations by fast computing machines. *The Journal of Chemical Physics, 21*(6), 1087–1092.
84. Aldridge, M., Baldassini, L., & Johnson, O. (2014). Group testing algorithms: Bounds and simulations. *IEEE Transactions on Information Theory, 60*(6), 3671–3687.
85. Elijah, O., Rahman, T. A., Orikumhi, I., Leow, C. Y., & Hindia, M. N. (2018). An overview of internet of things (IoT) and data analytics in agriculture: Benefits and challenges. *IEEE Internet of Things Journal, 5*(5), 3758–3773.
86. Kellam, & Barclay, W. (2020). The dynamics of humoral immune re-sponses following SARS-CoV-2 infection and the potential for rein-fection. *Journal of General Virology*, jgv001439.

87. Bonaccorsi, G., Pierri, F., Cinelli, M., Flori, A., Galeazzi, A., Porcelli, F., Schmidt, A. L., Valensise, C. M., Scala, A., Quattrociocchi, W., et al. (2020). Economic and social consequences of human mobility restrictions under COVID-19. *Proceedings of the National Academy of Sciences, 117*(27), 15 530–15 535.
88. Zhan, Y., Nishimura, J., & Kuroda, T. (2010). Human activity recognition from environmental background sounds for wireless sensor networks. *IEEJ Transactions on Electronics, Information and Systems, 130*(4), 565–572.
89. Sim, J. M., Lee, Y., & Kwon, O. (2015). Acoustic sensor based recognition of human activity in everyday life for smart home services. *International Journal of Distributed Sensor Networks, 11*(9), 679123.
90. Gupta, S., Morris, D., Patel, S., & Tan, D. (2012). Soundwave: Using the Doppler effect to sense gestures. In *Proceedings of the SIGCHI Conference on Human Factors in Computing Systems* (pp. 1911–1914).
91. Yang, Z., Zhou, Z., & Liu, Y. (2013). From RSSI to CSI: Indoor localization via channel response. *ACM Computing Surveys (CSUR), 46*(2), 25.
92. Wang, G., Gu, C., Inoue, T., & Li, C. (2014). A hybrid FMCW-interferometry radar for indoor precise positioning and versatile life activity monitoring. *IEEE Transactions on Microwave Theory and Techniques, 62*(11), 2812–2822.
93. Hernandez, J., McDuff, D., & Picard, R. W. (2015). Biowatch: Estimation of heart and breathing rates from wrist motions. In *2015 9th Interna-tional Conference on Pervasive Computing Technologies for Healthcare (PervasiveHealth)* (pp. 169–176). IEEE.
94. Murthy, R., Pavlidis, I., & Tsiamyrtzis, P. (2004). Touchless monitoring of breathing function. In *26th Annual International Conference of the IEEE Engineering in Medicine and Biology Society* (Vol. 1, pp. 1196–1199). IEEE.
95. Petkie, D. T., Benton, C., & Bryan, E. (2009). Millimeter wave radar for remote measurement of vital signs. In *2009 IEEE Radar Conference* (pp. 1–3). IEEE.
96. Chan, E. D., Chan, M. M., & Chan, M. M. (2013). Pulse oximetry: Under-standing its basic principles facilitates appreciation of its limitations. *Respiratory Medicine, 107*(6), 789–799.
97. Baker, S. B., Xiang, W., & Atkinson, I. (2017). Internet of things for smart healthcare: Technologies, challenges, and opportunities. *IEEE Access, 5*, 26 521–26 544.
98. Catarinucci, L., De Donno, D., Mainetti, L., Palano, L., Patrono, L., Stefanizzi, M. L., & Tarricone, L. (2015). An IoT-aware architecture for smart healthcare systems. *IEEE Internet of Things Journal, 2*(6), 515.
99. Jeong, S., Kuk, S., & Kim, H. (2019). A smartphone magnetometer-based diagnostic test for automatic contact tracing in infectious disease epidemics. *IEEE Access, 7*, 20 734–20 747.
100. Burns, G., Lioy, M., & Rongo, E. (2016) *Proximity detection of internet of things (IoT) devices using sound chirps*. Sep. 6 2016, US Patent9,438,440.
101. Liu, S., Jiang, Y., & Striegel, A. (2013). Face-to-face proximity estima-tion using bluetooth on smartphones. *IEEE Transactions on Mobile Computing, 13*(4), 811–823.
102. Vishwakarma, S., & Agrawal, A. (2013). A survey on activity recognition and behavior understanding in video surveillance. *The Visual Computer, 29*(10), 983–1009.
103. Pasku, V., De Angelis, A., De Angelis, G., Arumugam, D. D., Dionigi, M., Carbone, P., Moschitta, A., & Ricketts, D. S. (2017). Magnetic field-based positioning systems. *IEEE Communications Surveys & Tutorials, 19*(3), 2003–2017.
104. Shao, D., Liu, C., Tsow, F., Yang, Y., Du, Z., Iriya, R., Yu, H., & Tao, N. (2015). Noncontact monitoring of blood oxygen saturation using camera and dual-wavelength imaging system. *IEEE Transactions on Biomedical Engineering, 63*(6), 1091–1098.

**Dr A. Gasmi** is a physiologist with focus on physiological signal processing and variability of rhythmic biological systems. He is also a nutrition scientist and is currently the president of the Francophone Society of Nutritherapy and Applied Nutrigenetics in France and an active member of its bioinformatics and biosignals department. In addition, he is an associate scientist at the Inter-University Laboratory of Motor Biology at the University of Claude Bernard – Lyon 1 in France.

# Chapter 16
# Impact of Covid-19 Infodemic on the Global Picture

**Tapash Rudra and Sandeep Kautish**

## 16.1 Introduction

We remember centuries in memoir of events those mark significant indentations to the respective era. Humankind experienced a number of catastrophic events since the beginning including natural as well as anthropometric. The ongoing Covid-19 global pandemic is the combination of both to a considerable extent with an array of significant attributes. Indeed, the effects of the ongoing event have already made overwhelming impacts on the mankind as a whole.

Scientific community across the globe has been in the quest for the appropriate intervention of the Covid-19 pandemic. Scholarly works, research, and other associated events are going on day in and day out. To be fair enough, with the consistent monitoring and operational guidelines given by the World Health Organization (WHO), most of the facets of novel Covid-19 pandemic have been revealed including epidemiology, mode of transmission, and rate of prevalence, to name a few. However, since the very beginning of this monumental event, one aspect that people across the geographical periphery allowed to propagate exponentially like the novel Covid-19 itself is the "infodemic" [1]. To combat such a deadly epidemic, precise information is always a handful at the right juncture; unfortunately, however, it has been just the opposite. Dissemination of false information excelled several notch to the overall degree of the ongoing crisis.

One of the crucial attributes that immensely propagated the fallacious information within the community is the rumor in line with spread of novel SARS-CoV-2

T. Rudra (✉)
City University, Selangor, Malaysia

S. Kautish
LBEF Campus, Kathmandu Nepal; (In Academic Collaboration with Asia Pacific University of Technology & Innovation)
Kuala Lumpur, Malaysia



S. Kautish et al. (eds.), *Computational Intelligence Techniques for Combating COVID-19*, EAI/Springer Innovations in Communication and Computing,
https://doi.org/10.1007/978-3-030-68936-0_16

virus/Covid-19. It did not take too long for the scientific fraternity, however, to depict the trajectory of dissemination among the human beings of the novel pathogen are respiratory droplets and the surface they reside [2].

If we revert back to couple of centuries, the scenario was not that different what we are facing currently. The Spanish Flu/1918 H1N1 Influenza pandemic exhibited "physical distancing" as well in order to minimize the "spikes of infection" [3]. However, people of that time were in similar fallacy what we are now while facing the first global pandemic of the twenty-first century. In addition to that, people are more than in a jovial mood in certain parts of the world, and the policy makers have already started implementing lenient measures while it is still obscure whether the second or third wave of the pandemic is due or not [3].

### *16.1.1 Information Versus Misinformation*

It is well documented that SARS-CoV-2 virus adheres to RNA as genetic material. At the same regard, most RNA viruses are devoid of specific tools to repair the multiple gene copies. This leads to drastic malfunctions. By means of such manifestations, the novel SARS-CoV-2 virus is extremely unique regarding the degree of severity and the rate of propagation are concerned [4]. The novel Corona virus does have the abilities to repair the damaged RNAs during the replication of DNA. To be more precise, the novel SARS-CoV-2 virus corresponds less than ten mutations among the 30,000 loci within the genetic makeup. The paradox is still the novel SARS-CoV-2 virus has been rocketing along across the geographical boundaries [5].

The information is all about legitimacy. More importantly, the epidemic of such stature needs greater responsibility and awareness among the civilians. The abovementioned scientific factorials are noteworthy, keeping in mind that a cascade of misleading information on the same has provoked the global community in the negative direction, especially at the onset of the ongoing pandemic.

Within the span of around 1 month, from February to March, 2020, approximately 361,000,000 videos along with 19,200 articles have been propagated throughout the global periphery. In addition to it, around 550 million tweets including the terms such as "covid-19," "covid_19," "covid19," "coronavirus," and "corona virus" have been disseminated with an array of permutation and combinations [6]. The mentioned statistics is critical because most of the stories and information were fabricated and against the notion of scientific elements [7]. It is really obvious that since the beginning of the global pandemic the influence of fake and fallacious information has been the major obstacle to deal with. This kind of information not only has changed the mindset of the common people, but at the same time, it made the global crisis much more severe, almost demolishing the sustenance of the global health system as a whole.

### 16.1.2 Accelerated Disinformation and Social Media Hype

Exorbitant disinformation regarding the existing issues has been one of the booming topics across the global scholarly fraternity since quite a number of decades; however, the digitalized media has excelled the same into a new level [8–11]. Indeed, the pace has been galloping into a new orbit with the advent of the digital version of the social media including a handful of advanced applications. However, the progressive diminishing manual operations in tandem with the politically driven news propaganda have also triggered the rapid spread of the targeted stories/rumors [12–15].

According to the European Union (EU) commission alongside the European Action Plan (EAP) and Code of Practice (COP), the five essential points that should be implemented to combat the rapidly propagating disinformation are [15]:

- To improve on the level of transparency to sustain the digital media web.
- To authorize the legitimacy of the information.
- To standardize the protocols for monitoring the information before being shared by the media officials and subscribers.
- To develop proper strategies in order to sustain the integrity of the media ecosystem.
- To project consistent and outcome-based research to counter the influence of disinformation.

In line with the ongoing global Covid-19 pandemic, it is now becoming extremely crucial to imply the abovementioned strategies to restore the normalcy [16].

### 16.1.3 Conflict of Interest and Content Validation

Significant proportions of dispute around the ongoing pandemic have been the hallmark of the electronic media houses. The reason is primarily the lack of evidence-based techniques to filter out the disinformation. Moreover, there has been not enough privacy to contain with alongside the lenient General Data Protection Regulation [17–19]. The ongoing crisis has considerably opened up loopholes of the existing social media, especially the infrastructural fallacies are concerned. Right from the outbreak of the ongoing health crisis, lack of infrastructural support and monitoring of the news made the scenario several times worse as far as the spreading of disinformation is concerned. Scholarly works have demarcated how much the fake stories and rumors could be negatively directed from the originality [20, 21]. On the other hand, studies have also depicted how much crucial is the content of the news; otherwise, the actual factorials could be severely distorted [8]. The trustworthy information can only be drawn if there is proper content validation tools and that has exactly been lacking since the very beginning of the ongoing global pandemic.

### 16.1.4 Infodemic and the Role on the Global Picture

Colossal events such as global pandemics have always been known for taking millions of lives. The global pandemic during the period from 1918 to 1919 (Spanish Flu) took the death toll around 100 million globally, and only the United States experienced more number of casualties than the combined wars of the twentieth and twenty-first century [22]. Amidst the ongoing Covid-19 crisis, both the scientific fraternity and the modern-day historians are with similar waves of thoughts that we can learn a plenty from the past pandemics, even though the scenario is altogether different [23].

The 1918 H1N1 Influenza pandemic was primarily associated with three significant features that are accountable for the ongoing one as well. First and foremost, the civilians were measurably lethargic as far as the degree and depth of the infection. Second, they were very much apprehensive regarding the potential layouts to dismantle the spreading of the virus. Last but not the least, there was the lack of awareness about the mode of transmission of the causal pathogen across the community.

## 16.2 An Account of Literature Review on the Context of Infodemic

The onslaught of the ongoing global pandemic is indeed unprecedented and it will be in the years to come; however, the infodemic around it has been equally novel and catastrophic so far, as far as the dissemination of fallacious information is concerned. Series of debunked rumors has made the ongoing health crisis several times severe since the outbreak. The progressive disinformation and fabricated rumors took the health crisis to a new level. The Director General of WHO admirably mentioned "we're not just fighting an epidemic; we're fighting an infodemic."

Off late, numerous studies have been conducted in order to wipe out the negative aspects of infodemic among the public. One of the scholarly works emphasized that exponential spreading of disinformation could not only escalate the phobia among the public, but at the same time it could seriously damage the mental frames. Indeed, it could drastically produce prejudiced and eccentric attitude among the civilians. In reality, such things could maximize the level of disobedience, violation of the protocols, and off-course, downsizing the economy in the long run [24–26]. One of the major reasons for such phenomenon is the lack of evidence-based practice to nullify the effects of disinformation during the ongoing global pandemic [21, 27] (Table 16.1). However, it has enlightened the loopholes of the existing social media and at the same point pinpointed that media ecosystem should have the following to settle the clarity:

**Table 16.1** Annals of scientific papers off late on SARS-CoV-2 virus

| Serial number | Date | Name of the article | Name of the proposal |
|---|---|---|---|
| 1. | 18 January | Cheng VCC, Wong S-C, To KKW, Ho PL, Yuen K-Y. Preparedness and proactive infection control measures against the emerging Wuhan coronavirus pneumonia in China. J. Hosp. Infect. 2020. https://doi.org/10.1016/j.jhin.2020.01.010. | Wuhan coronavirus pneumonia |
| 2. | 20 January | Parry J. China coronavirus: Cases surge as official admits human to human transmission. Br. Med. J. 2020; 368:m236. https://doi.org/10.1136/bmj.m236. | China coronavirus |
| 3. | 21 January | Stop the Wuhan virus. Nature 2020; 577:450–450. https://doi.org/10.1038/d41586-020-00153-x | Wuhan virus |
| 4. | 22 January | Callaway E, Cyranoski D. China coronavirus: Six questions scientists are asking. Nature 2020; 577:605–7. https://doi.org/10.1038/d41586-020-00166-6 | China coronavirus |
| 5. | 22 January | Liu S-L, Saif L. Emerging Viruses without Borders: The Wuhan Coronavirus. Viruses 2020; 12:130. https://doi.org/10.3390/v12020130. | Wuhan coronavirus |
| 6. | 23 January | Callaway E, Cyranoski D. Why snakes probably aren't spreading the new China virus. Nature 2020. https://doi.org/10.1038/d41586-020-00180-8. | China virus |
| 7. | 24 January | Mahase E. China coronavirus: What do we know so far? Br. Med. J. 2020; 368:m308. https://doi.org/10.1136/bmj.m308. | China coronavirus |
| 8. | 28 January | Mahase E. China coronavirus: Mild but infectious cases may make it hard to control outbreak, report warns. Br. Med. J. 2020; 368:m325. https://doi.org/10.1136/bmj.m325. | China coronavirus |
| 9. | 29 January | Parry J. China coronavirus: Partial border closures into Hong Kong are not enough, say doctors. Br. Med. J. 2020; 368:m349. https://doi.org/10.1136/bmj.m349. | China coronavirus |
| 10. | 31 January | Callaway E. China coronavirus: labs worldwide scramble to analyse live samples. Nature 2020; 578:16–16. https://doi.org/10.1038/d41586-020-00262-7. | China coronavirus |
| 11. | 31 January | Mahase E. China coronavirus: WHO declares international emergency as death toll exceeds 200. Br. Med. J. 2020; 368:m408. https://doi.org/10.1136/bmj.m408. | China coronavirus |
| 12. | 31 January | Bassetti M, Vena A, Giacobbe DR. The novel Chinese coronavirus (2019-nCoV) infections: Challenges for fighting the storm. Eur. J. Clin. Invest. 2020: e13209. https://doi.org/10.1111/eci.13209. | Novel Chinese coronavirus |

(continued)

**Table 16.1** (continued)

| Serial number | Date | Name of the article | Name of the proposal |
|---|---|---|---|
| 13. | 31 January | Ralph R, Lew J, Zeng T, Francis M, Xue B, Roux M, et al. 2019-nCoV (Wuhan virus), a novel coronavirus: Human-to-human transmission, travel-related cases, and vaccine readiness. J. Infect. Dev. Ctries. 2020; 14:3–17. https://doi.org/10.3855/jidc.12425 | Wuhan virus |
| 14. | 3 February | Wu F, Zhao S, Yu B, Chen Y-M, Wang W, Song Z-G, et al. A new coronavirus associated with human respiratory disease in China. Nature 2020. https://doi.org/10.1038/s41586-020-2008-3. | WH-Human-1 coronavirus (WuhanHuman-1 coronavirus) |
| 15. | 4 February | Parry J. China coronavirus: Hong Kong health staff strike to demand border closure as city records first death. Br. Med. J. 2020; 368:m454. https://doi.org/10.1136/bmj.m454. | China coronavirus |
| 16. | 5 February | Jiang S, Xia S, Ying T, Lu L. A novel coronavirus (2019- nCoV) causing pneumonia-associated respiratory syndrome. Cell Mol. Immunol. 2020. https://doi.org/10.1038/s41423-020-0372-4. | PARS-CoV (pneumonia acute respiratory syndrome coronavirus) |
| 17. | 7 February | Cyranoski D. Did pangolins spread the China coronavirus to people? Nature 2020. https://doi.org/10.1038/d41586-020-00364-2. | China coronavirus |
| 18. | 11 February | Wang L-F, Anderson DE, Mackenzie JS, Merson MH. From Hendra to Wuhan: what has been learned in responding to emerging zoonotic viruses. Lancet 2020; 395: e33–4. https://doi.org/10.1016/S0140-6736(20)30350-0 | HARS-CoV (Han acute respiratory syndrome coronavirus) |
| 19. | 11 February | Gorbalenya AE, Baker SC, Baric RS, Groot RJ De, Gulyaeva AA, Haagmans BL, et al. The species and its viruses – a statement of the Coronavirus Study Group. BioRxiv 2020. https://doi.org/10.1101/2020.02.07.937862. | Acute respiratory syndrome coronavirus 2) |
| 20. | 12 February | Zhou T, Liu Q, Yang Z, Liao J, Yang K, Bai W, et al. Preliminary prediction of the basic reproduction number of the Wuhan novel coronavirus 2019-nCoV. J. Evid. Based Med. 2020. https://doi.org/10.1111/jebm.12376. | Wuhan novel coronavirus |
| 21. | 14 February | Jiang S, Shi Z-L. The first disease X is caused by a highly transmissible acute respiratory syndrome coronavirus. Virol. Sin. 2020. https://doi.org/10.1007/s12250-020-00206-5 | TARS-CoV (transmissible acute respiratory syndrome coronavirus) |
| 22. | 19 February | Jiang S, Shi Z, Shu Y, Song J, Gao GF, Tan W, et al. A distinct name is needed for the new coronavirus. Lancet 2020. https://doi.org/10.1016/S0140-6736(20)30419-0. | HCoV-19 (Human Coronavirus 2019) |

(continued)

**Table 16.1** (continued)

| Serial number | Date | Name of the article | Name of the proposal |
|---|---|---|---|
| 23. | 19 February | G. K.-M. Goh, A. K. Dunker, J. A. Foster, V. N. Uversky, rigidity of the outer Shell predicted by a protein intrinsic disorder model sheds light on the COVID-19 (Wuhan2019-nCoV) infectivity. Biomolecules. 10, 331 (2020). https://doi.org/10.3390/biom10020331 | Wuhan-2019-nCoV |
| 24. | 19 February | S. Kooraki, M. Hosseiny, L. Myers, A. Gholamrezanezhad, coronavirus (COVID-19) outbreak: What the Department of Radiology Should Know. J. Am. Coll. Radiol. (2020), https://doi.org/10.1016/j.jacr.2020.02.008. | NCIP (novel coronavirus-infected pneumonia) |
| 25. | 26 February | J. Xia, J. Tong, M. Liu, Y. Shen, D. Guo, evaluation of coronavirus in tears and conjunctival secretions of patients with SARS-CoV-2 infection. J. Med. Virol. (2020), https://doi.org/10.1002/jmv.25725. | NCP (novel coronavirus pneumonia) |

*Source*: As of 26 February 2020, the metadata of the relevant articles, retrieved from the PubMed

- Automated and algorithmically regulated information web.
- Sustainable infrastructure of the media web rather than quantity of content.
- Properly maintained repositories in order to propagate correct infodemic in masses.

### *16.2.1 The Influence of Infodemic in Worsening the Ongoing Pandemic*

The sharing of information has been ridiculously easy these days by the means of a handful of digital applications. The civilians across all the age groups have the options to surf and propagate the news at their ease [28]. Since the onset of the Covid-19 pandemic, electronic media houses have been the major contributors to swell up the illegitimate stories around the various aspects of it [29]. It is due to the dissemination of the misleading news/rumors among the public [30], without the scientific element and premature ways of filtering the contents [31]. Some of the rumors that initially have been dispersed like a rash regarding the ready-made remedies were the daily dose of oregano, use of bleaching agents and continuous use of saline suspension, etc. [31, 32]. Similar fabricated version of fake stories have been rampaging across the globe about the possible reasoning behind the emergence of the Covid-19 pandemic [33]. To say the least, these fallacious information have been multiplying at the back of the mind of the civilians leading to unwanted fear and stigmatization in the community. Furthermore, we cannot dislodge the influence of social media, especially, Facebook, Twitter, as well as YouTube to propagate the fake news throughout the global community at the onset of the ongoing pandemic. Lack of proper filtering process and various loopholes in the monitoring of transmission through the digital media about the news of Covid-19 pandemic were the other contributing factors. As a whole, the most frequently used applications such as Facebook, YouTube, and Twitter have been mishandled both by social networks and some section of netizens since the outbreak first started [34].

## 16.3 Principle Aids of Disinformation about Covid-19 Pandemic

There has been a handful of objects that considerably propagated the misleading news among the common people in the society about the Covid-19 pandemic:

- Numerous information from a variety of resources without scientific legitimacy.
- Sequential disturbances among the civilians leading to anxiety, depression, and trauma.
- Odd articles, blogs, or other publications from unauthentic sites without any protocol for quality control.
- Abundance of accessibility to write or post anything on anywhere irrespective of scientific depth.

### *16.3.1 Primary Things We Should Adhere to Counteract the Infodemic*

- The first and foremost task is to check the validity and authentication of the news related to pandemic before being shared even to the close ones. The mandatory thing is to evaluate the scientific truth of the information even if it is from the resource that is well known.
- At the same regard, it is very much critical to stop the propagation of any fake stories that might cause detrimental effects to the health system of the community. Serious and strict measures are needed to dislodge the origin of such misinformation, whenever found.
- Quality control of the data is of essential value as the information shall be utilized by mass after being dispersed on a large scale.
- The data related to any wing of the global pandemic including the origin, the mode of transmission, pathogenesis, potential therapeutics, or any other aspect must be covered up by relevant scientific references before being discharged to the global community.
- People should be responsible and realistic while participating in a social conversation regarding the discussion on the ongoing global pandemic. We have to be hundred percent confirmed about the reliability of the information before sharing to any social aids such as WhatsApp, Messenger, Facebook, etc. (Fig. 16.1).

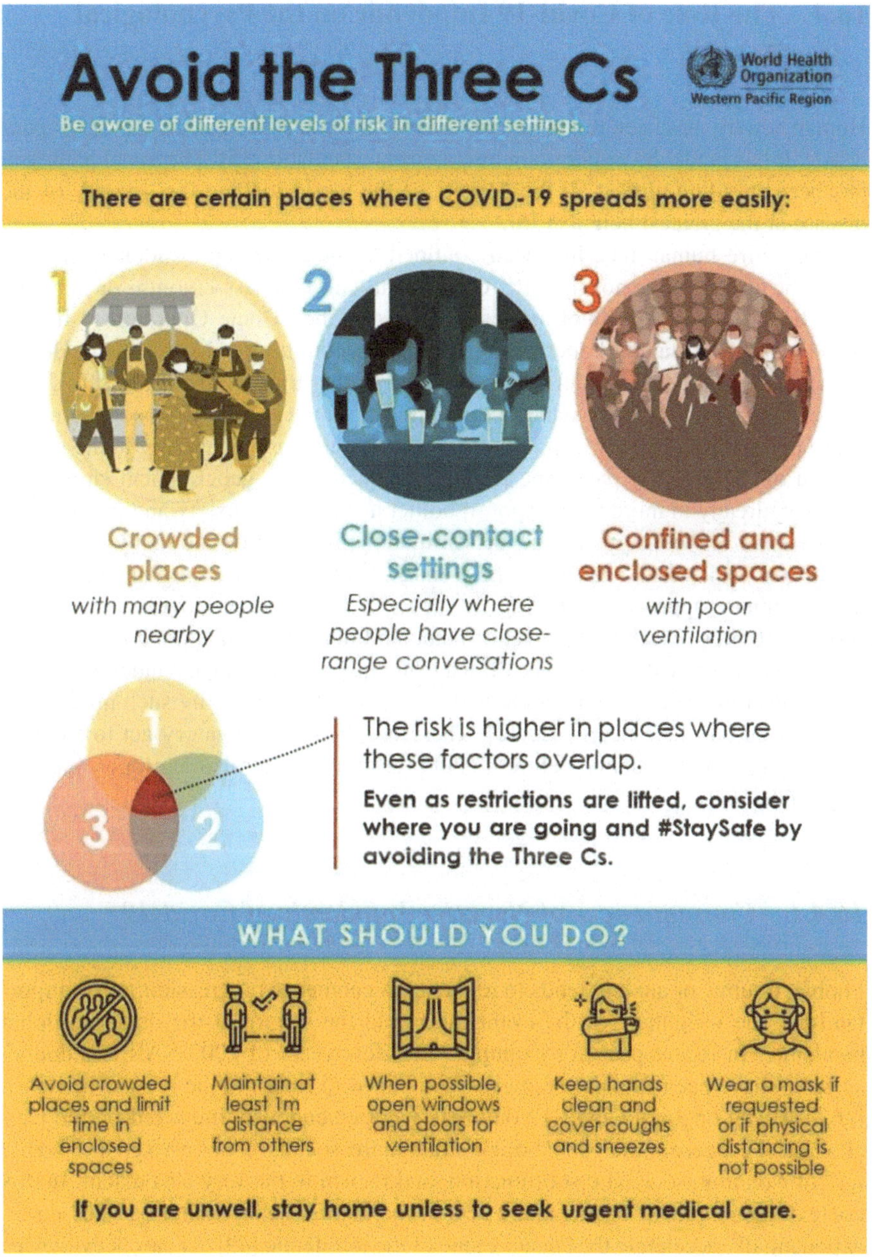


**Fig. 16.1** Necessary things for the civilians to look at. (Source: World Health Organization (WHO), Bulletin of Western Pacific Region, 2020)

## 16.4 The Role of Covid-19 Infodemic on the Psychological Aspects

Human activity has been reeling globally since the emergence of the Covid-19 pandemic. It has made the millennium into a virtual standstill [35]. The novel pathogen has been invading almost all the corners of the world making the severity of the disease at the greatest heights [36].

The entire human race has been confined to the respective residencies by the emphatic effects of the novel SARS-CoV-2 virus since the last 4 months or so by the periodical "Lockdowns" and implementations of the "Home Quarantine" in line with the relevant standard operation guidelines, recommended by the World Health Organization (WHO) in order to deaccelerate further transmission [37, 38]. Under such unprecedented circumstances, the mindset of the civilians has been the major cause of worries as plenty of psychological disorders are contributing to the global burden of the ongoing pandemic [39]. People across the geographical circumference are already in more than a spot of bother as far as the anxiety and psychological traumas are concerned. The dissemination of misinformation by means of digitalized social media has made the scenario even worse. In a long run this sort of non-pragmatic approach regarding the news of the ongoing Covid-19 pandemic should definitely escalate the level of panic and mass hysteria among the civilians [40]. Conclusive evidences can be drawn from the previous global pandemics where the mindset of the common people had been severely daunted by such misleading information and fake news [41, 42]. Therefore, it is an obligatory act to squeeze these misleading infodemic before it could reach to uncontrollable proportion [43–45] (Table 16.2).

### *16.4.1 Consequences of Negative Infodemic of Covid-19*

Phobia, trauma, or anxiety tends to replicate in geometric progression, more importantly, if the weightage of the event does hold the stature of the ongoing global pandemic. In recent past, for example, after few years of 2003 SARS epidemic, sufferers have been found extremely traumatized to return to the regular activities [46–48]. The ongoing Covid-19 outbreak has tremendously impacted on the psychological aspects of the people of all strata in the society. It has evoked the sizable fear of isolation, societal discrimination, and racism to the very best extent. In this context the nonpractical, premature acts of the digital media cannot be ruled out to exponentially accelerate the negative side of the infodemic [49]. Clear-cut evidences of criminal offence have been also depicted from certain corners from India in line with the influence of negative impact of infodemic [49, 50].

**Table 16.2** Effects of infodemic on the society and relevant recommendations

| Societal groups | Concerned issues | Recommendations |
|---|---|---|
| 1. Individuals tested positive for SARS-CoV-2 virus and the suspected ones for the same (home-quarantined) | Severe to mild anxiety<br>Trauma<br>PTSD | Continuous and thorough monitoring of the affected ones through medical interventions<br>Mental and emotional support from the family and friends to rule out the negative infodemic at bay [72]<br>Consistent encouragement from the concerned authorities [73] |
| 2. Healthcare professionals and caregivers | Enormous work pressure and stress<br>Depression<br>Non-guarantee of the jobs | Mandatory usage of PPE and other safety measures [72]<br>Continuous update on the authentic information to screen out whatever stigma existing at the back of the mind [73, 74] |
| 3. Children | Fear of getting infected<br>Agitation<br>Cognitive impairment | Development of thorough practice of maintaining the hygiene [75]<br>Encouragement of practicing free hand exercise during the stay at home on a regular basis [76] |
| 4. People over or around 60 years of age | Cognitive impairment<br>Agitation<br>Boredom | Regular physical exercise [77]<br>Exposure to relevant and authentic sources to lift the mental setup [78] |
| 5. Minorities | Constant anxiety of joblessness<br>Criminal offense | Security of providing the basic needs under such global crisis [79]<br>To make sure the affordability of healthcare commodities and protection of the basic human rights [80] |
| 6. Individuals having previously psychiatric issues | Addiction<br>Agitation<br>Violence | Online classes on psychological counselling and psychotherapies [81–88] |

### *16.4.2 The Isolation and Quarantine Saga*

In order to curtail down the progression of the novel Covid-19 virus, the policy makers across the world introduced the phenomenon of "Lockdown" in tandem with quarantine and isolation as the preliminary standard operation protocol [51]. However, the way lockdown has been implemented in certain parts of the Asian region has not only escalated the notion of mass hysteria but at the same regard magnified the misconception about the pandemic too. Moreover, the social media and the amount of vague, irrational information made the situation even worse as public were in constant dilemma which news to go for in practice [51–53]. It is quite staggering that the number of irrelevant rumors and misleading information has been disseminated regarding the thermal checking and usage of sanitization in the community through the aids of digital networking at the onset of the pandemic [44], although, it is a proven fact that body temperature is not at all the conclusive parameter to screen out Covid-19 patients. Such negative infodemic has increased the burden of psychological symptoms among the common people including the development of post-traumatic stress disorder (PTSD) and the associated ones [45–48]. On the contrary, it has been depicted that "Mandatory Lockdowns" as well as quarantine have been arrogantly disobeyed by certain sections of the community in India even in the designated high-risk zones for the Covid-19 [49]. The impact of negative infodemic along with the provocation by influential personals have been the principle factors behind such nuisance.

## 16.5 Social Media and Infodemic: The Crucial Passage of Play

The amplitude of conflicting information, news, and stories have been the most noticeable thing around the ongoing global health crisis. The digital media in various forms has been the flag bearer, and digital version of social media has already taken the responsibility to be the "global public health threat," especially, the manner they have propagated the negative infodemic of Covid-19 throughout the globe is concerned [50] (Fig. 16.2).

Off late, with the advent of advanced digital machineries and rapid interconnections, digital platform could be the vital tool for the fast and accurate monitoring of

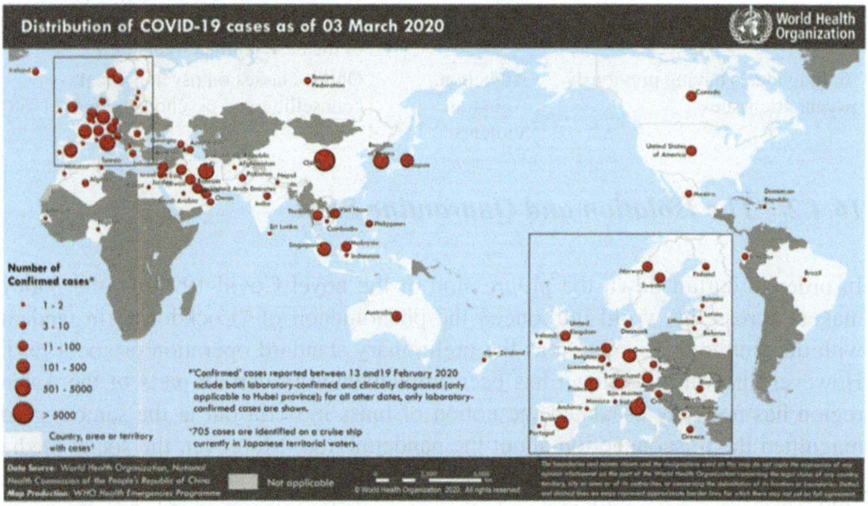


**Fig. 16.2** Geographical distribution of the COVID-19 infodemic (as of 29 February 2020). The pictorial view is depicted in the map of 58 countries and respective domains with low cumulative rates and negative perceptual bias in line with the notion of the origin of Covid-19 in the public. (Source: World Health Organization (WHO, 2020))

the ongoing global crisis, but in reality, since the onset of the ongoing pandemic, the "media web" contributed in the negative direction, which eventually doubled the degree of global trauma and depression among the civilians [51].

If we could revert back at the beginning, the onslaught of negative infodemic commenced few days after the first outbreak, and since then it has been galloping along to every corner of the global community as fast as the SARS-CoV-2 virus itself has been doing [52]. The World Health Organization (WHO) has shown the concern over the exponentially growing infodemic comprising of fake rumors and stories. The Director General of WHO asked the civilians across the globe to not only keep themselves safe, but at the same point, he appealed to curb down the metastasizing negative propaganda of infodemic [53].

One of the major reasons of the exponential growth of the negative infodemic is the unavailability of the exact number of death cases or the significant amount of conflicting figure among the sources. To be frank, this has been the principle feed for the social media to serve the common people by modifying and fabricating the reality into a fictitious figure. Soon after the emergence of the Covid-19 outbreak, most of the digital and social media engaged themselves in an "unhealthy rat race" and provoked the entire global community through the aids of blogs, videos, and other readily accessible digital applications [54]. Therefore, it is imperative to say that what we could have expected from the social media they just delivered the things in other way around.

With the influence of such fallacious and misleading information, certain section of the netizens even have been reported to simulate the symptoms of Covid-19 for the readily available popularity; however, such kind of non-civilian acts propelled the level of anxiety and hysteria among the innocent people [55]. Not only that, the misleading and simulating behavior made the mass extremely confused as they kept on seeing a variety of erroneous information through several audiovisual aids [56, 57].

On the other hand, some facets of social media took a different trajectory. They made the flamboyant collage between the various aspects of the ongoing pandemic and existing political issues and economic crisis, to name a few. These sections of media categorically designed and discharged the irrational blogs, fabricated links, and structured visual aids to achieve the ready-made publicity in the community [58]. It is worth mentioning that both the depth and degree of the ongoing Covid-19 pandemic have been excelled by such irresponsible stuffs. The social violence, disobedience, and consistent conflicting activities have been up and running by the influence of such negative infodemic [59]. In addition to that, common people have been reported to disobey the healthcare professionals regarding the Covid-19 therapeutic is concerned by the influence of constant fake propaganda of the digital social media [58–60].

### *16.5.1 Phenomenon of Racism: The Most Unwelcome Aspect*

Even before the emergence of the Covid-19 pandemic, the world across the geographical boundaries has been turbulent with a plenty of socioeconomic as well as political issues. In continuation to that, social and digital media added spices to even worsen the same [61–63]. The phenomenon of racism is one of the biggest threats of the twenty-first century. Since the very beginning, the social media has been extremely proactive to launch an anti-Chinese perception throughout the world. Corruptive news cuttings and provocation through the visual aids in Facebook, Messenger, as well as in WhatsApp have been the chief attributes used by the digital networking sites to negatively spread the infodemic and social discrimination and racism [64–66]. It is quite unfortunate to see such irresponsible acts from certain groups of netizens and media. In prolonged circumstances, these kinds of provocations should harm the integrity of the human kind as a whole. Therefore, it is high time to pull off the shocks for the policy makers as well as for the healthcare professionals to dislodge the notion of negative infodemic and restore the parity by taking robust actions.

## 16.6 Future Directives

- The Twenty-first century documented a variety of mental diseases across the geographical peripheries in line with the daily hustles and jostle. The ongoing health crisis, however, has added a new dimension to that [67].
- It should be of highest priority, therefore, for the social media to act meticulously to break the chain of negative infodemic to a further extent. The social media platforms should adhere to the basic guidelines given by the World Health Organization and convey the correct information about the ongoing crisis [65].
- The World Health Organization has launched news portals about the updates on the Covid-19 pandemic. The global media should use those references before passing the information to the public [66, 67].
- Since the very beginning of the ongoing pandemic, a significant number of fallacies have been manufactured about the potential therapeutics by some section of netizens in tandem with electronic media. This kind of irrational mindset could negatively influence the health professionals. Therefore, it should be imperative that policy makers of the respective country domains must take such things seriously into account to dislodge the misleading news/stories.
- Scientific fraternity around the globe have been deeply involved to design the appropriate remedies to combat the ongoing crisis. In view of the effects of convalescent plasma (CP) therapy against SARS [68], MERS, and 2009 HINI Influenza pandemic [69], health professionals have recommended the use of this technique for the ongoing one as well.

- The major reason behind the choice of this particular therapy is there are not enough proven therapeutics available for the Covid-19-specific treatment to secure the lives of the infected ones [68–70]. However, to captivate the efficacy of the CP therapy, healthcare professionals must take into account both the patient and the donor eligibility [71].
- However, more potent options have been also tried. The quest started with the application of anti-malarial drugs such as chloroquine and hydroxychloroquine. Since then other pharmaceuticals like ivermectin and remdesivir have been also implied in several clinical trials to find out the appropriate remedy.
- Before the ongoing Covid-19 pandemic, viruses like small pox severely catastrophized the societal image of the respective times. However, mankind came out from the very dark to the new dawn with the discovery of vaccines against such viruses.
- To discover the vaccine against novel SARS-CoV-2 is indeed a stiff mountain to climb, but humankind has done this in the past by discovering vaccines for similar kind of deadly diseases. In this regard the social media must be equally responsible to propagate the authentic news about the progressive events toward the possible development of the Covid-19 vaccine.
- Premature news cuttings, stories, and fabricated videos on the YouTube, Facebook, and other digital media platforms have already exponentially increased the inappropriate infodemic. Henceforth, media houses should be loyal and strict to filter out such nuisance to curb down the misleading news among the masses in future days to come.
- Apart from the conventional approach, medical science has been trying the level best to explore and incorporate ways that have been hitherto impossible to imagine. One of the booms of the modern-day computational biology in line with this is the implication of artificial intelligence (AI).
- Modern-day medical research has been revolving around these newly invented tools. Scientists and clinicians are in the process of amalgamation of traditional medical therapies in tandem with the artificial intelligence. In fact, the ongoing Covid-19 pandemic might be the potential target for the different wings of artificial intelligence to stamp the authority and come up with triumphs.
- Both the stakeholders and leading social media must encourage and highlight such new innovations to assure the civilians more prudently. We can be victorious against the rampaging pandemic, provided we shall be realistic. The responsibilities of the global electronic media must be of utmost importance in this regard (Fig. 16.3).

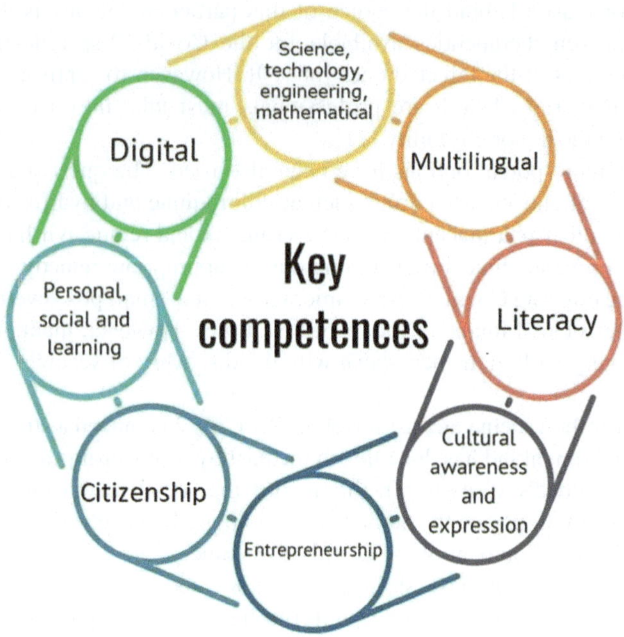


**Fig. 16.3** The principal attributes of the social media outreach

## 16.7 Conclusion

The onslaught of the ongoing global crisis has opened our eyes on how much a pathogen can contribute adversely on the overall mindset and psychology of the global community. Even though, we are in the twenty-first century, still the ongoing catastrophic event gave us the wake-up call that unless we will be pragmatic in our approach the sustenance of humankind is under ominous threat at any point of time.

Since the emergence of the ongoing pandemic, more than one million lives have been succumbed to death alongside another 45 million infected globally. However, the number of recoveries has been also increasing since the last few months with the implementations of robust guidelines and policies. This is a promising sign, even though, chances of resurgence should be given a vital importance. Any negligence around the possibilities of second and third waves of the pandemic might cause a serious blow toward the overall recovery. The policy makers of the respective countries along with the social media must be more proactive regarding this. The user-friendly digital versions of the social media should maintain the transparency about the latest updates on the existing pandemic is concerned. They should give authentic information among the masses.

The mental health of the civilians around the globe is at the dire straits right now. The condition of the socioeconomy is not different either. So, it is imperative for the people across the global community to contribute and act realistically to overhaul the ongoing crisis.

Thus far, the premature outlook of the digitalized social media has been the major escalating factor behind the spreading of misleading news around the ongoing pandemic. Therefore, it is high time to pull the shocks and convey the exact infodemic from the media platforms to resurrect the image as far as the overall dimension of the digital media is concerned.

## References


1. Zarocostas, J. (2020, February). How to fight an infodemic. *The Lancet, 395*(10225), 676.
2. Markel, H., Lipman, H. B., Navarro, J. A., Sloan, A., Michalsen, J. R., Stern, A. M., & Cetron, M. S. (2007). Nonpharmaceutical interventions implemented by US cities during the 1918–1919 influenza pandemic. *Journal of American Medical Association, 98*(6), 644–654.
3. Mueller, J., & Johnson, N. P. A. S. (2002). Updating the accounts: Global mortality of the 1918–1920 "Spanish": influenza pandemic. *Bulletin of the History of Medicine, 76*(1), 105–115.
4. Long, J. S., Mistry, B., Haslam, S. M., & Barclay, W. S. (2019, February). Host and viral determinants of influenza A virus species specificity. *Nature Reviews Microbiology, 17*, 67.
5. Lofgren, E., Fefferman, N. H., Naumov, Y. N., Gorski, J., & Naumova, E. N. (2007). Influenza seasonality: Underlying causes and modeling theories. *Journal of Virology, 81*(11), 5429–5436.
6. United Nations. (2020). UN tackles 'infodemic' of misinformation and cybercrime in COVID-19 crisis.
7. MIT Technology Review (Internet) (2020). How social media can combat the coronavirus 'infodemic'.
8. Benkler, Y., Faris, R., & Roberts, H. (2018). *Network propaganda: Manipulation, disinformation, and radicalization in American politics*. New York: Oxford University Press.
9. Dewey, J. (1927). *The public and its problems. Reprint 1946*. New York: Holt.
10. Lippmann, W. (1921). *Public opinion*. New York: Macmillan.
11. Lippmann, W. (1927). *The phantom public*. New Brunswick: Transaction Publishers.
12. Newman, N., Dutton, W., & Blank, G. (2014). Social media and the news: Implications for the press and society. In *In society and the internet: How networks of information and communication are changing our lives* (pp. 135–148). Oxford: Oxford University Press.
13. Newman, N., Fletcher, R., Kalogeropoulos, A., & Nielsen, R. K. (2019). *Digital news report*. Oxford: Reuters Institute for the Study of Journalism.
14. Nielsen, R. K., Fletcher, R., Newman, N., Brennen, S., & Howard, P. N.. (2020). Navigating the 'Infodemic': How people in six countries access and rate news and information about coronavirus. Reuters Institute for the Study of Journalism. https://reutersinstitute.politics.ox.ac.uk/infodemic-how-people-six-countries-access-and-rate-news-and-information-about-coronavirus
15. Vosoughi, S., Roy, D., & Aral, S. (2018). The spread of true and false news online. *Science (New York, NY), 359*(6380), 1146–1151.
16. Buning, M. D. C. (2018). A multi-dimensional approach to disinformation: report of the independent high level group on fake news and online disinformation, 1–40. Brussels: EU Commission. https://ec.europa.eu/digital-single-market/en/news/final-report-high-level-expert-group-fakenews-and-online-disinformation
17. Bechmann, A., & B. O'Loughlin. (2020). Democracy & disinformation: A turn in the debate, thinkers' programme, 1–30, 2020. Brussels: Royal Flemish Academy of Belgium for Sciences and the Arts.

18. Moeller, L. A., & Bechmann, A. (2019). *Research data exchange solution [report for the EU Commission]*. Brussels: SOMA.
19. Vreese, C., de Bastos, M., Esser, F., Giglietto, F., Lecleher, S., Pfetsch, B., Puschmann, C., Tromble, R., King, G., & Persily, N.. (2019). Public Statement from the Co-Chairs and European Advisory Committee of Social Science, 2019, Vol. 1." https://socialscience.one/blog/public-statement-europeanadvisory-committee-social-science-one
20. Lazer, D. M. J., Baum, M. A., Benkler, Y., Berinsky, A. J., Greenhill, K. M., Menczer, F., Metzger, M. J., et al. (2018). The science of fake news. *Science (New York, N.Y.), 359*(6380), 1094–1096.
21. Guess, A., Nagler, J., & Tucker, J. (2019). Less than you think: Prevalence and predictors of fake news dissemination on Facebook. *Science Advances, 5*(1), eaau4586.
22. Verity, R., Okell, L. C., Dorigatti, I., et al. (2020). Estimates of the severity of coronavirus disease 2019: A model-based analysis. *The Lancet Infectious Diseases, 20*(6), 669–677.
23. Morens, D. M., & Fauci, A. S. (2007). The 1918 influenza pandemic: Insights for the 21st century. *The Journal of Infectious Diseases, 195*(7), 1018–1028.
24. Mawson, A. R. (2005). Understanding mass panic and other collective responses to threat and disaster. *Psychiatry, 68*(2), 95–113.
25. Pearce, J. M., Lindekilde, L., Parker, D., & Rogers, M. B. (2019). Communicating with the public about marauding terrorist firearms attacks: Results from a survey experiment on factors influencing intention to "run, hide, tell" in the United Kingdom and Denmark. *Risk Analysis: An Official Publication of the Society for Risk Analysis, 39*(8), 1675–1694.
26. Sheppard, B., Rubin, G. J., Wardman, J. K., & Wessely, S. (2006). Viewpoint: Terrorism and dispelling the myth of a panic prone public. *Journal of Public Health Policy, 27*(3), 219–245.
27. Grinberg, N., Joseph, K., Friedland, L., Swire-Thompson, B., & Lazer, D. (2019). Fake News on Twitter during the 2016 U.S. presidential Election. *Science (New York, N.Y.), 63*(6425), 374–378.
28. Del Vicario, M., Bessi, A., Zollo, F., et al. (2016). The spreading of misinformation online. *Proceedings of the National Academy of Sciences of the United States of America, 113*(3), 554–559.
29. Lazer, D. M. J., Baum, M. A., Benkler, Y., et al. (2018). The science of fake news. *Science, 359*(6380), 1094–1096.
30. Vosoughi, S., Roy, D., & Aral, S. (2018). The spread of true and false news online. *Science, 359*(6380), 1146–1151.
31. Lewandowsky, S., Ecker, U. K. H., Seifert, C. M., et al. (2012). Misinformation and its correction: Continued influence and successful debiasing. *Psychological Science in the Public Interest, 13*(3), 106–131.
32. Chakravorti, B. (2020). As coronavirus spreads, so does fake news. Bloomberg Opinion, 5 February, 2020.Available at: www.bloomberg.com/opinion/articles/2020-02-05/as-coronavirus-spreads-sodoes-fake-news. Accessed 8 February 2020.
33. Taylor, J. (2020). Bat soup, dodgy cures and 'diseasology': The spread of coronavirus misinformation. The Guardian, 31 January, 2020. Available at: www.theguardian.com/world/2020/jan/31/bat-soupdodgy-cures-and-diseasology-the-spread-of-coronavirus-bunkum. Accessed 8 February 2020.
34. Aguilera, J. (2020). Xenophobia 'is a pre-existing condition'. How harmful stereotypes and racism are spreading around the coronavirus. Time, 1 February, 2020. Available at: https://time.Com/5775716/xenophobia-racism-stereotypes-coronavirus/. Accessed 8 February 2020.
35. Jones, D. S. (2020, March 12). History in a crisis – Lessons for covid-19. *The New England Journal of Medicine, 382*(18), 1681–1683.
36. Lai, C. C., Shih, T. P., Ko, W. C., Tang, H. J., & Hsueh, P. R. (2020). Severe acute respiratory syndrome coronavirus 2 (SARS-CoV-2) and coronavirus disease-2019 (COVID-19): The epidemic and the challenges. *International Journal of Antimicrobial Agents, 55*(10), 5924.
37. Rubin, G. J., & Wessely, S. (2020). The psychological effects of quarantining a city. *BMJ, 368*, m313.

38. Pulla, P. (2020). Covid-19: India imposes lockdown for 21 days and cases rise. *BMJ, 368*, m1251.
39. Kluge, H. N. P. (2020). Statement e physical and mental health key to resilience during COVID-19 pandemic. http://www.euro.who.int/en/health-topics/health-emergencies/coronavirus-covid-19/statements/statement-physical-and-mental-health-key-to-resilience-during-covid-19-pandemic. Accessed on 30th March, 2020.
40. Depoux, A., Martin, S., Karafillakis, E., Bsd, R. P., Wilder-Smith, A., & Larson, H. (2020). The pandemic of social media panic travels faster than the COVID-19 outbreak. *Journal of Travel Medicine, 27*(3), taaa031.
41. Sim, K., & Chua, H. C. (2004). The psychological impact of SARS: A matter of heart and mind. *CMAJ, 170*, 811.
42. Wu, P., Fang, Y., Guan, Z., Fan, B., Kong, J., Yao, Z., Liu, X., Fuller, C. J., Susser, E., Lu, J., & Hoven, C. W. (2009). The psychological impact of the SARS epidemic on hospital employees in China: Exposure, risk perception, and altruistic acceptance of risk. *Canadian Journal of Psychiatry, 54*, 302.
43. Shigemura, J., Ursano, R. J., Morganstein, J. C., Kurosawa, M., & Benedek, D. M. (2020). Public responses to the novel 2019 coronavirus (2019-nCoV) in Japan: Mental health consequences and target populations. *Psychiatry and Clinical Neurosciences, 74*, 281.
44. Lima, C. K. T., Carvalho, P. M. M., Lima, I. A. A. S., Nunes, J. V. A. O., Saraiva, J. S., de Souza, R. I., et al. (2020). The emotional impact of coronavirus 2019-nCoV (new coronavirus disease). *Psychiatry Research, 287*, 112915.
45. Zandifar, A., & Badrfam, R. (2020). Iranian mental health during the COVID-19 epidemic. *Asian Journal of Psychiatry, 51*, 101990.
46. Lee, S., Chan, L. Y., Chau, A. M., Kwok, K. P., & Kleinman, A. (2005). The experience of SARS- related stigma at Amoy Gardens. *Social Science & Medicine, 61*, 2038e46.
47. Person, B., Sy, F., Holton, K., Govert, B., & Liang, A. (2004). National center for infectious diseases/SARS community outreach team. Fear and stigma: the epidemic within the SARS outbreak. *Emerging Infectious Diseases, 10*, 358e63.
48. Siu, J. Y. (2008). The SARS-associated stigma of SARS victims in the post-SARS era of Hong Kong. *Qualitative Health Research, 18*, 729e38.
49. Verma, S., Mythily, S., Chan, Y. H., Deslypere, J. P., Teo, E. K., & Chong, S. A. (2004). Post-SARS psychological morbidity and stigma among general practitioners and traditional Chinese medicine practitioners in Singapore. *Annals of the Academy of Medicine, Singapore, 33*, 743e8.
50. Maunder, R., Hunter, J., Vincent, L., Bennett, J., Peladeau, N., Leszcz, M., et al. (2003). The immediate psychological and occupational impact of the 2003 SARS outbreak in a teaching hospital. *CMAJ, 168*, 1245.
51. Hawryluck, L., Gold, W. L., Robinson, S., Pogorski, S., Galea, S., & Styra, R. (2004). SARS control and psychological effects of quarantine, Toronto, Canada. *Emerging Infectious Diseases, 10*, 1206.
52. Brooks, S. K., Webster, R. K., Smith, L. E., Woodland, L., Wessely, S., Greenberg, N., et al. (2020). The psychological impact of quarantine and how to reduce it: Rapid review of the evidence. *Lancet, 395*, 912.
53. Li, W., Yang, Y., Liu, Z. H., Zhao, Y. J., Zhang, Q., Zhang, L., et al. (2020, March 15). Progression of mental health services during the COVID-19 outbreak in China. *International Journal of Biological Sciences, 16*, 1732.
54. Robertson, E., Hershenfield, K., Grace, S. L., & Stewart, D. E. (2004). The psychosocial effects of being quarantined following exposure to SARS: A qualitative study of Toronto health care workers. *Canadian Journal of Psychiatry, 49*, 403.
55. Barbisch, D., Koenig, K. L., & Shih, F. Y. (2015). Is there a case for quarantine? Perspectives from SARS to Ebola. *Disaster Medicine and Public Health Preparedness, 9*, –547.
56. Jeong, H., Yim, H. W., Song, Y. J., Ki, M., Min, J. A., Cho, J., & Chae, J. H. (2016). Mental health status of people isolated due to Middle East respiratory syndrome. *Epidemiology and Health, 38*, e2016048.

57. Liu, X., Kakade, M., Fuller, C. J., Fan, B., Fang, Y., Kong, J., et al. (2012). Depression after exposure to stressful events: Lessons learned from the severe acute respiratory syndrome epidemic. *Comprehensive Psychiatry, 53*, 15.
58. Mair-Jenkins, J., Saavedra-Campos, M., Baillie, J. K., et al. (2015). The effectiveness of convalescent plasma and hyper immune immunoglobulin for the treatment of severe acute respiratory infections of viral etiology: A systematic review and exploratory meta-analysis. *The Journal of Infectious Diseases, 211*(1), 80–90.
59. Duan, K., Liu, B., Li, C., et al. (2020). Effectiveness of convalescent plasma therapy in severe COVID-19 patients [published online ahead of print, 2020 Apr 6]. *Proceedings of the National Academy of Sciences of the United States of America*. 202004168. Available at: https://www.pnas.org/content/early/2020/04/02/2004168117 (accessed online on 13 April 2020). 60. DanaSparks. Convalescent plasma: A therapy for COVID-19? https://newsnetwork.mayoclinic.org/discussion/convalescent-plasma-a-therapy-for-covid-19/. Accessed online on 13 April 2020.
60. Roback, J. D., & Guarner, J. (2020). Convalescent plasma to treat COVID-19: Possibilities and challenges. *JAMA, 323*(16), 1561–1562. Published online March 27, 2020.
61. Chung, R. Y., & Li, M. M. (2020). Anti-Chinese sentiment during the 2019-nCoV outbreak. *Lancet, 395*, 686e.
62. Zhai, Y., & Du, X. (2020). Mental health care for international Chinese students affected by the COVID-19 outbreak. *Lancet Psychiatry, 7*, e22.
63. The New Indian Express. (2020). Bihar man beaten to death for informing Covid-19 medical help center about arrival of two people from Maharashtra. https://www.newindianexpress.com/nation/2020/mar/31/bihar-man-beaten-to-death-for-informing-covid–19-medical-help-center-about-arrival-of-two-people-fr-2123828.html; 2020. Accessed on 1st April, 2020.
64. Times of India. (2020). Covid-19: doctors gone to collect samples attacked in Indore. https://timesofindia.indiatimes.com/videos/news/covid-19-doctors-gone-to-collect-samples-attacked-in-indore/videoshow/74942153.cms;2020. Accessed on 2nd April, 2020.
65. The Economic Times. (2020). 11 Coronavirus suspects flee from a hospital in Maharashtra. https://economictimes.indiatimes.com/news/politics-and-nation/11-coronavirus-suspects-flee-from-a-hospital-in-maharashtra/videoshow/ 74644936.cms? From mdr; 2020. Accessed on 2nd April, 2020.
66. Sokolov, M. (2020). The pandemic infodemic: How social media helps [and hurts] during the coronavirus outbreak. The Drum 2020. https://www.thedrum.Com/opinion/2020/03/03/the-pandemic-infodemic-how-social-media-helps-and-hurts-during-the-coronavirus. Accessed on 30th March, 2020.
67. US-FDA Recommendations for Investigational COVID-19 Convalescent Plasma, update. April 8, 2020. Available at: https://www.fda.gov/vaccines-blood-biologics/investigational-new-drug-ind-or-device-exemption-ide-process-cber/recommendations-investigational-covid-19-convalescent-plasma. Accessed online on 13 April 2020.
68. Chen, Q., Liang, M., Li, Y., Guo, J., Fei, D., Wang, L., et al. (2020). Mental health care for medical staff in China during the COVID-19 outbreak. *Lancet Psychiatry, 7*, e15–e16.
69. Xiang, Y. T., Yang, Y., Li, W., Zhang, L., Zhang, Q., Cheung, T., et al. (2020). Timely mental health care for the 2019 novel coronavirus outbreak is urgently needed. *Lancet Psychiatry, 7*, 228–229.
70. Wang, G., Zhang, Y., Zhao, J., Zhang, J., & Jiang, F. (2020). Mitigate the effects of home confinement on children during the COVID-19 outbreak. *Lancet, 395*, 945.
71. Jiménez-Pavón, D., Carbonell-Baeza, A., & Lavie, C. J. (2020, March 24). Physical exercise as therapy to fight against the mental and physical consequences of COVID-19 quarantine: Special focus in older people. *Progress in Cardiovascular Diseases, 63*(3), 386–388.
72. Qiu, J., Shen, B., Zhao, M., Wang, Z., Xie, B., & Xu, Y. (2020). A nationwide survey of psychological distress among Chinese people in the COVID-19 epidemic: Implications and policy recommendations. *General Psychiatry, 33*, e100213.

73. Liu, S., Yang, L., Zhang, C., Xiang, Y. T., Liu, Z., Hu, S., et al. (2020). Online mental health services in China during the COVID-19 outbreak. *Lancet Psychiatry, 7*, e17–e18.
74. Tsai, J., & Wilson, M. (2020). COVID-19: A potential public health problem for homeless populations. *Lancet Publ Health, 20*(S2468), 30053–30050.
75. Kirby, T. (2020). Efforts escalate to protect homeless people from COVID-19 in UK. *The Lancet Respiratory Medicine, 20*(S2213), 30160.
76. Xiao, C. (2020). A novel approach of consultation on 2019 novel coronavirus [COVID-19]-Related psychological and mental problems: Structured letter therapy. *Psychiatry Investigation, 17*, 175.
77. Zhou, X., Snoswell, C. L., Harding, L. E., Bambling, M., Edirippulige, S., Bai, X., et al. (2020, March 23). The role of telehealth in reducing the mental health burden from COVID-19. *Telemedicine Journal and E-Health, 26*(4), 377–379.
78. Larson, H. J. (2018). The biggest pandemic risk? Viral misinformation. *Nature, 562*, 309.
79. Al-Garadi, M. A., Khan, M. S., Varathan, K. D., Mujtaba, G., & Al-Kabsi, A. M. (2016). Using online social networks to track a pandemic: A systematic review. *Journal of Biomedical Informatics, 62*, 1.
80. Shimizu, K. (2020). 2019-nCoV, fake news, and racism. *Lancet, 395*, 685.
81. Merchant, R. M., & Lurie, N. (2020, March 23). Social media and emergency preparedness in response to novel coronavirus. *JAMA, 323*(20), 2011–2012.
82. Asmundson, G. J. G., & Taylor, S. (2020). Coronaphobia: Fear and the 2019-nCoV outbreak. *Journal of Anxiety Disorders, 70*, 102196.
83. Ho, C. S., Chee, C. Y., & Ho, R. C. (2020). Mental health strategies to combat the psychological impact of COVID-19 beyond paranoia and panic. *Annals of the Academy of Medicine, Singapore, 49*, 155.
84. Soltaninejad, K. (2020). Methanol mass poisoning outbreak: A consequence of COVID-19 pandemic and misleading messages on social media. *International Journal of Occupational and Environmental Medicine, 11*, 148–150.
85. Tucci, V., & Moukaddam, N. (2017). We are the hollow men: The worldwide epidemic of mental illness, psychiatric and behavioral emergencies, and its impact on patients and providers. *Journal of Emergencies, Trauma, and Shock, 10*, 4.
86. Unadkat, S., & Farquhar, M. (2020). Doctors' wellbeing: Self-care during the covid-19 pandemic. *BMJ, 368*, 1150.
87. Piller, C. (2020). 'This is insane!' Many scientists lament Trump's embrace of risky malaria drugs for coronavirus. *Science*. https://doi.org/10.1126/science.abb9021. https://www.sciencemag.org/news/2020/03/insane-manyscientists-lament-trump-s-embrace-risky-malaria-drugs-coronavirus#.
88. Malta, M., Rimoin, A. W., & Strathdee, S. A. (2020). The coronavirus 2019-nCoV epidemic: Is hindsight 20/20? *EClinicalMedicine, 20*, 100289.

# Chapter 17
# COVIDz: Deep Learning for Coronavirus Disease Detection

**Mohammed Anis Oukebdane, Samir Ghouali, Emad Kamil Hussein, Mohammed Seghir Guellil, Amina Elbatoul Dinar, Walid Cherifi, Abd Ellah Youcef Taib, and Boualem Merabet**

## 17.1 Introduction

At the time of the study, the number of persons infected by the novel coronavirus (now known as COVID-19) exceeds 20,730,456, and deaths across the world from this disease are estimated to be 751,154, as reported by the World Health Organization (WHO) statistics [1]. In our days, if someone has a fever, dry cough and fatigue or even body nasal irritation, conjunctivitis, sore throat, nausea, loss of taste or odor, rash, or discoloration of hand fingers or feet, the first thing that will come into our

M. A. Oukebdane · A. E. Y. Taib · B. Merabet
Faculty of Sciences and Technology Mustapha Stambouli University, Mascara, Algeria

S. Ghouali (✉)
Faculty of Sciences and Technology Mustapha Stambouli University, Mascara, Algeria&
STIC Lab, University of Tlemcen, Tlemcen, Algeria
e-mail: s.ghouali@univ-mascara.dz

E. K. Hussein
Al Mussaib Technical College, Al Furat Al Awsat Technical University, Al Mussaib, Babil, Iraq
e-mail: emad_kamil72@atu.edu.iq

M. S. Guellil
Faculty of Economics, Business and Management Sciences, MCLDL Laboratory, University of Mascara, Mascara, Algeria
e-mail: m.guellil@univ-mascara.dz

A. E. Dinar
LSTE Laboratory, Faculty of Sciences and Technology Mustapha Stambouli University, Mascara, Algeria
e-mail: amina.dinar@univ-mascara.dz

W. Cherifi
InnoDev (Dev Software), Tlemcen, Algeria
e-mail: contact@innodev.dz



S. Kautish et al. (eds.), *Computational Intelligence Techniques for Combating COVID-19*, EAI/Springer Innovations in Communication and Computing,
https://doi.org/10.1007/978-3-030-68936-0_17

mind is COVID-19 [2]. Recently, another identified virus, originating from the severe acute respiratory syndrome coronavirus 2 (SARS-CoV-2) family, gives the impression that is profoundly undermining human lives [3]. Among CoV family including six infections' subtypes, Middle East respiratory syndrome (MERS)-CoV and SARS-CoV contribute to human respiratory disorders, and slow-reacting substance of anaphylaxis (SRS-A) dampers the activity of human cilia [4, 5]. Furthermore, extreme respiratory difficulties are linked to CoV disease [6], and breathing problems can lead to pneumonia, kidney problems, and fluid accumulation in human lungs [3]. Especially after it was officially announced as a global pandemic by WHO and the spread of true and false news about how it spreads, and based on the number of infections and that of deaths, most patients (about 80%) recover without the need to be hospitalized [7]. In terms of of the disease symptoms, about one in five people with the disease has difficulty in breathing which is a severe symptom [8]. Older people and those with other medical issues (heart, hypertension, diabetes, or malignancy) are bound to have genuine side effects [9]. Be that as it may, anyone and all will get COVID-19 and get seriously ill [10]. However, people of any age who develop a fever and/or cough associated with difficulty in breathing, chest pain/pressure, or loss of speech or difficulty moving should seek medical attention immediately [3].

WHO does not suggest self-prescription of drugs to combat COVID-19, it was necessary to find a simple technological means to be used in hospitals or by individuals who have not received trainings in the field of health in order to detect this disease, especially in remote areas and developing countries [11]. This is exactly what we focused our research on, to finally come out with software that can detect the virus in chest tomography scans. It returns the result, either infected or not, with a mention of it certainty on the result.

This paper is structured accordingly: Related works are discussed in Sect. 17.2. COVID-19 diagnosis and therapeutic care are in Sect. 17.3. Methods and materials are described in Sects. 17.4 and 17.5, respectively, with deep learning models and experimental setup parameters. In Sect. 17.6, success indicators and evaluations are comprehensive. Section 17.7 provides debate and conclusions derived from the proposed models. Finally, it outlines the interpretation and possible research.

## 17.2 Related Works

To diagnose COVID-19, different studies and several methods using X-rays are performed [12–14], and researchers use the deep neural network or deep Bayes-SqueezeNet [15–17]. In this work, COVID-19 disease is recognized and immediately identified from chest X-ray images by the CoroNet implementation of a deep structure neural network. The model uses a pre-trained unique structure with an ImageNet dataset trained end-to-end by collecting COVID-19 and pulmonary images from two different publicly available databases. However, in cases of COVID-19, accuracy rates vary from 93% to 98.2%, depending on the number of detection groups (normal pneumonia vs. bacterial pneumonia vs. COVID vs. viral pneumonia) or for three groups (normal vs. pneumonia vs. COVID). These rates clearly show that these models can be a very good way to diagnose against this virus, but this will only happen if they are effective with large data sets [18].

COVIDiagnosis is a framework focused on deep Bayes-SqueezeNet. Ferhat Ucar and Deniz Korkmaz described their approach as an offline rise in raw data as a three-stage method and training the SqueezeNet model developed in decision-making in the test process. The approach suggested classifies three classes of X-ray, called regular (normal), pneumonia, and COVID. COVIDiagnosis model achieved an accuracy of 98.3% which makes it the best proposed model till now [15].

COVID-Xpert is a COVID-19 case AI-controlled population screening with chest radiography images. They used DenseNet which they describe as follows: "DenseNet-121 is the framework for pre-training and fine-tuning AP and RF networks, and ShuffleNetV2, MobileNetv2, and SqueezeNet are the representative of MS networks for COVID-19 screening on smartphones." They achieved a remarkable accuracy of 88.9% [19].

COVID-Net is a modified deep convolutional neural network architecture used to detect COVID-19 cases from X-ray images. A human-machine synergistic structure approach is used in this analysis to generate COVID-Net. Furthermore, COVID-Net makes predictions using an explainability method in an attempt to not only gain deeper insights into critical factors associated with COVID cases, which can aid clinicians in improved screening, but also audit COVID-Net in a responsible and transparent manner to validate that it is making decisions based on relevant information from the CXR images, the accuracy of this model is 93.3% [20].

COVID-CAPS is a capsule network-based system for X-ray classification in COVID-19 events. The paper introduces an alternative simulation architecture focused on capsule networks, called COVID-CAPS, capable of managing small datasets. COVID-CAPS attained 95.7% accuracy, 90% sensitivity, 95.8% precision, and 0.97 area under a curve (AUC) [21].

COVID-ResNet is radiograph deep-learning system for screening COVID19. "This work introduces a 3-step methodology to fine-tune a ResNet-50 pre-trained architecture to boost model efficiency and minimize training time, we call it COVID-ResNet. It is accomplished by slowly re-sizing images to 128x128x3, 224x224x3, and 229x229x3 pixels and fine-tuning the network at each point. This approach, together with automatic learning rate selection, enabled us to achieve 96.23% (on all classes) accuracy on the COVIDx dataset with only 41 epochs" [22].

Since scientists aim to find the best manner and the most efficient way to help humanity in their war against COVID-19, we intend here to compare some solutions that have envisaged COVID-19.

## 17.3 COVID-19 Diagnosis and Therapeutic Care

### *17.3.1 Diagnostic Approach*

#### 17.3.1.1 Anamnesis

- The incubation period is 14 days following exposure. The median would be between 4 and 5 days after contact.
- Intrahospital contamination would have reached 41%.
- The average length of hospitalization for patients is between 17 and 25 days after the onset of the disease.
- Search for risk factors (especially obesity), history, and current treatment (diabetes, cardiovascular pathology, especially hypertension) [23].

#### 17.3.1.2 Biological Examinations

- Tests recommended in the emergency department: CBC, blood ionogram, renal function, liver workup, D-dimer, LDH, CPK, CRP, and blood cultures if fever.
- Normal MDT on admission for pneumonia may be elevated in more severe cases.
- Rapid diagnostic tests, molecular biology by RT-PCR by nasal swab or nasopharyngeal lavage [23].

#### 17.3.1.3 Imaging

- CT scan without injection in thin sections is the reference examination: frosted glass images, bilateral, predominant peripherally in the lower lobes with possible pleurisy and lymphadenopathies and interstitial syndrome.
- Lung ultrasound seems to be of interest in screening suspected patients.
- Chest X-ray: a sensitive technique that can be used as a default to perform a rapid pretest for abnormalities causing COVID-19 [23].

Here, we are devoted to this last point, i.e., detecting COVID-19 from chest X-ray images.

## 17.4 Methods and Materials

### *17.4.1 Python*

Python is a programming language of high general purpose, which was initially being mainly received as a screenplay for general purposes and was widely used as a web programming and script language of choice. Over the last decade, it may be an excellent resource for the academic programming world, and the language has been explosively extended in research and data processing applications since then. Python is a free-source language that helps anyone contribute and make available packages to other Python ecosystems. Python's academic community is relatively broad and used in numerous contexts, including market science, the development of algorithms, choice and derivative valuation, market simulations, and trading systems [24].

### *17.4.2 VGG-16*

A well-known and powerful neural network model, VGG-16, was used and developed during a competition set up by the ImageNet organization which aims to classify the content of images into 1000 everyday objects (sheep, hen, fork, castle, lamppost, various dog breeds, etc.). The VGG-16 was developed in 2014 and achieved the score of 92.7% accuracy.

It did not win the competition but stood out for its particularly good results given its very light architecture. The model shown below is a CNN network model proposed by K. Simonyan and A. Zisserman [25]. It makes it possible to reach 92.7% on the ImageNet database which contains 14 million images belonging to 1000 classes (Fig. 17.1).

A 224×224 RGB picture is the input for the cov1 layer. The image is passed by a stack of coevolutionary (conv.) layers, where filters were used with a very narrow reception area of 3×3 (which is the smallest size in which the notion of right/right,

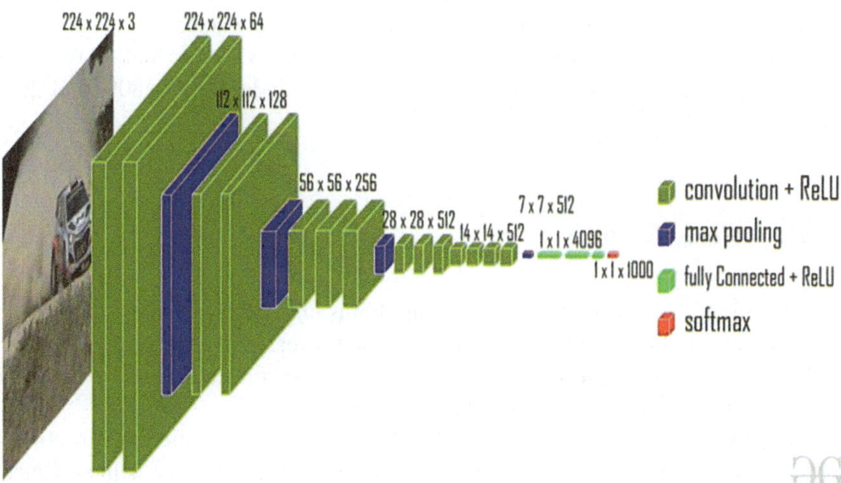


Fig. 17.1 VGG16 architecture [12]

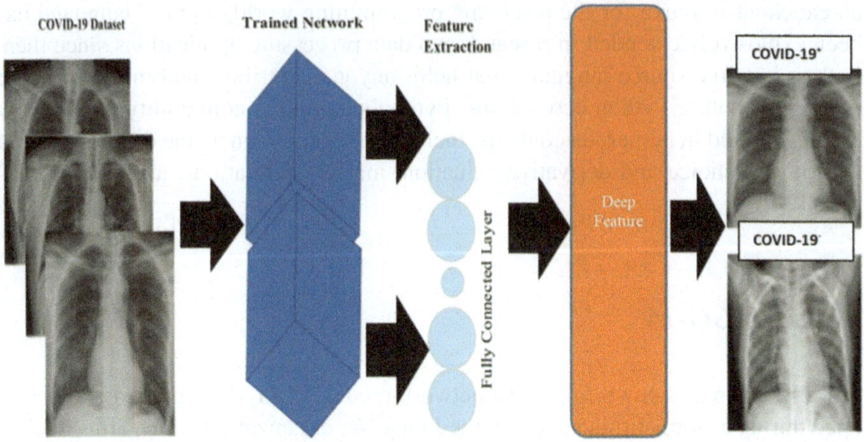


**Fig. 17.2** Proposed deep feature-based COVID-19 classification system

up/down, and center can be captured); in one configuration it also uses 1×1 [25]. The workflow of the proposed classification system is shown in Fig. 17.2.

### *17.4.3 Dataset*

In this work, the GitHub open-source repository has collected images of COVID-19 patients [26]. Our study was based on a dataset of 279 pictures of 139 COVID-19$^+$ and 140 COVID-19$^-$ patients. The size of each image was 128×128 pixels in this dataset. The choice of such a database makes our contribution more credible, based on comparisons made with works that have used the same database.

Figure 17.3 offers an allocated chest X-ray for COVID-19$^+$ and COVID-19$^-$ patients. The dataset was randomly divided into two independent, 80% and 20%, datasets for both training and testing.

### *17.4.4 Classification*

Deep learning is a part of machine learning that is enlivened by the usefulness of a human cerebrum [41] and is viewed as valuable for learning complex issues. Also, CNN is a sort of deep learning, which has indicated prominent execution in identification, characterization, and division assignments [27].

It is additionally revealed that CNN indicated promising outcomes in clinical applications, where a lot of information is accessible. Be that as it may, CNN's execution might be influenced when an adequate measure of information is not accessible. Particularly in clinical picture applications, there might be few marked

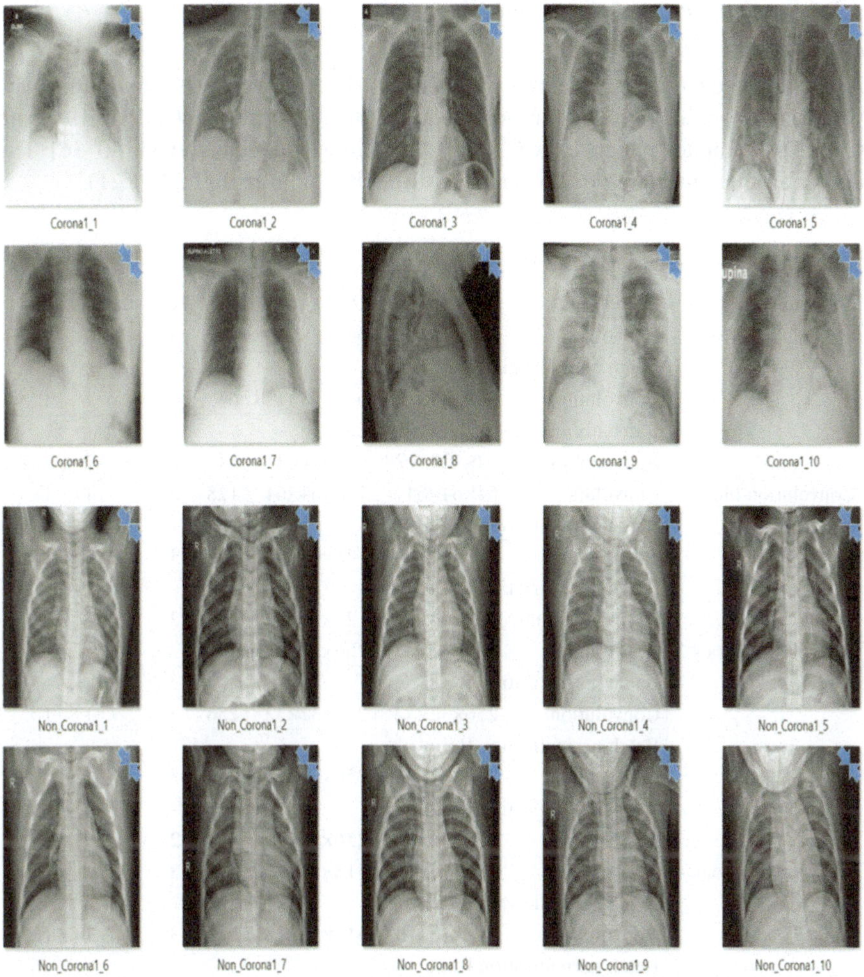


**Fig. 17.3** Representative chest X-ray images of (**a**) "COVID-19$^{+}$" and (**b**) normal "COVID-19$^{-}$" patients [13]

pictures accessible. Along these lines, the TL idea is generally abused to accomplish significant execution on a modest quantity of information, and it likewise diminishes the computational cost [28, 29]. During the preparation cycle, the system gets data from the pre-prepared framework through the TL method.

### 17.4.5 Implementation Details

As of now, the COVID-19 dataset is having restricted named tests, and in this way, we abuse TL-based tweaked pre-prepared systems for separating COVID-19⁻ from COVID-19⁺ tainted patients; the CNN system that we utilized is VGG [30–36]. The design architectures are professional and difficult to converge (Table 17.1).

**Table 17.1** Proposed custom VGG-16

| Layer number | Process unit | In | Out | Filt | Filt size | Str | 0Padd |
|---|---|---|---|---|---|---|---|
| Convolution block 1 | Convolution | 3×128×128 | 64×128×128 | 64 | 3 | 1 | 1 |
| | Batch normalization ReLu | | | | | | |
| | Convolution | 64×128×128 | 64×128×128 | 64 | 3 | 1 | 1 |
| | Batch normalization ReLu | | | | | | |
| | Max pooling | 64×128×128 | 64×64×64 | 64 | 2 | 2 | – |
| Convolution block 2 | Convolution | 64×64×64 | 128×64×64 | 128 | 3 | 1 | 1 |
| | Batch normalization ReLu | | | | | | |
| | Convolution | 128×64×64 | 128×64×64 | 128 | 3 | 1 | 1 |
| | Batch normalization ReLu | | | | | | |
| | Average pooling | 128×64×64 | 128×32×32 | 128 | 2 | 2 | – |
| Convolution block 3 | Convolution | 128×32×32 | 256×32×32 | 256 | 3 | 1 | 1 |
| | Batch normalization ReLu | | | | | | |
| | Convolution | 256×32×32 | 256×32×32 | 256 | 3 | 1 | 1 |
| | Batch normalization ReLu | | | | | | |
| | Convolution | 256×32×32 | 256×32×32 | 256 | 3 | 1 | 1 |
| | Batch normalization ReLu | | | | | | |
| | Max pooling | 256×32×32 | 256×16×16 | 256 | 2 | 2 | – |
| Convolution block 4 | Convolution | 256×16×16 | 512×16×16 | 512 | 3 | 1 | 1 |
| | Batch normalization ReLu | | | | | | |
| | Convolution | 512×16×16 | 512×16×16 | 512 | 3 | 1 | 1 |
| | Batch normalization ReLu | | | | | | |
| | Convolution | 512×16×16 | 512×16×16 | 512 | 3 | 1 | – |
| | Batch normalization ReLu | | | | | | |
| | Max pooling | 512×16×16 | 512×8×8 | 512 | 2 | 2 | – |
| Pooling | Average pooling | 512×8×8 | 512×7×7 | 512 | 2 | 2 | 3 |
| Layer 1 | Fuly connected | 25,088 | 4096 | 4096 | – | – | – |
| | ReLu dropout (0.5) | | | | | | |
| Layer 2 | Fuly connected | 4096 | 64 | 64 | – | – | – |
| | ReLu dropout (0.5) | | | | | | |
| Pooling layer | Average pooling | 512×8×8 | 512×7×7 | 512 | 2 | 2 | 3 |
| Layer 3 | Fuly connected | 64 | 2 | 2 | – | – | – |

## 17.5 Experimental Setup

All simulations were carried out on the Anaconda Prompt framework in a Toshiba (TM) i7-6600U CPU with a 2.80 GHz processor; the results as well as the display will be on a WEB browser. The training of the models approximately took about 18 hours (Fig. 17.4).

After accessing COVIDz, users will have to log in or register on the site if they do not have an account before, as shown in Fig. 17.5:

After having accounts, only registered users can carry out the forecasting process by clicking the "Take a COVID-19 Test" button (Fig. 17.6).

All that's left to do is download X-ray images, as done below in Fig. 17.7.

Then the image is analyzed and the results will be displayed on the interface and sent via the e-mail that was used during registration. Figures 17.8 and 17.9 below illustrate such an approach.

## 17.6 Performance Evaluation

For deep transfer learning models, six parameters have been used. Our method shows relevant results and measured quality metrics, including precision, sensitivity, specificities, recall, F-score and Matthews Correlation Coefficient (MCC). Accuracy in estimating the total number of assignments is defined in Eq. (17.1). Similarly, recall in Eq. (17.2) and specificity assess the proportion of right patients with COVID-19$^+$ and the percent of patients with COVID-19 (Eq. 17.3). Precision is shown in Eq. (17.4); the F-score in Eqs. (17.5) and (17.6) indicates the MCC. Table 17.2 below summarizes the statistical description for the different metrics and the confusion matrix, given in Fig.17.10.

$$\text{ACCUR} = \frac{\text{Predicted COVID}-19^{-} + \text{Predicted COVID}-19^{+}}{\text{Total}} \times 100 \quad (17.1)$$

$$\text{REC} = \frac{\text{Predicted COVID}-19^{+}}{\text{Total COVID}-19^{+}} \times 100 \quad (17.2)$$

$$\text{SP} = \frac{\text{Predicted COVID}-19^{-}}{\text{Total COVID}-19^{-}} \times 100 \quad (17.3)$$

$$\text{PRES} = \frac{\text{Predicted COVID}-19^{+}}{\text{Predicted COVID}-19^{+} + \text{Incorect Predicted COVID}-19^{+}} \times 100 \quad (17.4)$$

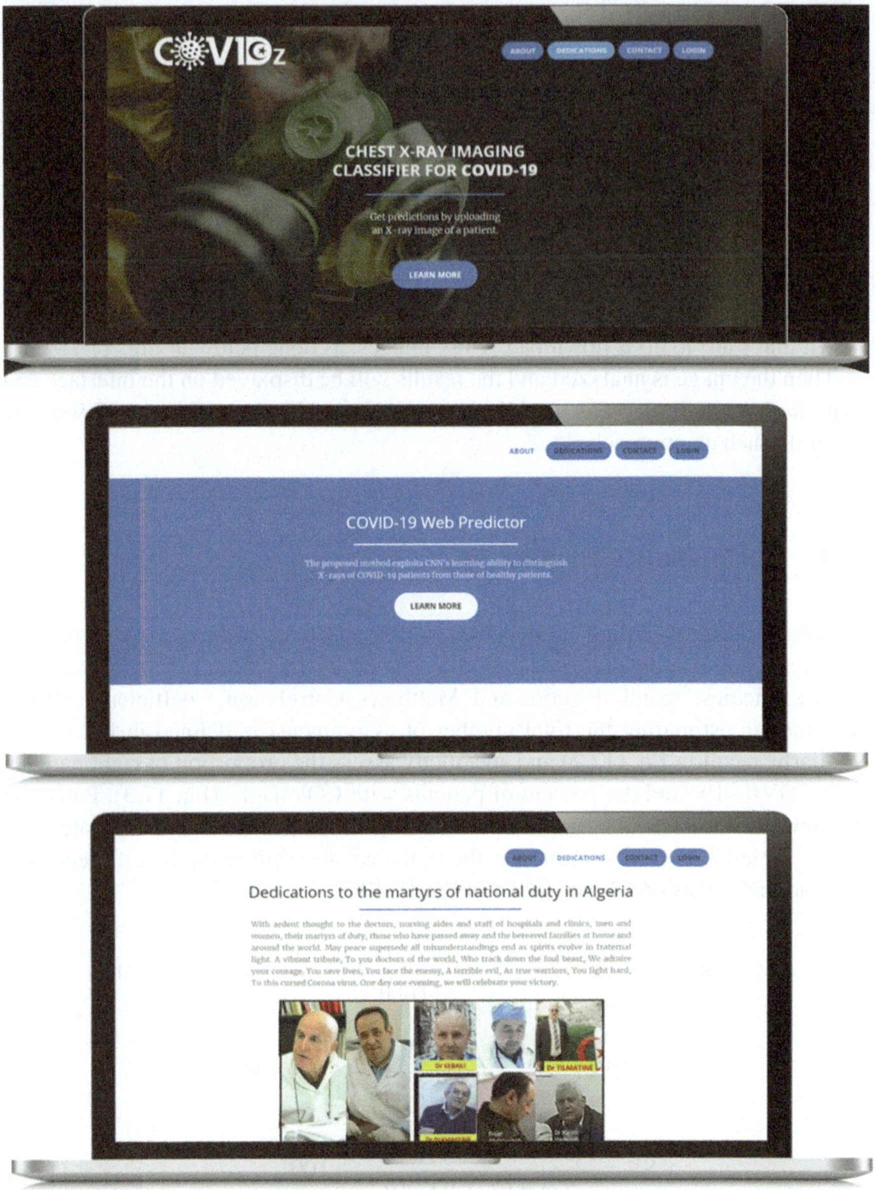


**Fig. 17.4** X-ray imaging classifier COVID-19 home page

$$F-\text{score} = 2 \times \frac{\text{PRES} \times \text{REC}}{\text{PRES} + \text{REC}} \tag{17.5}$$

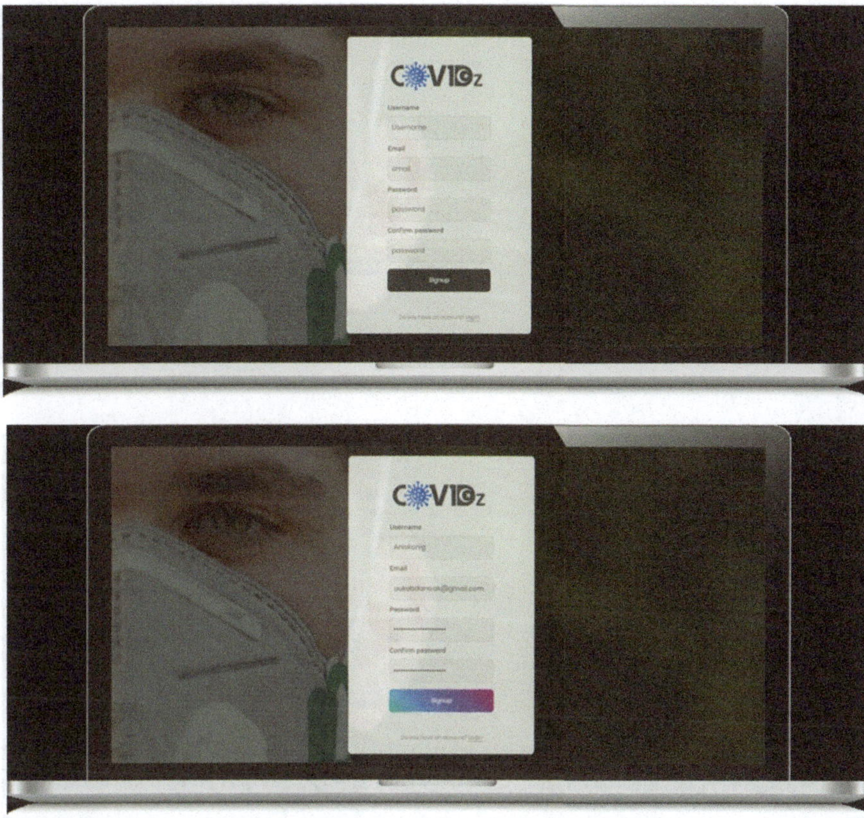


Fig. 17.5 Registration with personal information on COVIDz

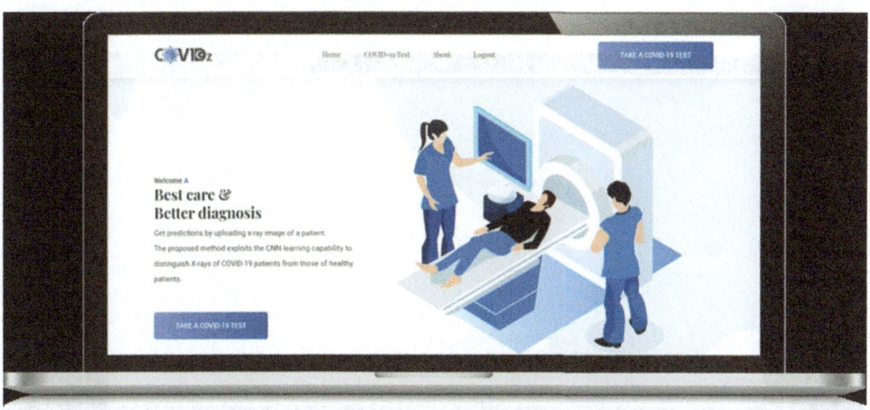


Fig. 17.6 Main page for subscribed users

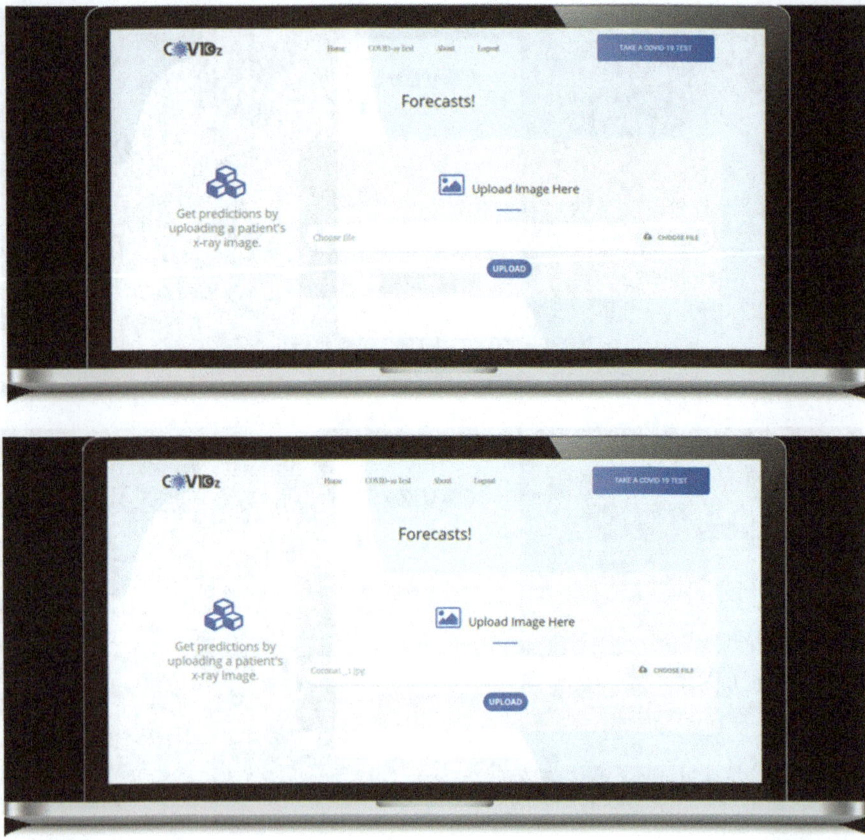


Fig. 17.7 Prediction page

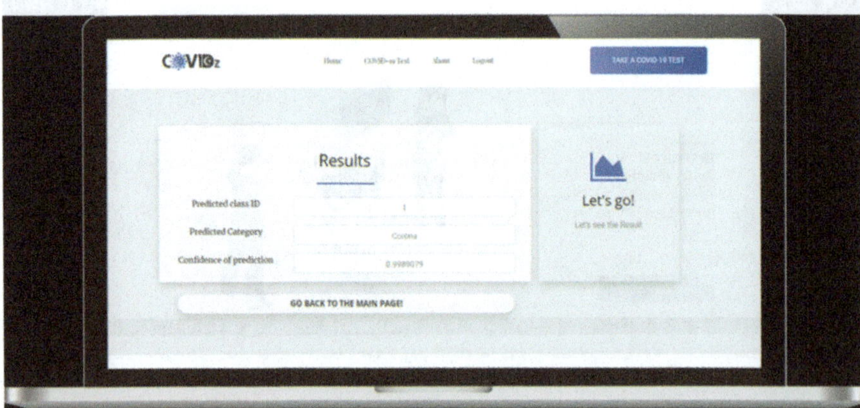


Fig. 17.8 Prediction result of an X-ray image

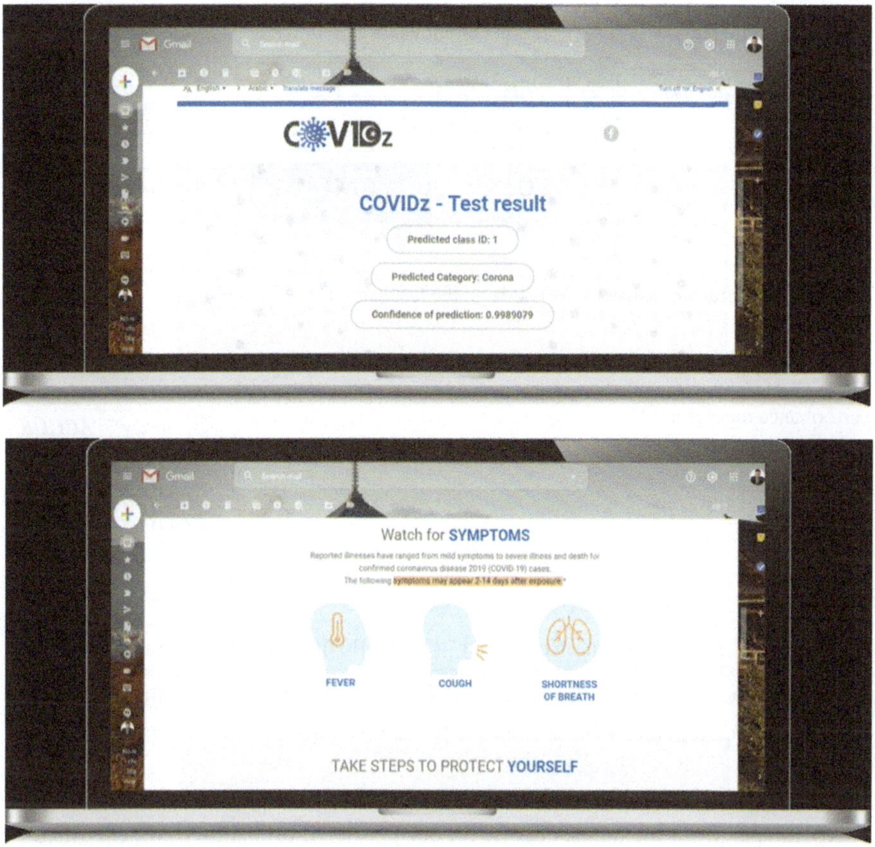


**Fig. 17.9** Automatic mail sending with details and some advices to be taken

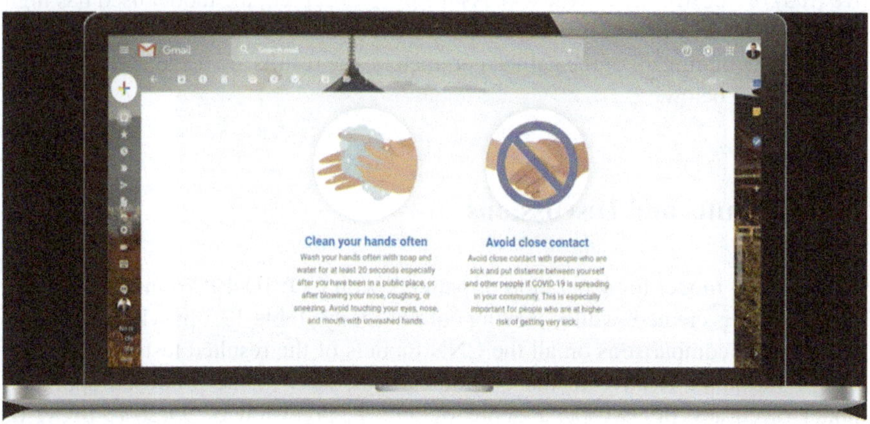


**Fig. 17.9** (continued)

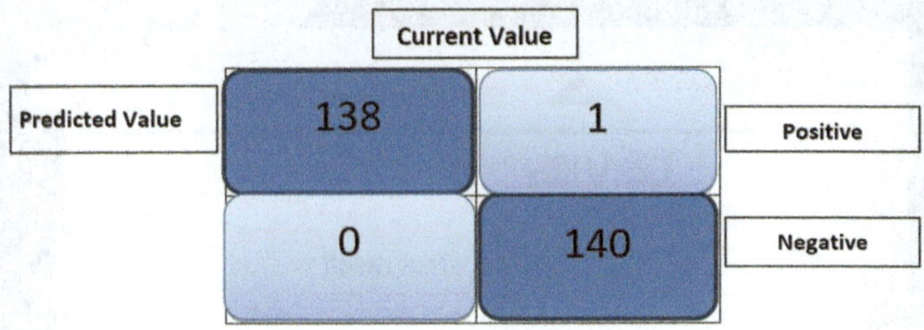


**Fig. 17.10** Confusion matrix for COVIDz on the test dataset

**Table 17.2** Various performance metrics used

| Metric | Symbol |
|---|---|
| *Accuracy* | *ACCUR* |
| *Recall* | *REC* |
| *Specificity* | *SP* |
| *Precision* | *PRES* |

$$\mathrm{MCC} \frac{(\text{True Positive} \times \text{True Negative}) - (\text{False Positive} \times \text{False Negative})}{\sqrt{\begin{array}{c}(\text{True Positive} + \text{False Positive})(\text{True Positive} + \text{False Negative}) \\ (\text{True Negative} + \text{False Positive})(\text{True Negative} + \text{False Negative})\end{array}}} \quad (17.6)$$

For a detailed visual analysis, the results given in Fig. 17.11 show 279 chest X-ray images from the dataset [26] with our predicted probability. Misclassified or unreasonable predictions sometimes can rely on reasonable explanations. By the aid of the class activation, we can investigate useful knowledge of the prediction regions. The probability values of the predictions are nearly 1.00 (whether for positive (red) or negative (green) cases). As it can be observed, the model used has high predicted anomaly probability scores for positive/negative patients.

After calculating all of the gained parameters, the results are listed and compared in Table 17.3 below.

## 17.7 Results and Discussions

A deep CNN model for separation of patients with COVID-19$^{+}$ from people using chest X-rays is created, while carrying out this study. Table 17.3 provides extensive performance comparisons on all the CNN models of the resulted tests, with excellent performance relative to those with the exactness of the proposed approach model (accuracy of 99.64%, F-score of 99,2%, precision of 99,28%, MCC of 99,28%, recall of 99,28%, and a specificity value of 100%, as Table 17.3 shows).

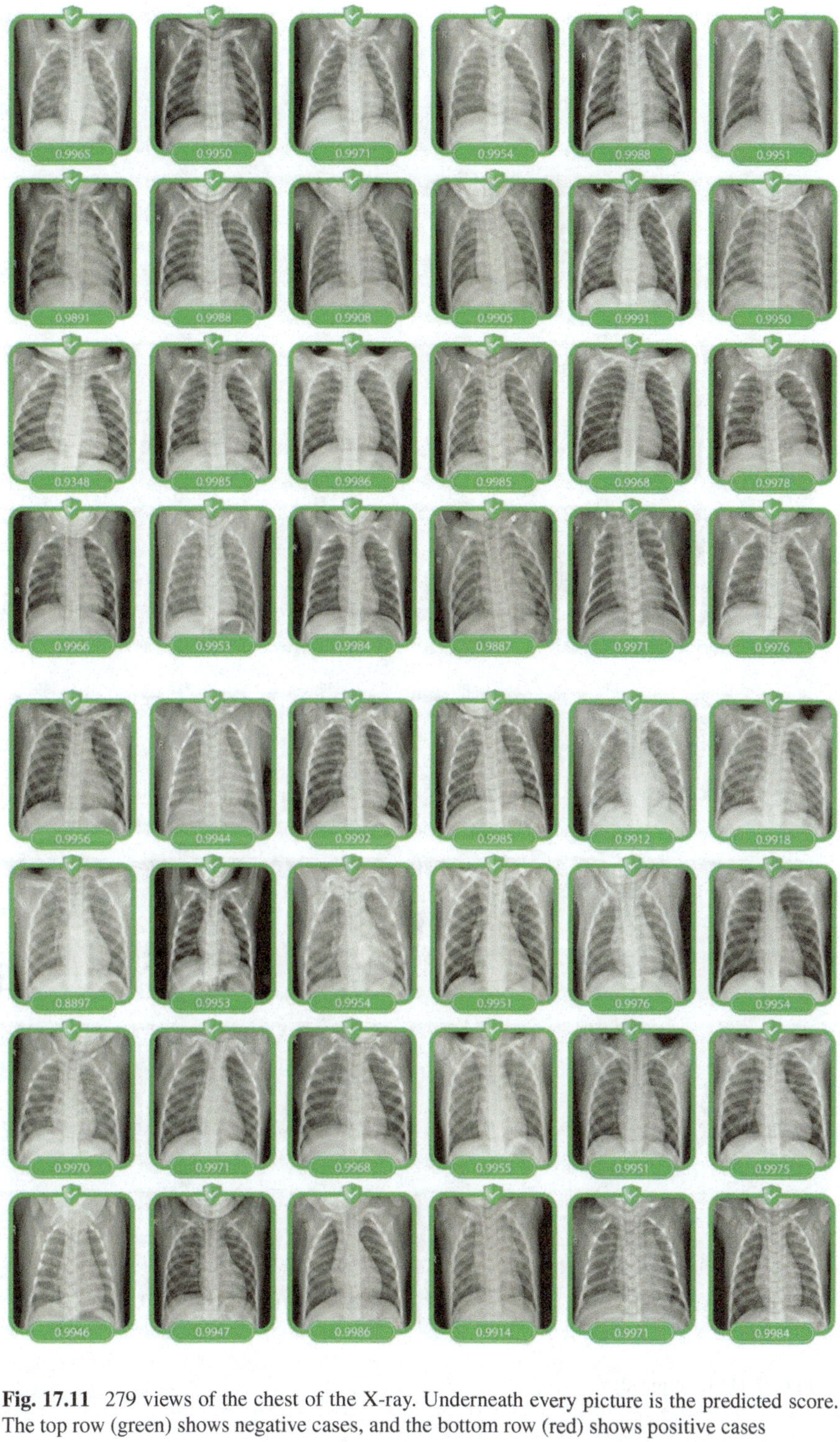


**Fig. 17.11** 279 views of the chest of the X-ray. Underneath every picture is the predicted score. The top row (green) shows negative cases, and the bottom row (red) shows positive cases

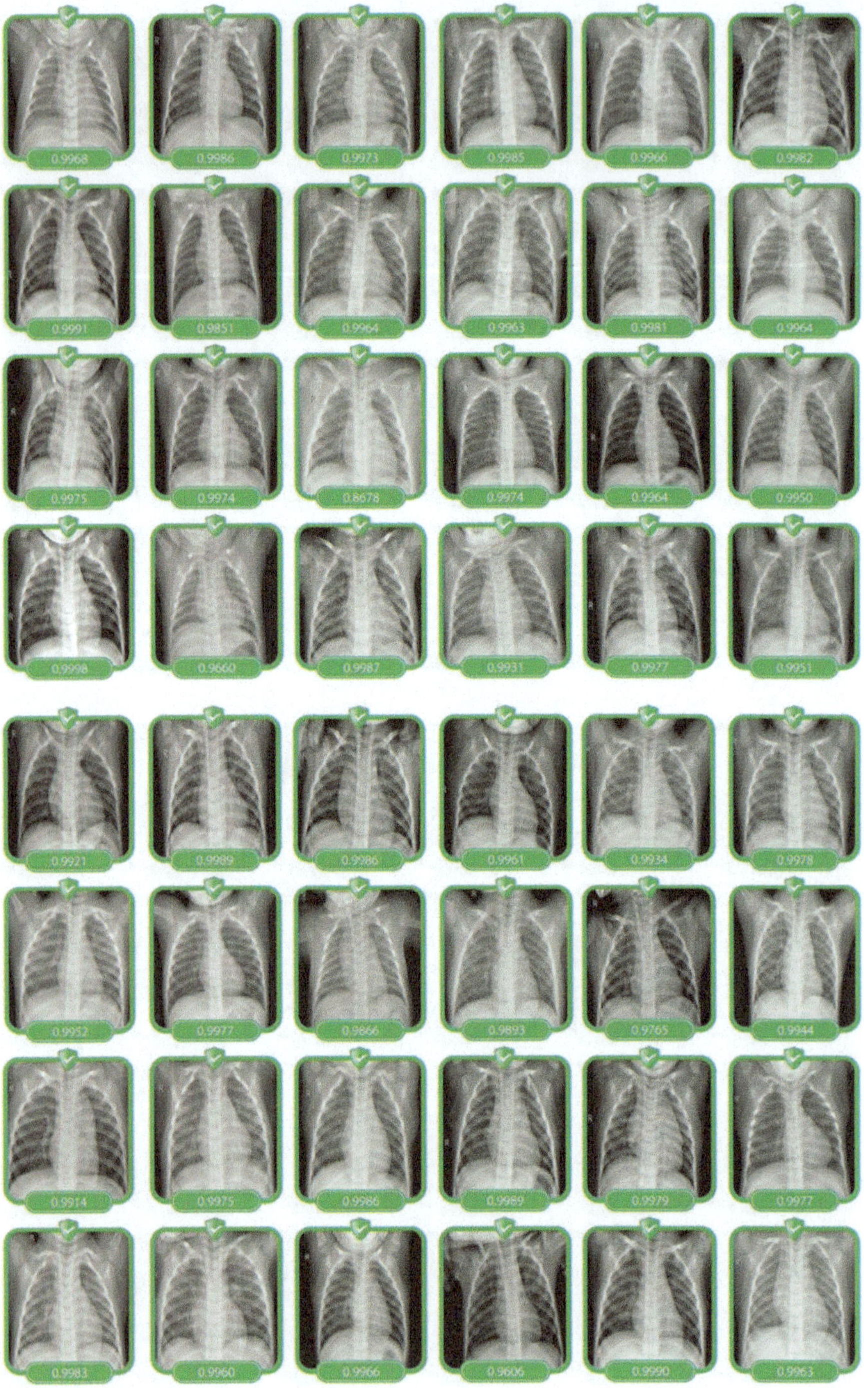


**Fig. 17.11** (continued)

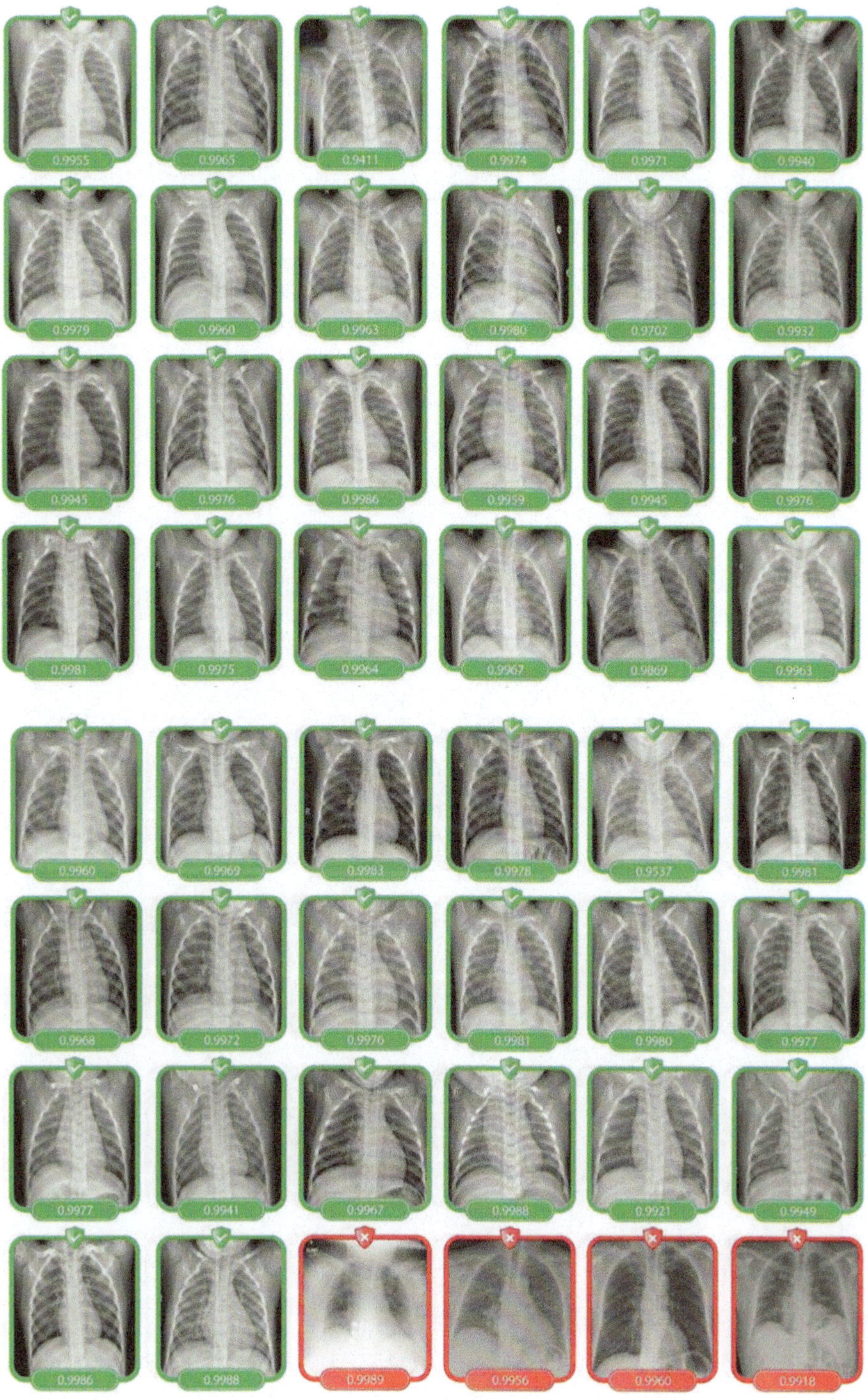


**Fig. 17.11** (continued)

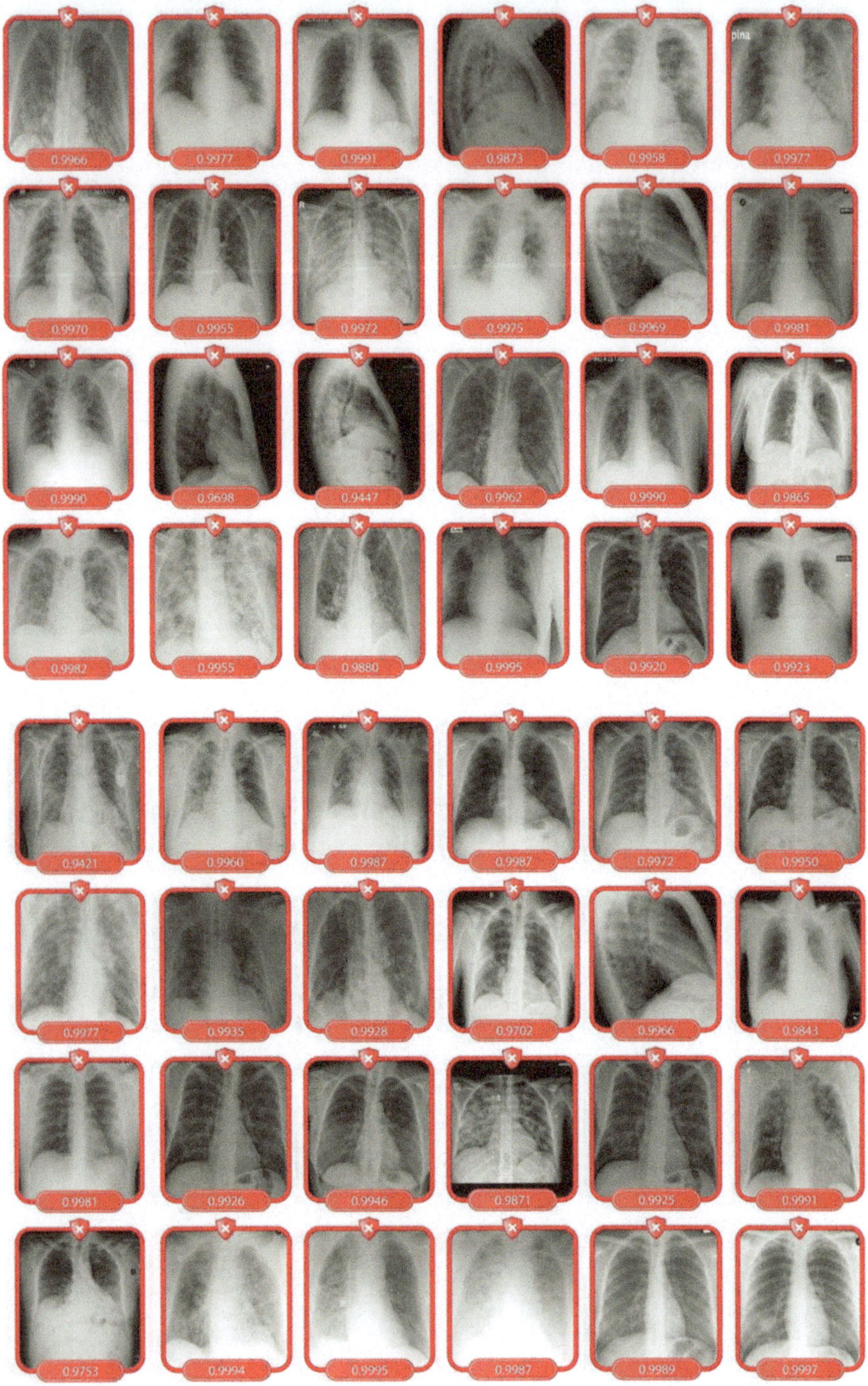


**Fig. 17.11** (continued)

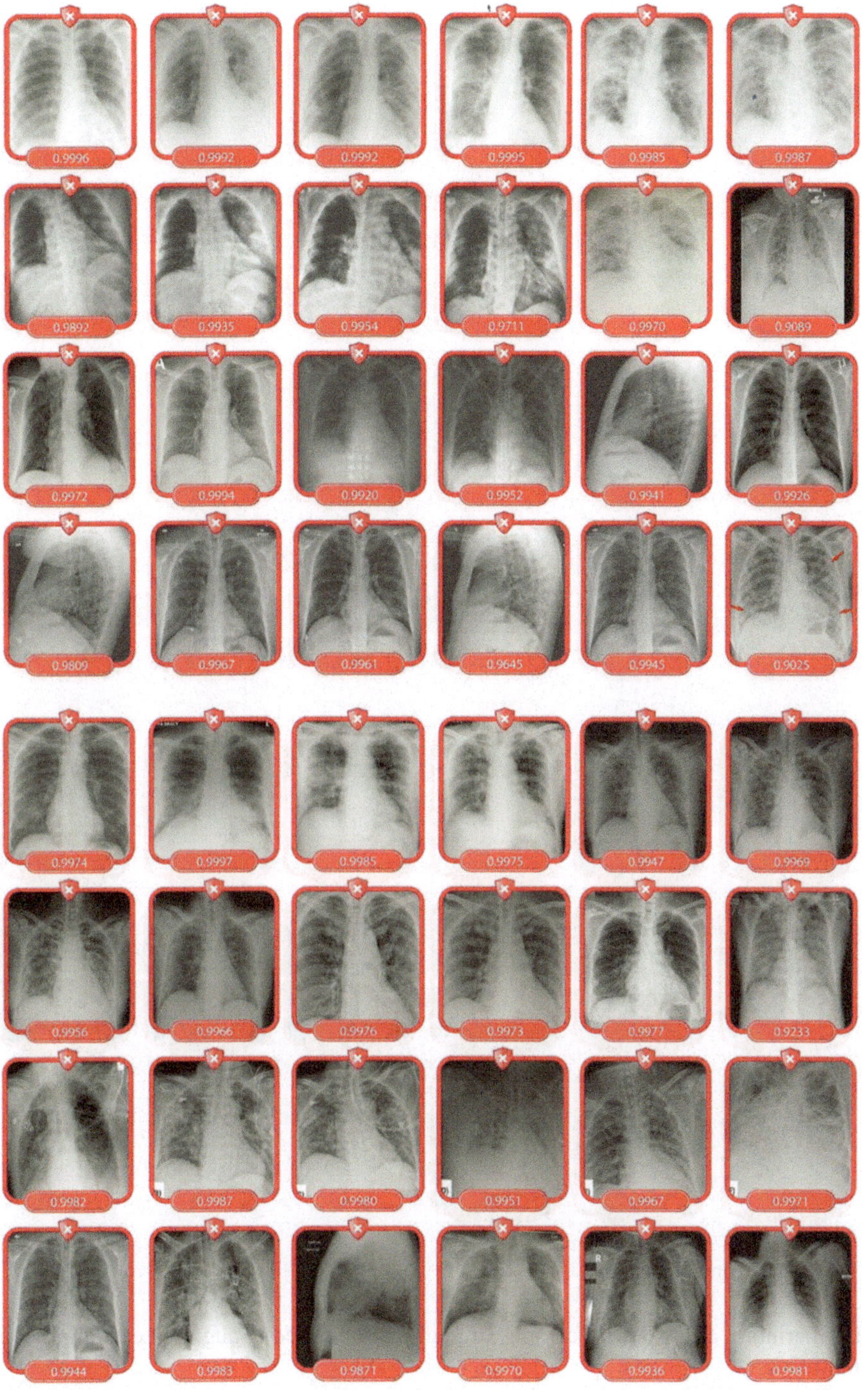


**Fig. 17.11** (continued)

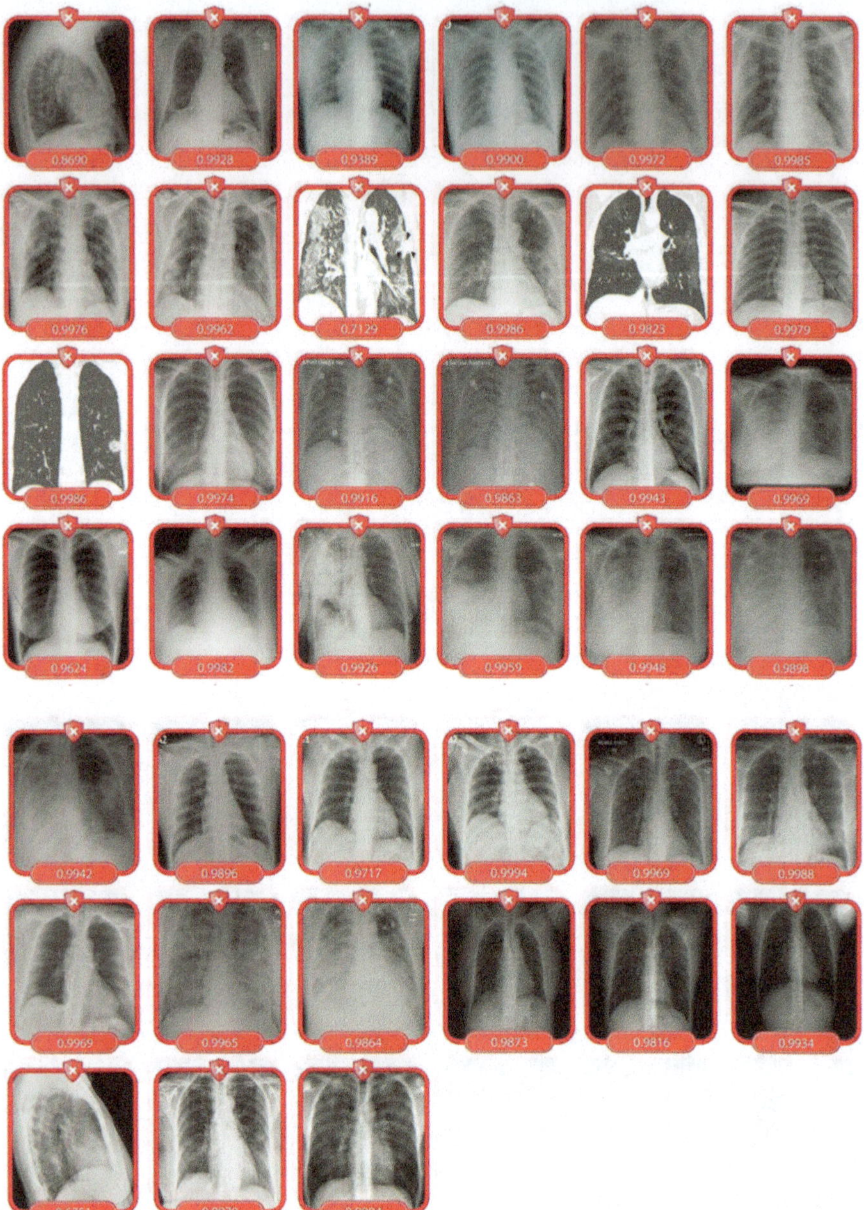


**Fig. 17.11** (continued)

Furthermore, a few pre-processing strategies are utilized to augment execution in a fair test set.

Our solution is not only used by a laboratory technician or an authorised person, but rather one of the centralised data technologies that can be used by any

**Table 17.3** Performance metrics comparisons

| Networks | Accuracy | F-score | MCC | Precision | Specificity | Recall |
|---|---|---|---|---|---|---|
| Alexnet | 50 | 0.66 | – | 100 | – | 50 |
| VGG19 | 91.67 | 0.91 | 0.83 | 93.33 | 93.33 | 90.32 |
| Google Net | 88.33 | 0.88 | 0.77 | 86.67 | 87.10 | 89.66 |
| Inceptionv3 | 95 | 0.95 | 0.90 | 100 | 100 | 90.91 |
| Resnet18 | 95 | 0.95 | 0.90 | 100 | 100 | 90.91 |
| Resnet50 | 95 | 0.95 | 0.90 | 100 | 100 | 90.91 |
| Squeeze Net | 78.33 | 0.80 | 0.58 | 90 | 86.96 | 72.97 |
| DenseNet201 | 95 | 0.95 | 0.90 | 100 | 100 | 90.91 |
| COVID-RENet | 96.67 | 0.97 | 0.94 | 100 | 100 | 93.75 |
| Our contribution "COVIDz" | 99,64 | 0,992 | 0,9928 | 99,28 | 100 | 99,28 |

practitioner. deep learning and AI are also used so that X-rays can be classified and detect infected area automatically.

## 17.8 Conclusion and Future Works

COVID-19, as a new pandemic of coronavirus, has affected humanity and continued as a challenge to produce disasters. Health monitoring is one of the primary measures that can be used to track pollution distribution in affected problem areas and track essential patients' well-being. Its importance in quick testing illustrates the need for quick, reliable, and accessible screening components. ML-based mechanized models, therefore, address a potential way of enhancing the screening efficiency with worthy effect and peculiarity [37, 38].

In the present article, we have proposed interpreting and examining chest X-ray images for a broad CNN grouping method for the differentiation of COVID-19$^{+}$ patients. Several clinical trials have shown that chest radiological images can track and monitor people affected by COVID-19. CNNs are incredible and powerful calculations that take explicit highlights in space from images using the algorithm of rear-propagation calculation [39, 40].

Chest images of COVID-19 patients have explicit marks, e.g., opacities of ground glass, rounded anatomy, and peripheral distribution of human lungs. It is worth mentioning that the proposed model, based on X-ray images, has exhibited efficient deep feature hierarchies.

The possible reason behind the improvement of such model is the coordinated use of normal and maximum concentration in the CNN architecture and the use of efficient calculation tools, such as Python and JavaScript. In perspective, we intend trying three various networks basing on neural models (like ResNet50, InceptionV3, and Inception-ResNetV2) in our future works.

**Acknowledgments** This work is supported by the General Directorate for Scientific Research and Technological Development (DGRSDT), Higher Education Ministry of Algeria, Algiers, Algeria. The authors would also like to thank Professor Abdelhakim Dinar from St. Peter's Neurology, Albany, New York 12204, and also STIC Laboratory, Faculty of Technology, University of Tlemcen, Algeria.

**Conflict of Interest** The authors have no conflict to disclose.

## References

1. World Health Organization. Coronavirus disease 2019 (covid-19): situation report, 207. 2020.
2. Satuna, R. K., Negi, A., & Satuna, R. (2020). Intuitive vision and indigenous immunity boosting approaches for COVID19: From the literature of Pandit Shriram Sharma Acharya. *Dev Sanskriti Interdisciplinary International Journal, 16*, 01–15. https://doi.org/10.36018/dsiij.v16i.162.
3. Roosa, K., Lee, Y., Luo, R., et al. (2020). Real-time forecasts of the COVID-19 epidemic in China from February 5th to February 24th. *Infectious Disease Modelling, 5*, 256–263. https://doi.org/10.1016/j.idm.2020.02.002.
4. Bisgaard, H., & Pedersen, M. (1987). SRS-A leukotriene's decrease the activity of human respiratory cilia. *Clinical Experimental Allergy, 17*(2), 95–103.
5. Yu, Y., Shi, Q., Zheng, P., Gao, L., Li, H., Tao, P., & Chen, H. (2020). Assessment of the quality of systematic reviews on COVID-19: A comparative study of previous coronavirus outbreaks. *Journal of Medical Virology*. https://doi.org/10.1002/jmv.25901.
6. https://www.lung.org/lung-health-diseases/lung-disease-lookup/pneumonia/symptoms-and-diagnosis. Accessed Aug 16, 2020.
7. Beigel, J. H., Tomashek, K. M., Dodd, L. E., Mehta, A. K., Zingman, B. S., Kalil, A. C., Hohmann, E., Chu, H. Y., Luetkemeyer, A., Kline, S., Lopez de Castilla, D., Finberg, R. W., Dierberg, K., Tapson, V., Hsieh, L., Patterson, T. F., Paredes, R., Sweeney, D. A., Short, W. R., Touloumi, G., Lye, D. C., Ohmagari, N., Oh, M., Ruiz-Palacios, G. M., Benfield, T., Fätkenheuer, G., Kortepeter, M. G., Atmar, R. L., Creech, C. B., Lundgren, J., Babiker, A. G., Pett, S., Neaton, J. D., Burgess, T. H., Bonnett, T., Green, M., Makowski, M., Osinusi, A., Nayak, S., Lane, H. C., & for the ACTT-1 Study Group Members. (2020. Massachusetts Medical Society). Remdesivir for the treatment of Covid-19 – Preliminary report. *The New England Journal of Medicine*. https://doi.org/10.1056/NEJMoa2007764.
8. Ruan, Q., Yang, K., Wang, W., Jiang, L., & Song, J. (2020). Correction to: Clinical predictors of mortality due to COVID-19 based on an analysis of data of 150 patients from Wuhan, China. *Intensive Care Medicine*. https://doi.org/10.1007/s00134-020-06028-z.
9. Holmes, E. A., O'Connor, R. C., Perry, V. H., Tracey, I., Wessely, S., Arseneault, L., & Bullmore, E. (2020). Multidisciplinary research priorities for the COVID-19 pandemic: A call for action for mental health science. *The Lancet Psychiatry*. https://doi.org/10.1016/s2215-0366(20)30168-1.
10. Murthy, S., Gomersall, C. D., & Fowler, R. A. (2020). Care for critically ill patients with COVID-19. *Journal of the American Medical Association*. https://doi.org/10.1001/jama.2020.3633.
11. Lee, V. J., Chiew, C. J., & Khong, W. X. (April 2020). Interrupting transmission of COVID-19: lessons from containment efforts in Singapore. *Journal of Travel Medicine, 27*(3), taaa039. https://doi.org/10.1093/jtm/taaa039.
12. Apostolopoulos, I. D., & Mpesiana, T. A. (2020). Covid-19: Automatic detection from X-ray images utilizing transfer learning with convolutional neural networks. *Physical and Engineering Sciences in Medicine, 43*, 635–640. https://doi.org/10.1007/s13246-020-00865-4.

13. Narayan Das, N., Kumar, N., Kaur, M., Kumar, V., & Singh, D. (2020). Automated deep transfer learning-based approach for detection of COVID-19 infection in chest X-rays. *IRBM*. https://doi.org/10.1016/j.irbm.2020.07.001.
14. Tsiknakis, N., Trivizakis, E., Vassalou, E. E., Papadakis, G. Z., Spandidos, D. A., Tsatsakis, A., Sánchez-García, J., López-González, R., Papanikolaou, N., Karantanas, A. H., Karantanas, A. H., et al. (2020). Interpretable artificial intelligence framework for COVID-19 screening on chest X-rays. *Experimental and Therapeutic Medicine, 20*, 727–735.
15. Ucar, F., & Korkmaz, D. (2020). COVIDiagnosis-Net: Deep Bayes-SqueezeNet based diagnostic of the coronavirus disease 2019 (COVID-19) from X-Ray images. *Medical Hypotheses*, 109761. https://doi.org/10.1016/j.mehy.2020.109761.
16. Islam, M. Z., Islam, M. M., & Asraf, A. (2020). A combined deep CNN-LSTM network for the detection of novel coronavirus (COVID-19) using X-ray images. *Informatics in Medicine Unlocked*, 100412. https://doi.org/10.1016/j.imu.2020.100412.
17. Turkoglu, M. (2020). COVIDetectioNet: COVID-19 diagnosis system based on X-ray images using features selected from pre-learned deep features ensemble. *Applied Intelligence*., Springer Science Media, LLC, part of Springer Nature. https://doi.org/10.1007/s10489-020-01888-w.
18. Khan, A. I., Shah, J. L., & Bhat, M. M. (2020). CoroNet: A deep neural network for detection and diagnosis of COVID-19 from chest X-ray images. *Computer Methods and Programs in Biomedicine, 196*, 105581. https://doi.org/10.1016/j.cmpb.2020.105581.
19. Xin, L., Chengyin, L., & Dongxiao, Z. (2020). COVID-MOBILEXPERT: On-device covid-19 screening using snapshots of chest x-ray. https://arxiv.org/pdf/2004.03042v2.pdf
20. Wang, L., & Wong, A. (2020). COVID-Net: A tailored deep convolutional neural network design for detection of COVID-19 cases from chest radiography images. ArXiv 2200309871.
21. Afshar, P., Heidarian, S., Naderkhani, F., Oikonomou, A., Plataniotis, K. N., Mohammadi, A., et al. (2020). COVİD-CAPS: A capsule network-based framework for identification of Covid-19 cases from X-Ray images. 1–4, 2020. ArXiv Prepr ArXiv200402696.
22. Farooq, M., & Hafeez, A. (2020). COVID-RESNET: A deep learning framework for screening of COVID19 from Radiographs.
23. Dominique, P., Maurice, R., & Albert, T.-D. (2019). Méga-guide pratique des urgences, de l'evidence based medicine à la pratique 2ème édition, Editeur: Elsevier Masson, pp. 984. ISBN: 9782294760938, EISBN: 9782294761645.
24. Taori, P., & Dasararaju, H. (2019). Introduction to Python. https://doi.org/10.1007/978-3-319-68837-4_29.
25. Simonyan, K., & Zisserman, A. (2015). Very deep convolutional networks for large-scale image recognition. In International Conference on Learning Representations (ICLR).
26. https://github.com/m-mohsin-zafar/shk_covid_pytorch. Accessed Aug 1, 2020.
27. Yamashita, R., Nishio, M., Do, R. K. G., & Togashi, K. (2018). Convolutional neural networks: An overview and application in radiology. *Insights Into Imaging, 9*(4), 611–629. https://doi.org/10.1007/s13244-018-0639-9.
28. Ahmed, U., Khan, A., Khan, S. H., Basit, A., Haq, I. U., & Lee, Y. S. (2019). Transfer learning and meta classification based deep churn prediction system for telecom industry. 1–10. http://arxiv.org/abs/1901.06091.
29. Wahab, N., Khan, A., & Lee, Y. S. (2019). Transfer learning based deep CNN for segmentation and detection of mitoses in breast cancer histopathological images. *Microscopy, 68*(3), 216–233. https://doi.org/10.1093/jmicro/dfz002.
30. Khan, A., Sohail, A., Zahoora, U., & Qureshi, A. S. (2019). A survey of the recent architectures of deep convolutional. *Neural Networks*, 1–68. https://doi.org/10.1007/s10462-020-09825-6.
31. Liu, X., Chi, M., Zhang, Y., & Qin, Y. (2018). Classifying high resolution remote sensing images by fine-tuned VGG deep networks. In: International Geoscience and Remote Sensing Symposium. https://doi.org/10.1109/IGARSS.2018.8518078.
32. Kieffer, B., Babaie, M., Kalra, S., & Tizhoosh, H. R. (2018). Convolutional neural networks for histopathology image classification: Training vs. Using pre-trained networks. In: Proceedings

of the 7th International Conference on Image Processing Theory, Tools and Applications, IPTA. https://doi.org/10.1109/IPTA.2017.8310149.
33. Szegedy, C., Wei, L., Yangqing, J., et al. (2015). Going deeper with convolutions. In: 2015 IEEE Conference on Computer Vision and Pattern Recognition (CVPR). 07, pp. 1–9. https://doi.org/10.1109/CVPR.2015.7298594
34. Simonyan, K., & Zisserman, A. (2015). Very deep convolutional networks for large-scale image recognition. *ICLR, 75*(6), 398–406. https://doi.org/10.2146/ajhp170251.
35. He, K., Zhang, X., Ren, S., & Sun, J. (2015). Deep residual learning for image recognition. *Multimedia Tools and Applications, 77*(9), 10437–10453. https://doi.org/10.1007/s11042-017-4440-4.
36. Huang, G., Liu, Z., Van Der Maaten, L., & Weinberger, K. Q. (2017). Densely connected convolutional networks. IEEE Conf Comput Vis Pattern Recognition, CVPR. 2261–2269. https://doi.org/10.1109/CVPR.2017.243.
37. Syeda, H. B., Syed, M., Sexton, K. W., Syed, S., Begum, S., Syed, F., Yu Jr., F. The role of machine learning techniques to tackle COVID-19 crisis: A systematic review. medRxiv 2020.08.23.20180158; https://doi.org/10.1101/2020.08.23.20180158.
38. Kashour, Z. T., Riaz, M., Garbati, M., Aldosary, O., Tlayjeh, H., Gerberi, D., Murad, M. H. M., Sohail, R., Kashour, T., Tleyjeh, I. M. (2020). Efficacy of chloroquine or hydroxychloroquine in COVID-19 patients: A systematic review and meta-analysis medRxiv 2020.07.12.20150110; https://doi.org/10.1101/2020.07.12.20150110.
39. Khan, A., Sohail, A., Zahoora, U., & Qureshi, A. S. (2019). A survey of the recent architectures of deep convolutional neural networks. 1–60. arXiv Prepr arXiv190106032.
40. Zhuge, Y., Ning, H., Mathen, P., et al. (2020). Automated glioma grading on conventional MRI images using deep convolutional neural networks. *Medical Physics, 47*(7), 3044–3053. https://doi.org/10.1002/mp.14168.
41. Rani, S., & Kautish, S. (2018, June). Association clustering and time series based data mining in continuous data for diabetes prediction. In 2018 Second International Conference on Intelligent Computing and Control Systems (ICICCS) (pp. 1209–1214). IEEE.

# Index

**A**
Aarogya Setu, 47, 308
Abacavir, 52
ABCpred tool, 170
Accelerometer, 316, 320
Acute kidney injury (AKI), 185
Acute respiratory distress syndrome (ARDS), 185
AdaBoost algorithm, 196
Affected SAARC countries, 18
Agglomerative approaches, 3, 12
AI-based health monitoring system, 325
AI-based radiological technologies, 46
AI-based robotic technologies, 53, 54
Alcohol-based sanitizer, 62
Allergenicity, 165
AlphaFold, 125, 244
AmpErase enzyme, 80
Analytical hierarchy process (AHP)
  M-AHP, 12, 14
  MCDM, 10
  Saaty's AHP, 13
  susceptibility risk index, 3, 10
Angiotensin-converting enzyme 2 (ACE2), 185, 194, 248, 249
Anthropometric, 333
Antigenicity, 164
Antiviral therapies, 292
Anxiety disorders, 207
Application programming interface (API), 47
Aptamer-based nano-biosensor, 90
Artificial intelligence (AI), 232, 238
  Aarogya Setu (mobile app), 47
  AI-driven algorithms, 47
  algorithm-based model, 46
  Alipay/WeChat, 48
  automated applications, 100
  automatic monitoring, 100
  clinical symptom matching, 308
  in COVID-19
    AI software, 51
    detection and diagnosis, 48
    drug development, 52, 53
    limitations, 55
    patients, 195, 196
    structural and molecular analysis, 52
  data-based trained model, 46
  and DS, 63
  intelligent agents, 276
  M-health, 309
Artificial Intelligence Markup Language (AIML), 278
Artificial Linguistic Internet Computer Entity, 278
Artificial neural network (ANN), 232
Asymptotic, 61
Asymptomatic carriers, 233
Atazanavir, 52
Augmented reality (AR)
  advancements, 203
  in anxiety disorders, 207
  for COVID-19
    patient education, 208
    physical therapies, 209
    psychological treatment, 209
  digital information tools, 225
  education, 204, 205
  gaming/entertainment, 204
  healthcare, 205
  HMD, 203



S. Kautish et al. (eds.), *Computational Intelligence Techniques for Combating COVID-19*, EAI/Springer Innovations in Communication and Computing,
https://doi.org/10.1007/978-3-030-68936-0

Augmented reality (AR) *(Cont)*
on mental health, 210
for psychological support, 209, 210
travel and tourism, 205
virtual shopping, 206
Augmented reality exposure-based therapy (AR-EBT), 207
Australian Census-based Epidemic Model (AceMod), 237
Authoritative sources, 292
Automated Venipuncture Device (AVD) robot, 53
Automatic annotations, 245

**B**
*Bacillus* Calmette-Guerin (BCG) vaccine, 2, 5, 7, 10–12, 14
Bat algorithm (BA), 146
Batch normalization (BN), 223
Bayesian probability network (BN), 308
Bernoulli sampling simulation, 322
Beta thalassemia heterozygote, 305
Big data analytics
comorbidity data integration, 190–192
high-throughput technologies, 189
multi-omics data, 189
organ-specific studies, 189
Bioinformatics approaches, 160–162
Biosensing, 320, 324
Biosensor, 89, 90
Biowatch accelerometer, 311
Blockchain
applications, 127
Blockchain 2.0, 126
Civitas, 128
COVID-19, 126
features, 126
IBM blockchain, 128
sectors, 126
technical and non-technical limitations, 128
utility, 126
Bluetooth and proximity sensors, 47
Bounding boxes, 107

**C**
CAD4COVID software, 50
C4.5 algorithm, 62, 65, 69–72
Centers for Disease Control and Prevention (CDC), 275
Centroid, 108
Chatbots, 62
architecture
generative model, 280, 281
mechanisms, 280
retrieval-based model, 281, 282
automatic communication, 275
challenges, 294
AI uncertainty, 295
Communiqué Elucidate, 294
gadget-to-human leap, 295
personalization, 295
style of Chatbot, 295
classification
construction, 280
goals achieved, 279
input distilling, 280
knowledge domain, 279
service provided, 279
in client service, 288
companies and organizations, 276
continuity, 299
for COVID-19
antiviral therapies, 292
"Clara" by CDC, 291
detection, symptoms, 289
evaluation, 289
in healthcare system, 289
individuals and organizations, 291
information device, 289, 290
interactions and guidance, 290
ongoing treatment, 292
precaution and anticipation, 291
protection and safety measures, 292
symptom screening, 291
on WHO, 290
customer awareness, 299
definition, 276
digital interactions, 276
digital portals, 275
in education
language study, 286
motivation builder, 287, 288
performance reviewer, 286
evolution
A.L.I.C.E., 278
ELIZA, 277
Jabberwacky, 277
SmarterChild, 278
Turing test, 277
on Facebook, 293
and functionality, 283
AIML design, 283
calibrations and collation, 286
instrumentation, 285
multilingualism, 286

paradigm identification using snippets, 284, 285
portal value assessment, 285
working, Chatbot, 287
HCI, 276
identity, 299
narrative, 300
objective-based responses, 299
and personal assistants, 278
response generation, 283
intent classification, 282
pattern-based heuristics, 281, 282
workflow, 284
responses, 298
situation awareness, 298
software program, 276
types
enterprise Chatbots, 279
entertainment Chatbots, 278
by WHO, 275
Chest radiograph, 88
Chest tomography, 356
Chest X-ray, 36, 231, 356, 358, 360, 361, 368, 369, 375
Chest X-ray image extraction, 231
Chloroquine, 159
C-ImmSim server, 175
Civitas, 128
Classifiers, 233–235, 245–249
Classification
CNN 3D classification types, 39
hybrid model, 40, 41
normal *vs*. COVID-19 cases, 33
normal *vs*. COVID-19 *vs*. pneumonia cases, 33
pneumonia *vs*. COVID-19 cases, 33
Climatic factors, 271
Climatic variables, 258
Clinical characteristics, 118
Clinical trial, 324
CLOMT technique, 316
Cloud Plus Terminal ("nCapp"), 310
CMake, 111
CNN models, 368
Codon adaptation index (CAI), 175
Cognitive behavior therapy (CBT), 207
Cognitive Internet of Medical Things (CIOMT), 306
Colossal events, 336
Comorbidity information, 196
Comorbidity network modeling, 191, 192, 194
Computational drug designing, 52
Computational methods, 170
Computational repurposing, 193
Computed tomography (CT), 88, 89, 231
Compute pairwise distance, 106, 108
Computer-aided peptide-based vaccine designing, 53
Computer-based healthcare system, 46
Computer program, 63
Compute Unified Device Architecture (CUDA), 110, 112, 113
Confirmed infected cases, 135
Constraint-handling techniques, 146
Content validation, 335
Contrast limited adaptive histogram equalization (CLAHE), 245
Conversational Chatbots, 279
Convolutional layer (Conv), 222
Convolutional neural networks (CNNs), 102, 103
advantages, 214
application area, 214
backbone X-ray, 245
backpropagation mechanism, 222
Bayesian-based CNN, 237
chest X-ray images, 240, 375
classifiers, 246
clinical applications, 360
control signals, 224
COVID-19 detection, 35
COVID-19 from X-rays, 33
COVID-Net, 357
CovNets and CNN GPU, 244
CT scan images, 240
CXR image prediction, 232
DCNN pretrained models, 244
deep neural network, 214
disadvantages, 214
EEG signals, 219
executable CNN networks, 246
human-computer interfaces, 214
imaging and computer vision, 232
InceptionV3, 35
layer, 222
medical image accuracy and performance, 233
1D-CNN-RF model, 221
on Porch image frameworks, 233
propagation, 224
pulmonary nodular characteristics, 29
pulmonary nodules, 28
ResNet and AlexNet ML techniques, 233
3D classification types, 39
three-dimensional ML technique, 233
VGG-16, 359
VGG model, 362
*Coronaviridae*, 117

Coronavirus
  on birds and mammals, 96
  Chatbots functionality (*see* Chatbots)
  moderate symptoms, 97
  preventive measure, 76
  upper respiratory tract, 61
  by WHO, 275
Coronavirus 2019 (COVID-19)
  AHP, 3
  AI-based drugs, 53
  AI-based model, 46
  blockchain-based applications, 128
  characteristics, 29
  chest CT scan and chest radiograph, 88, 89
  common symptoms, 98
  data types and resources, 186–188
  deaths, SAARC top 4 counties, 4, 5
  deep neural network method, 232
  diagnosis report development cycle, 37, 38
  diagnostic facilities, 76
  epidemic, 27
  exposure, 98
  factors for low death rate in SA
    average age, 9
    average temperature, 5, 6
    BCG vaccine, 5
    critical days, 6
    herd immunity, 9
    herd Immunity, 9, 10
  hybrid model, 40, 41
  incubation period, 75
  infection rates and population density, 259
  ML techniques and treatment, 234–235
  mortality rate, 62
  multi-organ association, 185
  Orbita, 293
  outbreak, 1
  pandemic outbreaks, 117
  PCR monitoring, 27
  and pneumonia cases, 33
  progression, 185
  quarantines, 1
  risk assessment, 72
  statistical data, 2
  structure, 27
  transmission rate, 2
  2019-nCoV, 75
  vaccine, 248, 249
  WHO COVID-19 Dashboard, 96
  worldwide confirmed cases, 136, 137
  Wuhan city, 117
  X-rays, 232, 235
COVID-19-affected countries, 17
COVID-CAPS, 357
COVID-19 comorbidities, 190–192
COVID-19 crisis, 62, 308
COVID-19 dataset
  case status, 67, 69
  confirmed cases, 68, 70
  description, 67
  environmental setup, 67, 68
  global map, 67, 69
COVIDiagnosis model, 357
COVID-19 global pandemic, 333
COVID-19 health crisis, 62
COVID-19 IgM/IgG antibody rapid test, 87, 88
COVID-19 infection, 159
  AI and IoT detection and tracing, 325
  airborne disease, 159
  cases and deaths, 159
  high mortality and transmission, 159
COVID-19 infodemic, *see* Infodemic
COVID-Net, 50, 235
COVID-19 outbreak, 118
COVID-19 pandemic, 1, 27, 224, 225
  AI-based drones and robotic technology, 54
  AI software, 51
  AR/VR technologies, 207
  challenges, 118
  collaborative and multidisciplinary research, 56
  face masks, 55
  MAE and TA, 54
  national and international organizations, 54
  poverty, 55
  social distancing, 54
  social media platforms, 54
  surveillance cameras, 54
COVID-ResNet, 357
COVID-19 risk factor
  age and gender, 68
  dataset description, 68
  patient symptom, 70
COVID-19 spreads
  direct, indirect and close contact, 137
  droplets, 137
  growth factor, daily new cases, 137
  nose discharges and saliva droplets, 62
  signs, 137
  touching, 137
  wearable sensors, 306
  Wuhan city of China, 159
COVID Symptom Study app, 51
COVID-Xpert, 357

COVIDz, 363, 368
CoVIg-19 Plasma Bot, 296
CovNet architecture model, 235, 236, 244
CRISPR, 82
Crowdsourcing, 188, 195
CT scan
  CNN, 29
  DL approach, 32
  DL architecture, 30
  feature extraction using transfer learning, 31
  intercept ROIs, 30, 31
  M-inception framework, 31
  nucleic acid-based identification, 32
  performance evaluation metrics, 31, 32
  precision, 33
  prediction, 31
  profound analysis method, 32
  PUIs, 32
  retrospective collection of datasets, 30
  standard CT photos, 29
CUDA Deep Neural Network (cuDNN) package, 110, 112

**D**

Data augmentation, 245
Data collection, 104
  Bluedot Insights, 104
  corona tracker API, 105
  HealthMap, 105
  kaggle.com, 105
  Microsoft Bing, 105
Data preprocessing, 245
Decision Tree Classifier, 233
Deep autoencoder, 211
Deep Bayes-SqueezeNet, 356, 357
Deep belief networks (DBNs), 213, 214
Deep Docking (DD) platform, 53
Deep learning (DL)
  AI technique, 196
  algorithms, 101
  applications, 101
  architecture, 211
  autoencoder, 211
  cardiac image processing, 309
  CNN (*see* Convolutional neural network (CNN))
  COVID-19 detection
    with CT images (*see* CT scan)
    X-ray scan (*see* X-ray images)
  to COVID-19 pneumonia, 39
    CT, 38
    diagnosis report development cycle, 37
    image data processing and augmentation, 37, 38
    VNET-IR-RPN method, 37
  DBNs, 213, 214
  GAN, 212, 215
  machine learning, 28, 63, 210
  in mental healthcare, 216, 217
  RBMs, 213
  RNN, 214, 215
  shallow and deep learning, 211
  single centralized data technologies, 374
Density-based spatial clustering of applications with noise (DBSCAN), 240
Deep neural networks (DNNs), 101, 103
Deep transfer learning models, 363
Diagnosis
  anamnesis, 358
  biological examinations, 358
  COVID-19, 46, 48, 50, 357
  imaging, 358
  ML implementation, 236–237
Diagnostic tests, 76
Differential evolution (DE), 146, 231
Digital assistants, 276
Digitalized media, 335
Discrete binary GSK optimization algorithm (DBGSK), 136, 146, 149–151, 153, 154
Discrete binary senior gaining and sharing stage, 146, 151, 154
Disseminated intravascular coagulation (DIC), 186
Distribution of coronavirus protective materials, 138
  disinfection fluids, 135
  heavy transport vehicle, 139
  hospitals and health centres, 139
  locations, store and hospitals, 145
  masks, 138, 139
  mathematical model for optimum distribution, 140–144
  medical gloves, 135
  medical masks, 139
  metaheuristic algorithms, 146
  "N95" respirator mask, 138
  optimum distribution, 136
  proposed formulation, 136
  respirator masks, 135
  transmission, 138
  and wearing masks, 138
Divisive approach, 12

Docking tools, 175
Drugs, 159
  development, 52, 53
  repurposing, 193, 194

**E**
Early detection algorithm (EDA), 297
EarlySense, 131
EEG signals
  depression diagnosis, 218
  EMD feature extraction method, 218
  stress levels, 218
Electroencephalogram (EEG)
  experimental analysis, 217
  monitoring process, 309
Electronic medical records (EMRs), 188, 190
ELIZA, 277
Embedded hardware, 110
Emerging technologies, 305
Empirical mode decomposition (EMD), 218
Enabled IoT
  data streaming, 306
  patients to Covid-19 recovery, 310, 311
Enterprise Chatbots, 279
Enterprise Data Warehouses (EDWs), 188
Entertainment Chatbots, 278
Environmental factors, 258
Enzyme-based biosensor pad, 83
Enzyme-linked immunosorbent assay (ELISA)
  antigen, 86
  enzymes and substrate, 86
  heterogeneous technique, 86
  homogeneous assay, 86
  nano-enabled IDμE, 320
  quantitative analysis technique, 86
  types, 86
Epidemic, 333, 334, 336, 342
Exorbitant disinformation, 335
Extracorporeal membrane oxygenation (ECMO), 292

**F**
False color composite (FCC), 260
Fast Fourier transform (FFT), 218
FDDB dataset, 102
5G networks, 309, 315
Femtomolar (FM) process, 319
Fog computing, 313
Fog layer, 306, 307, 313, 315, 316
Fractional Multichannel Exponent Moments (FrMEMS), 231

**G**
Gaining-sharing knowledge-based optimization algorithm (GSK), 136, 146–148
Gastrointestinal symptoms, 185
General Data Protection Regulation, 335
Generative adversarial networks (GANs), 212, 215, 237, 243, 244
Genetic algorithm (GA), 146
GenScript Rare Codon Analysis Tool, 175
GitHub open-source repository, 360
Google Bidirectional Encoder Representations from Transformer (BERT), 240
Google Deep Mind, 244, 246
Google Earth engine (GEE) platform, 260
Grey wolf optimizer (GWO), 146
"Ground-glass opacity" (GGO), 233

**H**
Handwashing, 62
Head-mounted display (HMD), 203
Healthcare
  Chatbots (*see* Chatbots)
  crisis, 257
  Data Repository, 188
  IoT, 119, 120
  systems, 188
Health managements, 283
HealthMap, 105
Herd immunity, 2, 9, 10
Hierarchical clustering
  dendrogram, 12
  gene expression pattern, 3
  LEACH, 4
  ML tool, 12
  physical parameters, 4
  unsupervised, 4
  web image search, 3
High-throughput technologies, 188, 189
1918 H1N1 Influenza pandemic, 336
Human activity, 342
Human-computer interaction, 276
Human-computer interface, 217
Human coronaviruses, 159
Hybrid DL frameworks, 40
Hyperimmune globulin (H-Ig), 296

**I**
IDE-based biosensor, 325
IEDB MHC-I binding prediction tool, 171
ImageNet, 35, 36
Immune dynamics simulation, 175

Immunoinformatics
B-cell epitope prediction, 170
conformational B-cell epitope prediction, 166
epitope, 166, 171
linear B-cell epitope, 166
MHC-I binding, 171
population coverage calculation, 172
reverse vaccinology, 160–162
T-cell epitope prediction, 170
tools, 166–169
vaccines, 161
Immunosorbent assay, *see* Enzyme-linked immunosorbent assay (ELISA)
Industry IoHT (IIoHT), 131
Industry status, 131
Infodemic
colossal events, 336
evidence-based practice, 336
geographical distribution, 344
information *vs.* misinformation, 334
mandatory thing, 340
media ecosystem, 336
misleading news, Covid-19 pandemic, 340
negative aspects, 336
ongoing global pandemic, 336
on psychological aspects
isolation and quarantine saga, 343, 344
lockdowns, 342
negative infodemic, 342
panic and mass hysteria, 342
sharing of information, 339
social conversation, 340
on social media, 335, 344–346
on the society, 343
in worsening the ongoing pandemic, 339–340
Input distilling, 280
In silico cloning, 175
Intelligent agents, 276
Interactive AR, 203
Interactive VR, 203
Internet-connected hospitals, 117
Internet of COVID Things (IoCT)
AI-based IoCT applications, 124, 125
AlphaFold, 125
blockchain-based applications, 126–128
medical equipments, 121
ML algorithms, 125
proposed category, 122
security challenges, 129
smart thermometers, 122, 123
testing kits, 122
wearables, 123, 124, 129, 132
Internet of Health Things (IoHT), 131
Internet of Medical Things (IoMT), 121
biosensing chip applications, 325
enable integrated healthcare appliance, 308
"POC LFIA" device, 306
testing methods, 305
Internet of Things (IoT), 48, 66
to Covid-19 pandemic, 118
airport screening, 313
BlueDot, 313
Fog and Cloud layer integration, 315
Fog computing, 313
functional significance, 315
spatiotemporal mapping, 314
execution processes, 118
healthcare, 118–120
IoMT, 121
IoT-based applications, 119
M-health, 309
"nCapp", 310
nano-biosensing system, 306
performance metrics, 324
smartphone applications, 118
IoT applications
accelerometer, 316
AI apps, 318
bio-cyber interface, 319
big data and virtual reality, 318
bio-market, 319
care coordination and system management, 326
CLOMT technique, 316
communicator architecture, 317
EHR systems, 326
electrochemical biosensor, 320
in 5G, 315
fog layer, 315, 316
health status code tool, 307
HIV retroviral drugs, 317
low-level disease detections, 318
MAPE-K model, 317
quality of health, 326
speech monitoring, 316
3D scanning, 318
voice-enabled pathological detecting tool, 316
wearable IoT sensors, 315
WESN (Wi-Fi-Bluetooth-GPS), 317
IoT infrared thermography (IRT) camera, 311
IoT visualization tools, 320–322
Isothermal amplification
LAMP (*see* Loop-mediated isothermal amplification (LAMP))

**J**
Jabberwacky, 277
Java Codon Adaptation Tool (JCAT), 175
Jetson Nano, 110–113
Junior gaining-sharing knowledge stage, 146–149, 151, 154

**K**
Kaggle, 105
KNN classifier, 231

**L**
LifeSignals (a Silicon Valley startup), 123
Linear discriminant analysis (LDA), 218
Lockdowns
  on air pollutants, 268, 270
  atmospheric pollutants, 271
  break of economic activities, 257
  COVID-19 pandemic, 264
  in Delhi, 262, 264
  measures, 257, 264
  in New York, 262
  physical distancing, 258
  preventive measures, 270
  social distancing, 270
Long short-term memory (LSTM), 103
Loop-mediated isothermal amplification (LAMP)
  advantages, 80
  COVID-19 diagnosis, 80
  diagnostic tool, 80
  disadvantages, 81
  field survey, 80
Lopinavir, 159
Low-energy adaptive clustering hierarchy (LEACH), 4
LSTM-GRU architecture modeling technique, 47

**M**
Machine learning (ML)
  AceMod, 237
  and advanced bio-computational techniques, 46
  and AI, 28
  algorithms, 232
  alignment-free ML, 244
  applications for COVID-19
    case analysis and forecastination, 66
    image pattern analysis, 67
    prediction, 65
    risk level analysis, 66
    social distance identification, 65
  COVID-19 with ML, 232
  data molecules for COVID-19 prediction, 241, 242
  data sets, 238
  DCNN pretrained models, 244
  diagnostic and prognostic analysis, 231
  DL (*see* Deep learning (DL))
  GAN model, 243, 244
  Google Deep Mind, 244, 246
  in healthcare, 248, 249
  image/video classification tool, 243
  LSTM ML tool, 240
  map measuring techniques, 244
  modeling, 232
  patient diagnostic and drug suggestion, 62
  process
    data collection, 63
    data preparation, 64
    evaluation model, 64
    model selection, 64
    parameter tuning, 64
    prediction, 64
    predictive model, 63
    steps, 64
    training, 64
  SIR model, 241
  time series modeling, 242
Mandatory lockdowns, 344
Manta Ray Foraging optimization, differential evolution (MRFODE), 231
Masks, 138, 139
Max pooling layer (MaxPool), 223
Medical IoT (MIoT), 50
Medical masks, 139
Medical sensing methodologies, 320
Memory-based T-cell-based cell-mediated immunity, 161
Mental health
  AR/VR impact, 207, 210
  COVID-19 pandemic, 209
  deep learning, 217
Mental illness, 216
Metabiota, 47
Metagenomic sequencing, 85
MHC-I binding, 171
M-health, 309
Microarray, 83, 84
Microfluidic network, 319
microSD, 110, 112, 113
Microsoft Bing, 105

Microsoft's Coronavirus Self-Checker Bot, 294
Middle East respiratory syndrome (MERS), 97
Middle East respiratory syndrome-coronavirus (MERS-CoV), 61, 160
Mild-to-moderate proteinuria, 185
Mitigation, 258
ML-assisted COVID-19 healthcare system, 62
  AI, 63
  C4.5 algorithm, 65
  computer program, 63
  ML challenges in COVID-19, 65
  ML process, 63
Mobile applications, 121, 122, 129, 130
Mobile AR, 203
Mobile cloud computing model (MCC), 316
Modified AlexNet model (MAN), 245
Modified AutoEncoder (MAE), 54
Modified inception (M-Inception), 31
Molecular assay techniques
  COVID-19, 76
  microarray, 83, 84
  mNGS, 84
  nucleic acid, 76
  programmed RNA-targeted analysis, 82
  rolling circle amplification, 83
  RT-PCR technique (*see* Reverse transcription-polymerase chain reaction (RT-PCR))
  TMA, 81, 82
Molecular docking, 53, 174
Molecular dynamics (MD) simulations, 175
Molecule Transformer-Drug Target Interaction (MT-DTI), 52
Monitoring mass gatherings, 100
Multilayer perceptron (MLP), 232
Multilingualism, 286
Multi-omics-based molecular data, 189, 192
Multiple analytical hierarchy process (M-AHP), 10, 12, 14, 19–23

**N**

Nano Jetpack image, 110, 112
Nano SD image, 112
Natural language processing (NLP), 47, 104, 276
Nervous system, 186
NetMHCIIpan 3.0 prediction tool, 171
Network IOMT process, 308
Neural networks, 100
Neurons, 100
Next-generation sequencing (mNGS), 84
NHS WhatsApp Bot, 293
Nonlinear binary constrained optimization, 136, 154
Non-nested generalized exemplar (NNGE), 308
Novel coronavirus 2019, 28
N pixel, 108
"N95" respirator mask, 138
NVIDIA's Jetpack, 112

**O**

Obstructive sleep apnea (OSA) device, 309
Omics datasets, 193
Ongoing health crisis, 335, 336, 346
Ongoing pandemic, 335, 339–340, 342, 345, 346, 348, 349
Online databases, 186
Online tools, 164, 165, 170
OpenCV, 110
Open-domain Chatbot, 62
Open-Source-COVID-19, 188
Operational Land Imager (OLI) sensor's data, 259, 260
Orbita Chatbot, 293
Orthopedic IOMT, 305

**P**

Paper-based diagnostic tools, 90
Particle swarm optimization (PSO) algorithm, 146
PCR-based molecular testing tool, 321
Person under investigations (PUIs), 32
Personal health records (PHRs), 188, 190
Personalized treatment, 189, 196
Physical distancing, 334
Plasma therapy, 296
Pneumonia, 135
Point-of-care diagnostic tests, 89
Polymerase chain reaction (PCR), 76, 305, 313, 320, 321
  RT-PCR (*see* Reverse transcription-polymerase chain reaction (RT-PCR))
Position-specific scoring matrix (PSSM) method, 171
Post-calibration, 261
Pre-calibration, 261
Precision, 357, 363, 368
Predictive modelling, 258, 260, 266–268, 271
Pre-lockdown, 268, 270, 271
Programmed RNA-targeted analysis, 82

ProPred-I and IMTECH tools, 171
Protection expansion protected extension (PEPX) design method, 235
Protective materials for COVID-19, 154
Protein interactive network (PPIN), 308
Public health, 125
Python (programming language), 109, 358, 359, 375

**Q**
Quadratic inequality, 143
Quality of service (QoS), 316
Quarantine, 305

**R**
Racism, 346
Raman spectrophotometer (RNA), 319
Random forest (RF), 196, 234, 245, 248, 249
Random pooling, 321
Rapid testing kit, 87, 88
Receiver operating characteristics (ROC), 234, 235
Rectified Linear Unit (ReLU), 223, 246
Recurrent convolution neural network (R-CNN), 106
Recurrent neural networks (RNN), 102, 103, 214, 215
Reinforcement learning, 41
ReLU-based deep learning image visualization technique, 232
Remdesivir, 159
Remote patient monitoring, 297
Repurposable drugs, 194
Repurposed drugs, 193
Residual neural network (ResNet) template, 35
Restricted Boltzmann machines (RBMs), 103, 213
Reverse transcriptase polymerase chain reaction (RT-PCR), 48, 232, 233, 289
  advantages, 77
  COBAS 6800/8800, 77, 79
  disadvantages, 77
  DNA/RNA, 76
  DNA sequence, 76, 77
  LAMP method, 80, 81
  primers, 77
  SARS-CoV-2, 77
  Taq polymerase, 77
Reverse vaccinology, 160–162
  adhesion-like properties, 165
  allergenicity and toxicity, 165
  antigenicity prediction, 164
  bioinformatics approaches, 162
  conservation of domains, 166
  functional protein, 162
  to host proteins, 166
  physicochemical property analysis, 165
  retrieval of proteome, SARS-CoV-2, 162
  signal peptides, 166
  subcellular localizations, 165
  targets protein/antigen, 162
  tools, 162, 164
  transmembrane helix, 166
Rhabdomyolysis, 186
Risk assessment, 72
Risk factor (RF), 6, 10, 12, 14, 17, 18
Ritonavir, 159
RNA-based assay, 231
Rolling circle amplification, 83

**S**
SAARC nations, 1, 2
Sandwich ELISA, 87
SARS-CoV-2
  neurological diseases, 186
  outbreak, 46
  virus, 334, 337–339
Self-practices, 98
Senior gaining-sharing knowledge stage, 146–148, 151
Serologic assay
  advantages, 87
  direct assay, 86, 87
  ELISA, 86 (*see also* Enzyme-linked immunosorbent assay (ELISA))
  IgM, 84
  indirect, 87
  sandwich ELISA, 87
  sensitivity, 85
  serum/plasma, 84
  viral infection diagnostic technique, 85
Severe acute respiratory syndrome (SARS), 97, 117
Severe acute respiratory syndrome coronavirus (SARS-CoV), 61
  beta-coronavirus, 160
  bioinformatics strategies for peptide-based vaccines, 162
  geographic regions, 162
  immunoinformatics-based vaccines, 162
  and MERS-CoV, 160
  potential candidate peptide-based vaccines, 162, 163

reverse vaccinology (*see* Reverse vaccinology)
in silico approach, 161
Severe acute respiratory syndrome coronavirus 2 (SARS-CoV-2), 45, 288, 289
Single-shot detector (SSD), 106
Slow-reacting substance of anaphylaxis (SRS-A), 356
SmartBots interactive agents, 276
SmarterChild, 278
Smart thermometers, 122, 123
Social control, 104, 106, 114
Social distancing, 50–51, 53–55, 65, 66, 99, 118, 305
Social distancing detector algorithm, 106
Social media
digital media, 344
Facebook, 339
facets, 345
and infodemic, 344, 345
irrational information, 343
loopholes, 336
ongoing crisis, 335
principal attributes, 348
racism, 346
Twitter, 339
"unhealthy rat race", 345
user-friendly digital versions, 348
YouTube, 339
Socio-urban factors, 270, 271
Specific high-sensitivity enzymatic reporter unlocking (SHERLOCK) platform, 82
Structural proteins, 75
Structural vaccinology, 160, 162
on binding grooves, 159
homology modeling, 172
MD simulation, 175
molecular docking, 172
on pockets/active sites, 172
protein-ligand docking, 174
protein-protein docking, 174
tools, 172, 173
Support vector machines (SVMs), 50, 195, 196, 232–235, 240, 241, 245, 260, 272, 317
Suppression, 258
Surface-enhanced Raman scattering (SERS) phenomena, 319
Susceptibility risk index, 3, 10
Susceptible-infected-recovered-deceased (SIRD) model, 239
Susceptible-infected-recovered (SIR) model, 195, 238–242
SVM kernel functions, 261
SVM machine learning, 267
Swab testing, 48

**T**
Teaching-learning-based optimization (TLBO), 146
Telehealth, 118, 129
Telemedicine, 129, 132
Temperature, 258
Text mining algorithms, 186
3D clustering method, 37
3D printers, 50
Topological AutoEncoder (TA), 54
Toxicity assessment, 165
Traditional machine learning technique, 101
Transcription-mediated amplification (TMA), 81, 82
Trivial solution, 141
Turing test, 277
2D deep CNN, 237

**U**
Universal Language Model Fine-Tuning (ULMFiT) tool, 240
Unsupervised learning mechanism, 101
Urban density, 260, 264, 270, 271
UVD robots, 53

**V**
Ventilated spaces, 136
Versatile datasets, 64
VGG-16 (neural network model), 359, 362
Virtual assessment tool
CoVIg-19 Plasma Bot, 296
Microsoft, 296
plasma therapy, 296
teams bots for internal maintenance, 297
voice-enabled bot, 297
on webpage, 296
*See also* Chatbots
Virtual environment, 111
Virtual reality (VR)
in anxiety disorders, 207
for COVID-19
outbreak, 219
patient education, 208
physical therapies, 209
psychological treatment, 209
definition, 203
digital information tools, 225

Virtual reality (VR) *(Cont)*
education, 204, 205
gaming/entertainment, 204
healthcare, 205
HMD, 203
on mental health, 210
for psychological support, 209, 210
travel and tourism, 205
virtual shopping, 206
Virus disinfection, 137
VisMol system, 205

**W**
Water cycle algorithm (WCA), 146
Wearable devices, 297
Wearable sensors, 310
Wearables, 123, 124, 129, 132
WhatsApp, 109
WHO (World Health Organization), 95, 97, 105, 108
WHO COVID-19 Dashboard, 96
WHOOP (Boston-based technology startup), 123
Wireless sensor network (WSN), 3, 4, 315, 325

**X**
XGBoost algorithm, 50
X-ray, 88, 231
CNN approach, 33
COVID-19 detection
DL, 34
ImageNet, 35, 36
pre-trained COVID-19 cases, 36
research, 35
ResNet template, 35
X-ray radiography (CXR), 232–234
Xvision Spine System (XVS), 205

**Y**
YOLO (You Only Look Once) object detection, 106–108, 114

**Z**
Zika outbreak, 242

The manufacturer's authorised representative in the EU is Springer Nature Customer Service Centre GmbH, Europaplatz 3, 69115 Heidelberg, Germany. If you have any concerns regarding our products, please contact ProductSafety@springernature.com

Printed and bound by CPI Group (UK) Ltd, Croydon, CR0 4YY
22/09/2026
02221048-0004